THE SAFETY BIOHACKER

Comprehensive Treatise on Biosecurity

Class 0 Architecture for Longevity and Elite Performance

Andrea Bancalà

"To those who have decided to stop being passengers of their own biology and have chosen to become its Pilots. Because survival is not a hope, but a deliberate work of engineering."

Andrea Bancalà

TABLE OF CONTENTS

FOREWORD: THE SAFETY OFFICER'S CODE

- From Workplace Safety to Life Safety.
- Risk Analysis: Why DIY biohacking is a system in crisis.
- The "Zero Biological Accidents" Philosophy.

PART 1: FOUNDATIONS & BARRIERS (Remediation)

- **Chapter 1:** Air and Water Engineering (Radon, PM2.5, Osmosis).
- **Chapter 2:** The Invisible Saboteurs (Detox from Smoking, Alcohol, Metals).
- **Chapter 3:** The Oral Gateway (Amalgams, NICO, Oral Microbiome).
- **Chapter 4:** Nutrition, Microbiome, and Bio-Economy (Intestinal Barrier and Smart Spending).

PART 2: SYNCHRONIZATION & ENERGY (The Engine)

- **Chapter 5:** Chronobiology and Sleep (Circadian Rhythms and Glinphatic Flushing).
- **Chapter 6:** Photobiomodulation (Red Light, NIR, and UV).
- **Chapter 7:** The Metabolic Engine (VO2 Max, Zone 2, and Strength).

- **Chapter 8:** Thermodynamics and Safety (Hot/Cold and the Safety Curve).

PART 3: STRUCTURE & DEFENSE (The Hardware)

- **Chapter 9:** Bio-Electromagnetism and Grounding (Cell Voltage and EMF).
- **Chapter 10:** Structural Engineering (Fascia, Posture, and Tensegrity).
- **Chapter 11:** Office Biohacking (Ergonomics and Survival in Office Work).
- **Chapter 12:** Bio-Integrated Dermatology (Skin as an endocrine organ).

PART 4: MOLECULAR OVERCLOCKING (The Software)

- **Chapter 13:** The Endocrine System (Men and Women, Testosterone, Thyroid, and Cycle Syncing).
- **Chapter 14:** Neuro-Engineering (Focus, Dopamine, and Stress Management).
- **Chapter 15:** Molecular Longevity (Autophagy, Sirtuins, NAD+).
- **Chapter 16:** Elite Diagnostics & Bio-Privacy (DNA, Longevity Dashboard, and Genetic Data Security).
- **Chapter 17:** Peptides and Bioregulators (The frontier of signaling).

- **Chapter 18:** Bio-Harmony and Social Epigenetics (Co-regulation and Impact on the Family).

PART 5: CLINICAL FRONTIERS (Extra-Safety)

- **Chapter 19:** Regenerative Medicine (Stem Cells, Exosomes, Apheresis).
- **Chapter 20:** Crisis Management & Resilience (The "Safety Kit" for acute emergencies).

PART 6: STRATEGIC INTEGRATION (Execution)

- **Chapter 21:** Elite Supplements and Peptides in Detail (The Ones You Really Need)
- **Chapter 22:** The Chronobiology of Integration (The Hourly Master Plan).
- **Chapter 23:** The Best Supplements and Therapeutic Dosages for Elite Biohackers (Complete List).
- **Chapter 24:** The Roadmap (Annual Routine).
- **Chapter 25:** Biohacking for the Masses (The ROI of Health Even for Those on a Zero Budget).

PART 7: THE GENDER DIFFERENCE IN BIOHACKING

- **Chapter 26:** The Data Error (Why women are not "little men").

- **Chapter 27:** Cycle Syncing (Synchronizing the Infradian: Food, Sport, Work).
- **Chapter 28:** Bio-Security and Contraception. (Endocrine Secrets)
- **Chapter 29:** The Second Spring (Perimenopause, Menopause, and Bioidentical HRT).

PART 8: TOWARDS ZERO INJURIES

- **Chapter 30:** Human 2.0 (Digital Twins & AI Safety Guard).
- **Chapter 31:** Zero Injuries (The Philosophy of Predictive Maintenance).

PART 9: SPECIES HORIZONS: SPECULATIVE BIO-SECURITY

- **Chapter 32:** The Horizon of Events (Transhumanism and Future Risk Management)

PART 10: EPILOGUE

- **Chapter 33:** The 10 Commandments of the Safety Biohacker

---

ACKNOWLEDGEMENTS

NOTE ON THE AUTHOR

SCIENTIFIC VALIDATION AND BIBLIOGRAPHIC ARCHITECTURE OF THE "SAFETY BIOHACKER" PROTOCOL: FORENSIC ANALYSIS OF MOLECULAR MECHANISMS AND CLINICAL EVIDENCE

LEGAL DISCLAIMER AND BIO-SAFETY PROTOCOL

APPENDIX A: SAFETY BIOHACKER TECHNICAL GLOSSARY

APPENDIX B: HEMATOLOGICAL AND BIOMETRIC AUDIT PROTOCOL

APPENDIX C: SUPPLY BRAND HANDBOOK

CALL TO ACTION

FOREWORD

THE SAFETY OFFICER'S CODE: SURVIVING THE PERFECT STORM

My name is Andrea Bancalà. In my professional life, I deal with chemical, biological, and radioactive safety at the National Institute of Health in Rome.

There, my world is governed by a ruthless binary code: **Safety** or **Risk**. There are no "maybes," no "let's hope."

There are standard operating procedures (SOPs), risk analyses, and emergency protocols.

My job is to predict the unpredictable, analyze invisible threats, and ensure that complex systems continue to operate, protecting the most precious commodity there is: human life.

Seeing national epidemiological data every day has given me a brutal perspective that most people ignore: **the population is not "aging," it is simply "deteriorating" due to lack of maintenance.**

I am writing this book because the gap between what the scientific elite knows and what the population does is an abyss that swallows vitality and years of life.

My institutional and moral role compels me not to stand by and watch.

I am fascinated by the promise of extending human life and enhancing cognitive performance to overcome the limits imposed by nature.

In recent years, I have read thousands of scientific papers and personally tested many protocols.

But the deeper I went down the White Rabbit's hole, the more I noticed a fracture.

A systemic error so big that it was invisible to everyone.

The world of biohacking, born for excellence, had turned into a **biological gamble**.

I see managers taking nootropics for concentration while their brains are intoxicated with heavy metals.

I see athletes seeking recovery with cryotherapy while their intestinal barrier is a sieve.

I see ordinary people installing "Formula 1 software" on oxidized, inflamed, and structurally compromised "hardware" (the body).

The result is not optimization, it is **accelerated entropy**.

It's like watching someone try to break a speed record in a vintage Ferrari that leaks oil and has a rusty chassis.

The inevitable conclusion is not the finish line, but a crash at the first corner.

It was at that moment that I understood my mission: there was a lack of a **Safety Officer** figure within the world of Biohacking.

THE PERFECT STORM: WHY THIS BOOK, WHY NOW?

We are not living in normal times; we are in the midst of a **Perfect Storm**.

Never in the history of humanity has our body been subjected to such a total and simultaneous siege:

1. **The Environmental Siege:** We breathe fine particulate matter (PM2.5) and radon gas, we drink water that carries microplastics and drug residues.
2. **The Digital Siege:** We are the first generation constantly immersed in a bath of electromagnetic frequencies (EMF) and artificial blue light that confuse our circadian rhythms, preventing deep nighttime repair.
3. **Psychological Siege:** Our nervous system is trapped in a state of chronic alertness that shuts down regeneration processes.

In this "Class 1" risk scenario, seeking health by following grandma's advice ("eat a little of everything") or Internet fads is not only ineffective, it is **dangerous**.

You cannot "hope" to age well these days; hope is not a strategy.

You have to engineer your survival.

WHO THIS BOOK IS NOT FOR

Before we continue, we must be honest with each other: this book is not for everyone.

I want to be brutally honest, as I would be during a security audit.

- **Put this book down if** you are looking for a magic pill that will fix years of abuse to your body in a week.
- **Put this book down if** you think health is just a matter of "luck" or "genetics" and you're not willing to take radical responsibility for your biology.
- **Put this book down if** you are content with "not dying."

Our mission here is different.

We don't want to just survive or drag ourselves to the end of our days.

We want **Apex Vitality**, we want to reach 80 with the energy, mental clarity, and physical strength of a 40-year-old, we want to live in a body that is not a burden but a competitive advantage.

We don't sell dreams here, we sell **Biological Engineering**.

This is a manual for those who have decided that "normal" is not enough, for those who look at the statistics on chronic diseases and say, ***"Not me. Not today. Not ever."***

GROUND ZERO: THE "SAFETY BIOHACKER" METHOD

"The Safety Biohacker" is not a collection of tricks, it is a **Complete Operating System**.

It applies the logic of workplace safety to your personal biology.

We use the Deming cycle, **PDCA (Plan-Do-Check-Act)**, to transform your health from an improvised art to an exact science.

Our approach is sequential and non-negotiable; you can't build the roof if you don't have the foundation.

Here is the eight-step process for achieving Class 0 biosecurity:

- **STEP 1: REMEDIATION (Risk Assessment).** Before adding, we remove. You will learn how to secure the air you breathe and the water that hydrates you, eliminate "invisible saboteurs" such as heavy metals and toxins, remediate the "oral construction site," and seal the intestinal barrier. We will build on clean ground.

- **PHASE 2: THE ENGINE (Engineering).** We will restart your metabolism, synchronize your circadian rhythms with Solar Logic, teach you how to "eat light" with photobiomodulation, and use thermodynamics to forge unshakeable resilience through hormesis.

- **PHASE 3: THE HARDWARE (Maintenance).** We will strengthen your physical and bioelectrical structure, explore cellular voltage, fascial tensegrity, and posture, applying survival protocols for the modern office (Occupational Safety) and treating the skin as a vital endocrine organ.

- **PHASE 4: THE SOFTWARE (Overclocking).** We push the molecular accelerator, optimize the endocrine system and neuro-engineering for indestructible focus, activating the pathways of molecular longevity (Sirtuins, NAD+, Autophagy). We integrate elite diagnostics, peptide signals, and social harmony for a bug-free source code.
- **PHASE 5: THE CLINIC (Advanced Defense).** We enter the heavy laboratory for structural repair. You will discover the frontiers of regenerative medicine—stem cells, exosomes, and apheresis—and learn "Crisis Management" to handle any acute emergency with a tactical Safety Kit.

- **STEP 6: EXECUTION (Strategic Integration).** The operational "Master Plan." We will translate theory into precise timetables for integration, elite therapeutic dosages, and annual routines, including the MVP ( ) protocol to maximize health ROI even with zero budget.

- **STEP 7: SPECIFICITY (Gender Safety).** We will correct the "Gender Data Gap" by adapting each protocol to female physiology. From infradian rhythm synchronization (Cycle Syncing) to contraceptive biosecurity, to the management of the "Second Spring" (Menopause).

- **STEP 8: THE FUTURE (Predictive Maintenance).** Towards Zero Accidents. We will use AI and Digital Twins to monitor your telemetry in real time and move from reactive to predictive medicine, projecting ourselves towards the horizons of transhumanism and future risk management.

YOUR BIOLOGICAL BUSINESS PLAN: THE BIO-ECONOMY

There is one last fundamental point.

Biohacking is often portrayed as an elitist hobby for Silicon Valley billionaires, but that is not my vision.

Consider this manual as the **Business Plan for your existence**.

Health is the only asset that, if it defaults, renders all other real estate or financial investments useless.

You will learn about the **Bio-Economy**: you will discover that biohacking is the smartest financial investment you can make.

Spending resources today on smart prevention (often at no cost, such as sunshine, breathing, or fasting) will save you a fortune in medical care and "lost years of life" tomorrow.

In this book, you will always find two parallel paths:

1. The **"Apex Way"**: The ultimate technological solution for those with no budget constraints.
2. **The "Safety Officer Way"**: The practical, smart, and economical solution based on pure physiology.

My goal is to give you the keys to your operating system, regardless of your bank account. I want you to be independent, competent, and, above all, **safe**.

THE PACT

If you are still reading, it means you are ready. I am committed to providing you with the most detailed maps, the most rigorous data, and the safest protocols that science and experience can offer.

You only need to contribute one thing: the **Discipline of Execution**.

Knowledge without action is just another useless piece of data in your brain. Longevity is not a destination you arrive at by chance; it is a process of continuous, deliberate, and strategic maintenance.

If you are tired of being a passive passenger in your own decline and want to take control to build an impregnable biological fortress, turn the page.

Put on your helmet. We are about to enter the most important construction site of your life: your body.

Dr. Andrea Bancalà *Safety Officer & The Safety Biohacker*

PART 1: FOUNDATIONS & BARRIERS (The Cleanup)

Operational Objective: Zero Risk

The Concept: Imagine you want to build the tallest skyscraper in the world.

Most people start by worrying about the color of the windows or the decor of the penthouse (supplements, nootropics).

This is a fatal mistake.

If the ground you're building on is toxic or unstable, the skyscraper will collapse before it reaches the third floor.

In **Phase 1**, we won't try to make you "run faster"; we'll try to release the handbrake that you've been pulling for years without knowing it.

The Battle Plan: In this section, we will apply the **Environmental and Internal Remediation** Protocol:

1. **Chapter 1:** We will secure the air you breathe and the water that hydrates you.

   These are your primary "inputs"; if they are corrupt, the whole system is corrupt.

2. **Chapter 2:** We will identify and eliminate the "Invisible Saboteurs": heavy metals, plastics, and voluntary toxins that act like viruses in your biological software.

3. **Chapter 3:** We will explore the "Oral Construction Site," and you will discover why the mouth is the gateway to systemic diseases.
4. **Chapter 4:** We will seal the most important frontier: the intestinal barrier.

Don't skip this part.

Elite performance is impossible in a toxic body.

First we clean, then we build.

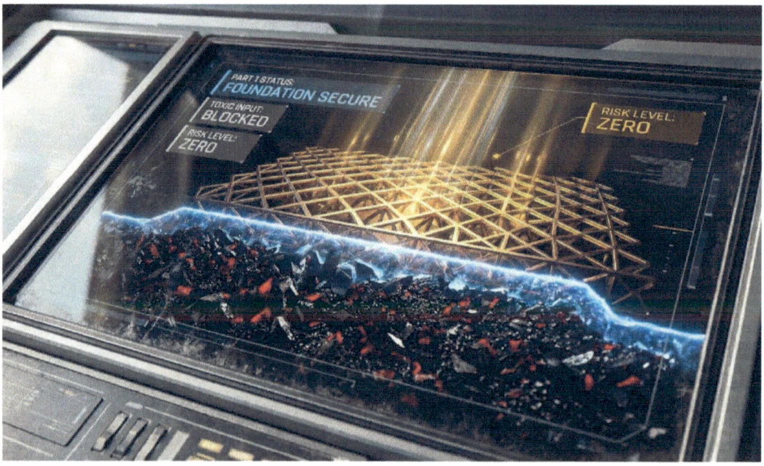

CHAPTER 1

AIR AND WATER ENGINEERING: THE VECTORS OF LIFE

"If the indoor environment is five times more polluted than the outdoor environment, every breath is an open breach in your defensive perimeter."

Most people begin their health journey by buying exotic supplements or joining a gym.

From a biosecurity standpoint, this is a critical procedural error.

It's the equivalent of polishing the bodywork of a Formula 1 car while the engine is sucking in sand and the cooling system is taking in contaminated water.

As **a Safety Officer**, I apply a fundamental rule: **the quality of the input determines the quality of the output**.

You introduce approximately **11,000 liters of air** and at least **2-3 liters of water** into your system every single day.

These are not passive elements of survival; they are the **primary carriers of chemical information**.

Every molecule you inhale or ingest sends a signal to your cells: "We are safe, repair" or "We are under attack, defend."

If these flows are corrupted by fine particulate matter, endocrine disruptors, or heavy metals, your immune system will be perpetually engaged in a defensive war, diverting vital energy (ATP) from DNA repair processes and longevity.

In this chapter, we will transform your home into a **Class 0 "Clean Room"** by balancing elite technology, fluid physics, and rigorous maintenance protocols.

PART 1: AERO-TOXICOLOGY AND ATMOSPHERIC REMEDIATION

1.1 Risk Analysis: The Chemistry of the Invisible

Indoor air is not empty; it is an aerosol of particles and gases that interact directly with your blood.

Here are the enemies that a Safety Biohacker must neutralize, analyzed at the molecular level:

1. **PM 2.5 (Fine Particulate Matter): The Vascular Killer**
   This is not simply "dust"; we are talking about particles < 2.5 microns that bypass the protective cilia of the bronchi and enter directly into the bloodstream.

- **The Mechanism:** The body recognizes them as invaders and triggers a storm of inflammatory cytokines (**IL-6 and TNF-alpha**), causing endothelial oxidative stress (stiffening of the arteries) and neuroinflammation.

2. **VOCs (Volatile Organic Compounds): Domestic Off-Gassing**
   Furniture, paints, and detergents release gases such as formaldehyde and benzene, a process called *off-gassing*.

- **The Risk:** VOCs saturate the liver's detoxification systems (**Phase 1 and 2 of the liver**) while you sleep, preventing nighttime regeneration and detoxification.

3. **CO_2 (Carbon Dioxide): Silent Hypoxia**
   In a closed room, CO_2 quickly rises above 2,000 ppm.

- **Physiology:** This level induces **mild respiratory acidosis** in the blood, the pH drops slightly, causing nighttime awakenings, headaches, and that morning "brain fog" sensation that many confuse with sleep deprivation.

4. **Radon Gas: Radiation from Below**
   The invisible radioactive killer that rises from the ground is classified as a Group 1 carcinogen. You cannot see or smell it: you must measure it.

TECHNICAL BOX: THE DANGER OF MYCOTOXINS

Please note: a HEPA filter captures mold spores, but not always gaseous mycotoxins. If you smell a musty odor, there is a bio-safety problem (Sick Building Syndrome).

In these cases, ventilation or PCO (photocatalysis) technology is required to destroy the toxic molecule at a chemical level.

1.2 The Biological Filter: Nasal Breathing and Nitric Oxide

We can have the best filters in the world, but if you breathe through your mouth, the safety system fails. The nose is not just a conduit; it is a sophisticated biological system.

- **Filtration and Heating:** The nasal turbinates trap particulate matter and bring the air to the ideal temperature.
- **The Magic of (NO):** The paranasal sinuses produce **nitric oxide (NO)**, an antiviral and bronchodilator gas. By inhaling through your nose, you bring this gas into your lungs, improving blood oxygenation by 15-20%.
- **Apex Action:** At night, the mouth tends to open. Biohackers use **mouth taping** (a microporous patch on the lips) to force nasal breathing and ensure 8 hours of filtered air.

  If you don't trust Mouth Taping because you're afraid your nose will close and you'll have oxygen deprivation, use a nasal dilator (external patch or internal device) to ensure your nasal passages remain clear while you sleep.

1.3 Solution Engineering: Technology and Ions

To purify the air, we use a layered approach:

- **HEPA H13/H14 filtration:** The minimum standard for the bedroom (99.95%+ retention).

- **Activated Carbon:** Kilograms, not grams, to absorb chemical VOCs.
- **Hygrometric Management:** Maintain humidity at **40-60**%.

  Below 40%, your mucous membranes dry out and viruses pass through; above 60%, mold proliferates.

SAFETY NOTE: An air purifier without a built-in or external laser sensor is a blind system. You cannot manage what you cannot measure correctly, so make sure you have data feedback (display or app) to know if the system is working.

AIR VITAMINS: NEGATIVE IONIZATION

It is not enough to remove the "bad" (particulate matter); you have to add the "good."

In closed offices, the air is charged with **positive ions** (generated by screens and devices) that cause lethargy.

In nature (forests, waterfalls), the air is rich in **negative ions**.

A Safety Biohacker seeks to restore this regenerating electrical charge by using high-quality bipolar ionizers (without ozone) or simply by ventilating during a thunderstorm and walking barefoot (grounding).

Safety Officer's note on monitoring: > "For an accurate risk analysis, CO_2 and PM2.5 sensors should not be placed near windows or on the floor.

They must be placed in the **Breathing** Zone: at head height on the bedside table or desk , as this is where critical gas exchange

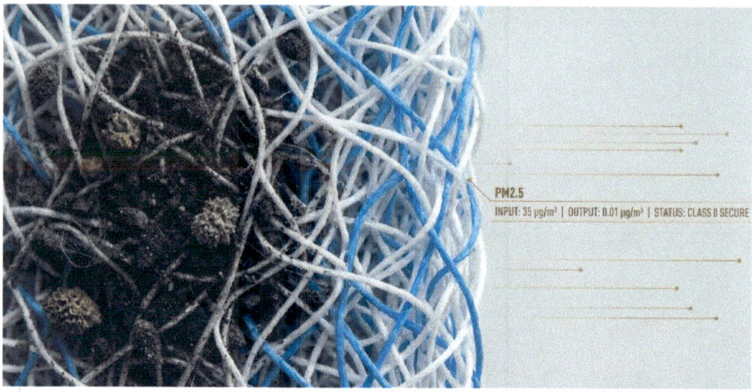
PM2.5
INPUT: 35 µg/m³ | OUTPUT: 0.01 µg/m³ | STATUS: CLASS 0 SECURE

takes place, and this is where we must measure air compliance."

PART 2: APPLIED HYDROLOGY AND BIO-COMPATIBILITY

2.1 Water as a Chemical Solution

Today, water is contaminated with **nanoplastics** (up to 240,000 particles/liter), **PFAS** ("immortal" endocrine disruptors), and **chlorine** (which kills the microbiome and forms carcinogenic trihalomethanes). But purity is not enough; water must be **alive**.

SAFETY BOX: THE SKIN SIEGE

The shower is chlorine's **Trojan horse**. Many people filter their drinking water but ignore the water they wash with.

During a hot shower, the pores of the skin dilate, absorbing chlorine and heavy metals like a sponge.

Worse still, the heat vaporizes the chlorine (gas), which is inhaled directly into the lungs and enters the bloodstream instantly.

The fact: A 10-minute shower can be equivalent to the toxic absorption of 4 liters of unfiltered drinking water. A shower filter is not optional; it is mandatory PPE (Personal Protective Equipment).

2.2 ORP and Hydrogen: The Electronic Frontier

Here we enter the physics of water.

- **ORP (Oxidation-Reduction Potential):** Tap water has a positive ORP (+200/400 mV), so it "steals" electrons (it is an oxidant).
- **Healing Water:** We want water with a negative ORP (-200/-400 mV). This water acts as an electron donor, neutralizing free radicals.
- **The Solution:** The addition of **molecular hydrogen (H2)** transforms water into a powerful selective antioxidant that reduces inflammation.

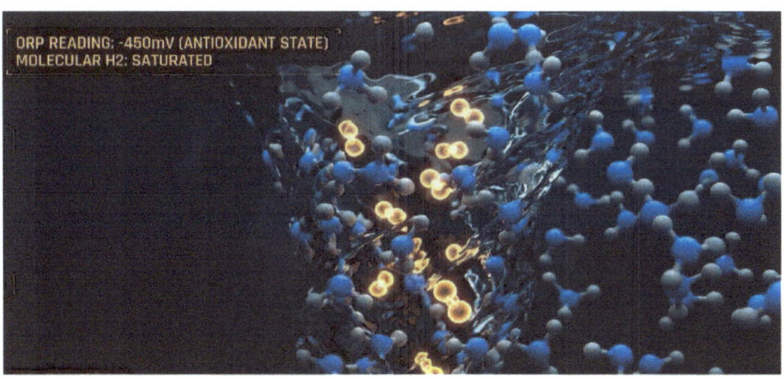

2.3 The Gold Standard: Osmosis, Kinetics, and Deuterium

1. **Reverse Osmosis (RO):** Removes 99% of physical contaminants by pushing water through a 0.0001 micron membrane.

2. **Remineralization:** Crucially, RO water is "empty" and acidic; it must be replenished with electrolytes to prevent bone demineralization.

3. **Vortexing (Water Kinetics):** In addition to chemistry, physics matters.

   In nature, water moves in vortexes, not straight pipes. Vortexing water (with special devices or jugs) breaks up large molecular "clusters," improving surface tension and making it more bioavailable to cells.

4. **Frontiera Apex (Deuterium):** Low-deuterium water (DDW, <130 ppm) is the latest hack for maximizing the efficiency of mitochondrial nanomotors (ATP synthase) by reducing friction at the atomic level.

THE LAW OF THE FILTER: If you don't buy a filter for your water, you become the filter, and your kidneys and liver will be forced to process what technology could have stopped upstream.

THE OPERATING PROTOCOL: FROM THEORY TO PRACTICE

PHASE 1: AUDIT (Measure)

- **Air Monitor:** Laser for PM2.5, CO2, and VOC (Target: CO2 < 800 ppm).

- **Radon Audit:** Dosimeter at the lowest point in the house.
- **Water Test:** TDS meter (Target RO: < 30 ppm pre-minerals).

STEP 2: THE "ZERO PRICE PROTOCOL" (Democratic Biohacking)

If you can't invest in equipment today, do this to achieve 80% of the result:

- **Air (NASA Plants):** Fill your home with **Sansevieria** (Mother-in-law's Tongue), which produces oxygen at night and absorbs formaldehyde.
- **Water (Boiling & Decanting):** If you drink from the tap, leave the water in an open jug for 30 minutes or bring it to a boil. This evaporates most of the chlorine (but does not remove metals or plastics).
- **Water (Binchotan):** Use original Binchotan charcoal sticks in glass, they absorb impurities and release minerals at a negligible cost.
- **Tactical Ventilation:** Open everything for 5 minutes every 3 hours, CO2 drops to zero at no cost.

PHASE 3: APEX PROTOCOL (Elite Technology)

- **Air:** HEPA H13-H14 purifier + Activated Carbon (kg) + Environmental Probiotics + Ionizer.

- **Water:** Under-sink reverse osmosis + Molecular Hydrogen Generator + Vortexer + Chlorine filter for the shower.
- **Bio-Filter:** Mandatory nighttime mouth taping and, for safety, internal or external device to keep the nasal passages open.

PHASE 4: OPERATIONAL MAINTENANCE (The Safety Cycle)

An elite biohacker knows that a dirty filter is more dangerous than no filter at all.

- **The Risk:** If a HEPA filter is not changed, it becomes a breeding ground for bacteria and mold; if an osmosis membrane breaks, the TDS rises without you noticing, exposing you to contaminant spikes.
- **The Action:**
  - **Calibration:** Check outdoor CO2 sensors every 6 months to reset the zero.
  - **Replacement:** Create a digital calendar for filter changes; don't wait for the warning light to come on or the water to change taste.
  - **Sanitization:** Clean humidifier tanks and water bottles regularly to prevent bacterial biofilm.

SAFETY OFFICER'S ADVICE

"Security is layered. Don't rely on just one system. Filter your water, but don't drink it from plastic. Filter the air, but breathe through your nose. Biohacking isn't about buying expensive gadgets, it's about creating redundant security that protects your biology even when one system fails."

✅ SAFETY CHECKLIST: MODULE 1

Chapter validation. If you don't have 5 green check marks, the system is at risk.

- [ ] **AUDIT:** Have you measured Radon and CO2?
- [ ] **BIOLOGY:** Do you breathe through your nose at night (Mouth Taping)?
- [ ] **WATER:** Have you eliminated plastic bottles?
- [ ] **FILTRATION:** Do you use Osmosis, Binchotan, or certified filters?
- [ ] **SHOWER:** Do you have a chlorine filter (inhalation risk)?
- [ ] **ORP:** Do you supplement hydrogen and use "living" water (H2+Vortex)?
- [ ] **MAINTENANCE:** Do you have an active schedule for changing filters (air/water)?

Safety Status:

🔴 **RED:** Open mouth, plastic water, stale air.

🟢 **GREEN:** Clear nose, Osmosis + Hydrogen, Active monitoring and Scheduled maintenance.

CHAPTER 2

THE INVISIBLE SABOTEURS: SYSTEMIC TOXICOLOGY AND ADVANCED REMEDIATION PROTOCOLS

"You can't 'overclock' a system that's on fire. Before seeking extreme performance, we must restore organic clearance."

In biohacking, I often see the "Summator" mistake: people adding expensive supplements to a toxic lifestyle, hoping that the good will cancel out the bad.

Biology doesn't work by addition, but by **subtraction of interference**.

The key concept that a biohacker must master is **Total Toxic Load (Body Burden)**.

Your body is like a barrel, filling up with stressors every day: heavy metals, alcohol metabolites, endocrine disruptors, herbicides.

As long as the level is low, the system manages, but when the barrel overflows, you don't have "a few symptoms": you have a systemic collapse with chronic inflammation, autoimmunity, and adrenal fatigue.

If your body is busy managing these threats, it will never have the energy resources (ATP) to activate longevity genes; **it is stuck in "Emergency Management" mode.**

In this chapter, we will defuse the Saboteurs that are silently rewriting your genetic code.

PART 1: VOLUNTARY "SUICIDE" (Smoking and Alcohol)

1.1 Smoking: The Destruction of the Source Code

I will not talk about the lungs or the risk of cancer, those are well-known facts, let's talk about **Damage Engineering**.

Smoking is not a vice, it is an industrial production of **DNA adducts**. Tobacco toxins (polycyclic aromatic hydrocarbons) are electrophilic: they desperately seek electrons and snatch them from your DNA, chemically binding (covalent bond) to the nitrogenous bases.

This creates a physical obstruction on the double helix that prevents proper cell replication.

- **The Pro-Oxidant Effect (The Integration Paradox):** If you smoke and take multivitamins, you may accelerate the damage.

  In a smoke-saturated lung environment (high oxygen tension and free radicals), some antioxidants such as beta-carotene or high-dose Vitamin E undergo a *pro-*

oxidant shift; instead of extinguishing the fire, they become fuel.

A Safety Officer knows not to throw water on a chemical fire: first, remove the oxygen (stop smoking).

1.2 Alcohol: The Great Metabolic Deception

Alcohol is the **gerontogen** (age generator) par excellence.

The problem is not intoxication (neurological effect), it is the metabolite: **acetaldehyde**.

1. **Molecular Glue:** Acetaldehyde is 30 times more toxic than ethanol and acts by creating *cross-links* between proteins.

   Imagine your collagen and elastin fibers (skin, blood vessels) as loose rubber bands; acetaldehyde "glues" them together into a rigid tangle, which is accelerated structural aging.

2. **Glymphatic Sabotage:** Even a moderate dose of alcohol in the evening suppresses REM sleep and fragments deep sleep.

   It is during these phases that the glymphatic system "opens the taps" to wash toxic proteins (beta-amyloid) out of the brain. Drinking in the evening means waking up with a "dirty" brain.

3. **The NAD+ Bottleneck:** To break down alcohol, the liver consumes enormous amounts of **NAD+**, the same molecule that sirtuins need to repair DNA. Drinking alcohol means stealing fuel from longevity to pay the price of detoxification.

PART 2: THE INVISIBLE INVASION (Metals, Plastics, and Chemicals)

2.1 Heavy Metals: False Friends (Molecular Mimicry)

Heavy metals (mercury, lead, cadmium, aluminum) do not destroy cells by exploding; they deceive them.

They use **molecular mimicry** to replace essential minerals in enzymes:

- **Lead** replaces calcium in bones and neurons.
- **Cadmium** displaces zinc from DNA repair enzymes.
- **Mercury** has a deadly affinity for the sulfhydryl groups of mitochondria, blocking the electron transport chain.

THE SELENIUM SHIELD: THE MOLECULAR PPE

Mercury has an extreme chemical affinity for selenium. When it enters the body, it "sequesters" selenium reserves, preventing the production of glutathione peroxidase (the brain's main antioxidant) and causing neurotoxicity.

Apex Action: Always ensure that the selenium:mercury ratio is in your favor. Never consume large fish without supplementing with selenium or eating two Brazil nuts. Selenium acts as a molecular handcuff, neutralizing mercury before it reaches your mitochondria.

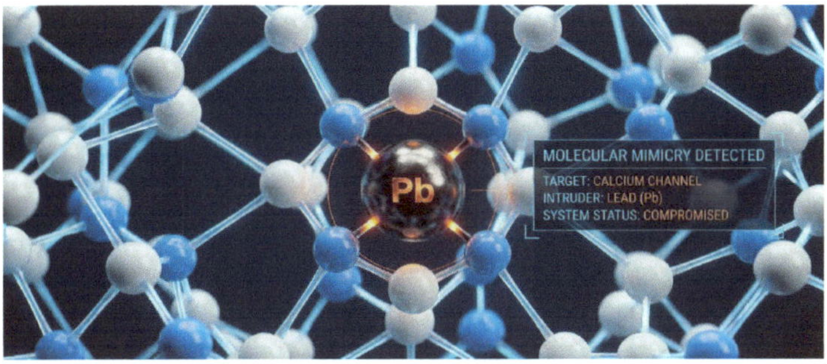

Pb
MOLECULAR MIMICRY DETECTED
TARGET: CALCIUM CHANNEL
INTRUDER: LEAD (Pb)
SYSTEM STATUS: COMPROMISED

TECHNICAL BOX: THE BLOOD LIMIT

"I had my blood tested and the metals are fine." Wrong.

The blood is just a highway; the body quickly moves metals from the blood to "storage" tissues (bones, fat, brain) to protect vital organs. A clean blood test does not rule out chronic tissue toxicity. To see the truth, you need a mineralogram (hair) or a provocation test.

SPECIFIC SHIELD: SILICA VS ALUMINUM

Aluminum (found in deodorants and cookware) is a neurotoxin linked to neurodegenerative diseases.

The Elite Antidote: **Orthosilicic Acid** (Silica).

It is the natural antagonist of aluminum: it binds to it in the blood, forming an inert compound that is easily excreted by the kidneys.

Apex Action: Drinking mineral water rich in silica (>30 mg/L) or using horsetail/orthosilicic acid supplements is the biosecurity strategy to protect the brain from aluminum accumulation.

TOXIC SYNERGY: THE "OPEN DOOR" EFFECT (Toxins + EMF)

Modern toxicology meets physics: there is evidence that chronic exposure to electromagnetic fields (EMFs) increases the permeability of the blood-brain barrier (BBB).

The Impact: If your brain barrier is "open" due to nighttime Wi-Fi, heavy metals in the blood have free access to neurons.

Apex Action: Chemical toxicity is amplified by electromagnetic vulnerability, so never start a metal detox protocol in an EMF-saturated environment.

2.2 Plastics and Xenohormones: Endocrine Hacking

We live in the Plastic Age, microplastics act as **Xenohormones** (alien hormones).

- **PFAS (Forever Chemicals):** Indestructible fluorinated compounds, they have a half-life in the human body of years.
- **BPA and Phthalates:** They mimic estrogen, bind to cell receptors intended for your hormones, sending false signals of "growth" or "fat accumulation."

MARKETING TRAP: THE DECEPTION OF "BPA-FREE"

Warning: companies often replace Bisphenol A (BPA) with **BPS (Bisphenol S)** or **BPF**. Recent studies show that these substitutes are just as potent as endocrine disruptors.

Apex Action: Don't trust "greenwashing." The only safe plastic is the kind that doesn't come into contact with your hot food. Switch completely to glass or steel.

2.3 Glyphosate: Structural Infiltration

Glyphosate is structurally similar to the amino acid **glycine**.

The body can be tricked into inserting glyphosate into protein chains instead of glycine, creating defective collagen and compromising the integrity of the intestinal barrier (leaky gut).

2.4 Personal Care Audit (Transdermal Bio-Security)

The skin is a permeable "customs barrier" that has no metabolic filters.

When you eat a poison, the liver has a chance to filter it (First Pass), but when you rub it on your skin, it enters the bloodstream directly.

- **The Safety Officer's Rule:** *"If you can't eat it, don't put it on your skin."*

  If the INCI of your deodorant looks like an industrial chemistry treatise, it is a flaw in your safety system.

PART 3: THE BIOCHEMISTRY OF CLEANSING (The Liver and the Intestines)

Detoxification

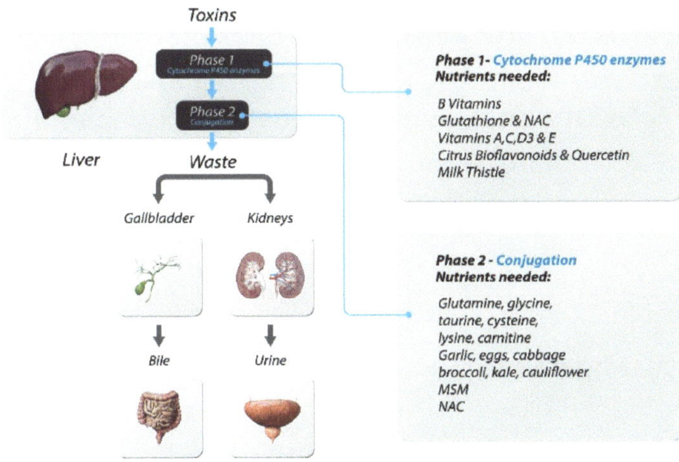

The liver works like a 3-step assembly line. If one step gets blocked, detoxification becomes intoxication.

1. **STAGE 1 (Activation - Cytochrome P450):** The "Cutter."

   The liver oxidizes the toxin, creating an intermediate metabolite that is often **more toxic and reactive** than the original toxin (free radicals).

THE PARADOX OF CAFFEINE

Many biohackers abuse coffee. But caffeine is a powerful inducer of Phase 1 (via the CYP1A2 enzyme).

If you have a genetic mutation that slows down Phase 2 (MTHFR) and you drink 5 coffees a day, you are "pumping gasoline" into a Phase 1 that breaks down poisons faster than you can pack them.

Apex Action: During chemical remediation, drastically reduce caffeine so you don't create a toxic traffic jam in your liver.

2. **PHASE 2 (Conjugation):** "Packaging."

   The toxic metabolite is combined with molecules such as glutathione or methyl groups to make it water-soluble and safe.

   - ***Genetic Risk (MTHFR):*** If you have an MTHFR mutation, your Phase 2 is slow. If you stimulate Phase 1 but Phase 2 is blocked, you accumulate toxins.

   Safety Note: Genetics is not destiny, it is an indication of load. Knowing your MTHFR polymorphism is not meant to scare you, but to let you know how much extra protection you need to provide to your disposal system.

THE SAFETY KPI: HOMOCYSTEINE

If methylation (Phase 2) is blocked, **homocysteine** rises in the blood. This molecule is not just a marker; it is an endogenous toxin that "scratches" the endothelium of the arteries and destroys collagen.

Apex Action: Check your levels. If they are above **9-10 μmol/L**, your Phase 2 is stalled. This is a sign that your disposal system is overheating.

3. **PHASE 3 (Transport and Elimination):** The "Courier."

   Expulsion via bile into the intestine.

THE LUBRICANT OF PHASE 3: BILE

It is not enough to package the waste; the conveyor belt must keep moving.

If your bile is thick and sticky ("bile sludge"), toxins remain trapped in the liver, causing inflammation.

Apex Action: Supplementing with **taurine**, **choline,** or bile salts (**TUDCA**) is essential for thinning the bile and ensuring that the toxic load reaches the intestine for final expulsion.

THE FINAL SABOTEUR: BETA-GLUCURONIDASE

In the intestine, "bad" bacteria produce the enzyme **Beta-Glucuronidase**, which "unwraps the package" prepared by the liver, releasing the toxin again, which is then reabsorbed.

Solution: Calcium D-Glucarate (which inhibits the enzyme) and prebiotic fibers.

THE OPERATING PROTOCOL: DETOX & PROTECTION

Before taking action, memorize the **Safety Officer's Golden Rule**:

DRAINAGE BEFORE MOBILIZATION

If you use a powerful chelator to "loosen" metals from tissues, but your excretory organs (kidneys, intestines, liver) are clogged, the metals will redistribute to the brain and kidneys, causing acute damage.

The Mandatory Sequence:

1. Open the drains (Hydration, Fluid Bile, Bowel Regularity).
2. Clean the intestines (Binders).
3. Only at the end, mobilize the metals.

CRISIS MANAGEMENT: THE HERXHEIMER REACTION

If you experience headaches, nausea, or skin rashes during a detox protocol, it is not "the detox working"; it is your system collapsing. This is called **a healing crisis**.

It means that you are mobilizing toxins faster than you can expel them.

Emergency Protocol: Stop the mobilizers immediately, double the Binders (Charcoal/Zeolite) and massive hydration. Safety is not a race.

PHASE 1: TURN OFF THE TAPS (Elimination at the Source)

1. **Safe Cooking:** Get rid of scratched Teflon. Use stainless steel, cast iron, or glass instead.
2. **Smart Fish:** Stop eating predators (tuna), yes to small blue fish.
3. **Clean Cosmetics:** Use apps to scan the INCI.
4. **Thermal Hygiene:** Avoid handling receipts (BPA).

PHASE 2: OPEN THE DRAINS (Physiological Support)

1. **Mineral & Silica Hydration:** Silica-rich water for aluminum.
2. **Sweating (Sauna):** The gold standard for expelling phthalates and metals.
3. **Glycine Saturation:** Consume **collagen/glycine** to protect yourself from glyphosate.

4. **Bile Flow:** Taurine or bitter foods to stimulate bile.

DEMOCRATIC BIOHACKING: THE MAGNESIUM BATH

Don't have a sauna or thousands of dollars to spend? A hot bath with **500g of Epsom salts (magnesium sulfate)** is your affordable "external kidney." The heat stimulates sweating, while the sulfate provides bioavailable sulfur, an essential fuel for Phase 2 liver function.

PHASE 3: TACTICAL CHELATION (Binders & Inhibitors)

- **Chlorella/Zeolite:** Use **Zeolite** for heavy metals (thanks to its electrical charge) and **Activated Carbon** for organic toxins (mold, pesticides). Diversify the Binders for 360° defense.
- **NAC (N-Acetylcysteine):** To recharge hepatic glutathione.
- **Calcium D-Glucarate:** To inhibit toxic reabsorption (Beta-Glucuronidase).

OPERATIONAL SAFETY: THE 2-HOUR RULE

Warning: Binders (carbon, zeolite) are "blind"; they absorb everything, including life-saving drugs and valuable nutrients.

- ***Apex Action:*** Always take them at least **2 hours before or after** medications, supplements, or meals rich in nutrients or , otherwise they will sequester the good along with the bad.

SAFETY OFFICER'S WORD

"True detox is not a juice diet, it is bioengineering: understanding the kinetics of the Hepatic Phases and respecting your own genetics. If you remove metals from tissues with aggressive chelators without having binders in the intestine or without blocking Beta-Glucuronidase, you are only moving the poison from the bones to the brain. Patience is your safety."

✅ SAFETY CHECKLIST: CHAPTER 2

Chapter validation. If you don't have 5 green ticks, you are under chemical attack.

- [ ] **KITCHEN:** Have you replaced scratched Teflon pans with steel/cast iron ones?
- [ ] **FISH:** Have you eliminated your regular consumption of large predators (tuna)?
- [ ] **COSMETICS:** Have you checked the INCI of the products you put on your skin?
- [ ] **PLASTIC:** Do you use glass containers to store and heat food (even if they are "BPA-free")?
- [ ] **DRAINAGE:** Do you take saunas or Epsom salt baths at least twice a week?
- [ ] **SUPPORT:** Do you take silica for aluminum or taurine for bile?
- [ ] **STEP 3: Do** you supplement with fiber or calcium D-glucarate to prevent toxic reabsorption?

Safety Status:

🔴 **RED:** You cook with Teflon, use industrial cosmetics, and suffer from constipation.

🟢 **GREEN:** Inert materials, clean INCI, complete liver support.

CHAPTER 3

THE ORAL GATEWAY: THE SENTINEL OF THE SYSTEM (BIOLOGICAL DENTISTRY)

"A doctor who ignores the patient's mouth is like an engineer who inspects a skyscraper while ignoring its foundations."

There is a dangerous divide in modern medicine: we treat the body as a holistic unit, but leave the mouth to dentists, as if it were an entity separate from biology.

The anatomical truth is brutal: **the mouth is the main gateway for chronic diseases**.

As a Safety Officer, I apply the theory **of Focal Infection**: a localized infectious focus (a devitalized tooth, inflamed gums) can spread bacteria and toxins to distant organs (heart, kidneys, joints) through the bloodstream, triggering pathologies that appear to have no cause.

In this chapter, we will move from "mechanical" dentistry (repairing the hole) to "biological" dentistry (biocompatibility and systemic safety).

PART 1: TIME BOMBS (Root Canals, NICO, and Meridians)

1.1 The Paradox of Mummification (Root Canal)

Root canal treatment is the only medical procedure that involves leaving a **dead** organ inside the body.

If your liver died, or your finger became gangrenous, the surgeon would remove it immediately to avoid sepsis, but with teeth, we do the opposite: we "mummify" them.

- **The Architecture of Risk:** A tooth is not solid; dentin is traversed by kilometers of microscopic **dentinal tubules** (if unrolled, the tubules of a front tooth measure 4 km).
- **The Bacterial Bunker:** When the nerve is removed and the main canal is sealed, it is physically impossible to sterilize these lateral microtubules. The trapped bacteria, deprived of oxygen and unreachable by white blood cells, mutate, become anaerobic, and begin to produce powerful toxins such as **thioethers** and **mercaptans**.
- **The Systemic Impact:** These toxins seep into the bloodstream 24/7, inhibiting key enzymes essential for energy production.

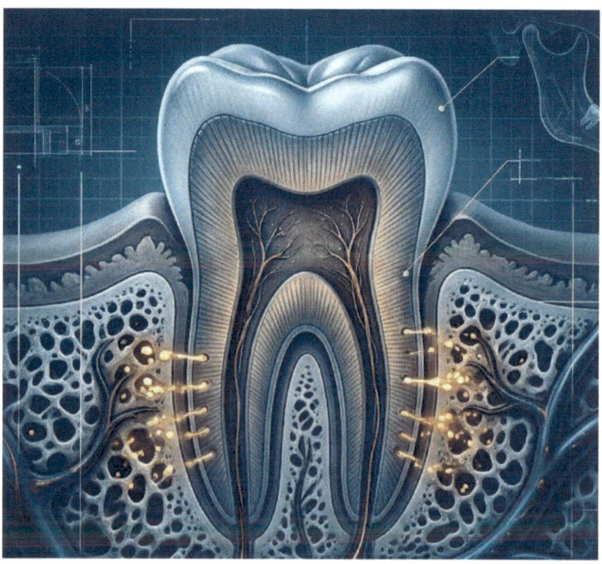

1.2 The Tooth-Organ Map (The Bio-Electrical Connection)

In biological medicine, each tooth acts as a "fuse" on a specific electrical circuit (meridian). If the tooth is infected or metallic, the circuit short-circuits.

- **Clinical Examples:**
  - **Incisors:** Connected to the kidneys and bladder, infections here are often linked to chronic cystitis.
  - **Canines:** Connected to the liver and gallbladder.
  - **Premolars:** Connected to the lungs and large intestine.
  - **Molars:** Connected to the stomach and pancreas.
- **Apex Action:** If you have a chronic problem with an organ that won't heal, check the corresponding tooth. Often, by healing the tooth, the organ improves "miraculously."

1.3 Silent Cavitations (NICO)

Often, where a wisdom tooth was extracted years ago, the bone does not heal perfectly. A **cavity** (NICO) forms: a pocket of necrotic bone and fat, invisible on normal X-rays.

- **The Cytokine Factory:** These areas are biological factories of **RANTES (CCL5)**, an aggressive pro-inflammatory cytokine linked to chronic fatigue, ALS, multiple sclerosis, and breast cancer.

- **Safety Audit:** A 2D overview does not see them. A 3D **CBCT (Cone Beam)** is needed to identify these immunological "black holes."

THE SYSTEM MONITOR: hs-CRP (HIGH-SENSITIVITY C-REACTIVE PROTEIN)

You can't claim to be a confident biohacker if you don't monitor systemic inflammation.

Silent infections in the mouth (NICO, periodontitis) are the number one cause of chronic elevation of high-sensitivity C-reactive protein (hs-CRP).

The Longevity KPI: If your value is above **1.0 mg/L** despite a perfect diet and healthy lifestyle, the flaw is almost certainly in the Oral Gateway; an infected mouth is a constant fire consuming your longevity resources.

PART 2: CHEMICAL, ELECTRICAL, AND MATERIAL WARFARE

2.1 Amalgam: The Toxic Reactor

Silver fillings **are 50% mercury**, which is not a stable material. It releases mercury vapors every time you chew, drink hot beverages, or grind your teeth.

The vapor passes through the mucous membranes and reaches the brain, accumulating as a neurotoxin.

SAFETY PROTOCOL: S.M.A.R.T.

Removing an amalgam filling without protection is worse than keeping it in. Demand the **S.M.A.R.T.** (Safe Mercury Amalgam Removal Technique) protocol:

1. Rubber dam (isolation).
2. High-volume suction + Clean-Up.
3. External nasal air source (oxygen).
4. Cold cutting (to avoid vaporizing the mercury).

2.2 Galvanic Conflict: The "Battery in the Mouth"

The mouth is a moist, salty environment. If you have different metals (e.g., an amalgam filling and a gold or titanium bridge), saliva acts as an electrolyte, creating a real battery.

- **The Impact:** A measurable electric current is generated (galvanism), which forces the accelerated release of metal ions into the tissues and disrupts brain electrophysiology, as the mouth is only a few centimeters from the temporal lobe.
- **Apex Action:** An elite biohacker asks the dentist to measure the galvanic currents. If they exceed **100 mV** or **3 μA**, your nervous system is under constant electrical interference, and you need to remediate.

2.3 Materials Engineering: Titanium vs. Zirconia

For years, titanium has been the standard for implants.

But a Safety Officer looks at the long-term data.

- **The Titanium Risk:** In addition to galvanism, titanium acts as an **"antenna"** for electromagnetic fields (Wi-Fi, 5G), which can cause local tissue overheating. It is also subject to corrosion and peri-implantitis.
- The **Apex Solution (Class 0): Zirconia** implants are made of inert, biocompatible, white (aesthetic) and, above all, **non-conductive** ceramic. They do not create antennas or batteries and are the ultimate choice for safety.

2.4 The Brain Assassin: *P. Gingivalis*

The bacterium *Porphyromonas gingivalis* (which causes periodontitis) produces toxic enzymes called **gingipains**.

These travel from the mouth to the brain, destroying neurons and increasing the production of beta-amyloid plaques (Alzheimer's).

- **Safety Rule:** If your gums bleed, the blood-brain barrier is under attack.

PART 3: MICROBIOME, CHEMISTRY, AND STRUCTURE

3.1 The Mouth as an Ecosystem (The Nitric and Intestinal Axis)

The mouth is home to the second most complex microbiome after the gut.

MOUTHWASH: THE SILENT KILLER OF BLOOD PRESSURE

Specific bacteria (nitrate reducers) live on the back of the tongue and convert plant nitrates into nitrites, precursors **of nitric oxide (NO)**.

NO is the most powerful vasodilator in the body.

The Sabotage: Using antibacterial mouthwashes (chlorhexidine or alcohol-based) is like cutting the brakes on a car: you kill these bacteria, NO production plummets, and your blood pressure rises immediately.

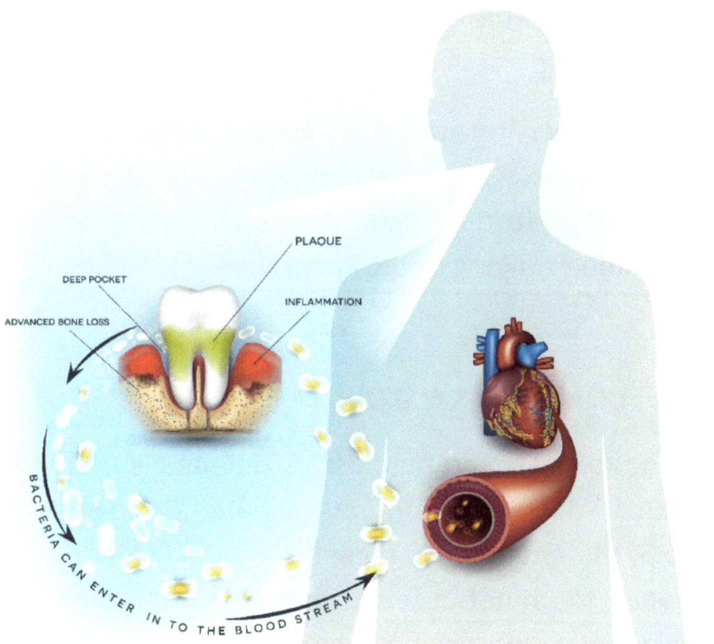

THE MOUTH-GUT BRIDGE: THE BACTERIAL CASCADE

We swallow about 1.5 liters of saliva per day. If the mouth is colonized by pathogenic bacteria (periodontitis), we are literally "seeding" inflammation in the intestine 24 hours a day.

Apex Action: It is impossible to heal a leaky gut or dysbiosis if the upstream "source" is contaminated. Gut health starts above the neck.

3.2 Fluoride vs. Hydroxyapatite: Biomimetics

- **The Fluoride Risk:** Neurotoxic and endocrine disrupting.
- **The Apex Alternative: Hydroxyapatite** (micro or nano). This is the substance that teeth are made of (97% of enamel). It does not poison bacteria, but **repairs** enamel by filling micro-scratches.

THE CHEMICAL PPE: XYLITOL

In addition to passive repair, active defense is needed. Xylitol (wood sugar) acts as **a "molecular bait."** Cariogenic bacteria such as *S. Mutans* eagerly ingest it, mistaking it for sugar, but are unable to metabolize it and starve to death. It also stimulates salivation, raising the pH.

Apex Action: Using 100% xylitol sprays or gum after meals is a tactical countermeasure to decimate the enemy bacterial population without using antibiotics.

PH AUDIT: SURFACE SAFETY

The hardware (enamel) has a precise breaking point: **pH 5.5**. Below this threshold, minerals begin to dissolve.

The 4-Hour Rule: If you eat small snacks frequently, keep your mouth in a constant state of acidity. Saliva needs time to recharge minerals. Wait at least 4 hours between meals to allow the self-repair system to activate.

3.3 Nutritional and Postural Orthodontics (Mewing)

Crooked teeth and a narrow palate are not bad luck, they are a sign of "structural malnutrition" and poor posture.

- **The X Factor and the Mineralization Square:**

Dental architecture requires the **Mineralization Square**: D3 + K2 + Magnesium + Calcium.

Without this protocol, your "foundations" will remain fragile.

- **Oxygen Breach Syndrome (OSAS) and Mewing:**

A narrow palate is a flaw in the ventilation system. If the space is reduced, during sleep the tongue slips back, closing the airways (**Obstructive Apnea**). This causes intermittent hypoxia.

Apex Action: Practice **Mewing**.

Keep your tongue stuck to the palate to expand the airways and prevent hypoxia.

3.4 Mechanical Stress: Bruxism

Many biohackers focus on chemistry but forget about mechanics.

- **Hardware Failure:** Nighttime grinding (bruxism) is an alert signal from the nervous system or compensation for apnea.
- **The Toxic Risk:** If you still have amalgam fillings, bruxism increases the release of mercury vapors from friction by **1,000**%.
- **Apex Action:** A protective mouthguard is mandatory **mechanical PPE** to protect oral architecture.

THE OPERATING PROTOCOL: AUDIT & REMEDIATION

PHASE 1: RADIOLOGICAL AND ELECTRICAL AUDIT

1. **CBCT (Cone Beam 3D):** Mandatory. To look for NICO and silent infections.
2. **Galvanic Test:** Measurement of currents in the mouth (Target: < 100 mV).
3. **Meridian Check:** Correlates your problematic teeth with your suffering organs.

PHASE 2: REMEDIATION AND BIOSAFETY

1. **Amalgam Removal:** S.M.A.R.T. Protocol only.

2. **Metal Replacement:** Switch from Titanium to **Zirconia**.

3. **Ozone Therapy:** To sterilize tubules and cavitations.

4. **Neural Therapy:** The Electrical Reset. Scars (extractions, surgeries) can act as neurological "disturbance fields." Make sure your dentist uses procaine to "reset" the electrical potential of scars and eliminate remote interference.

STEP 3: DAILY MAINTENANCE (Apex Routine)

- **Morning:**
    - **Tongue Scraping:** Remove the toxic coating (Ama).
    - **Oil Pulling:** 10 minutes with coconut oil.
- **Evening:**
    - **Floss/Interdental brush:** Non-negotiable.
    - **Biomimetic Toothpaste:** Hydroxyapatite.
    - **Xylitol:** Gum/spray after meals.
    - **Oral probiotics:** e.g., *S. Salivarius K12*.

SAFETY OFFICER'S WORD

"A biological dentist is not a luxury, but a partner in survival. Oral prevention is the best financial investment of your life (Bio-Economy). A professional hygiene session and a check-up cost less than a dinner out, but reduce the risk of ending up in intensive care for heart or neurodegenerative problems in twenty years by 50%. This is the ROI (Return on Investment) of longevity."

✅ SAFETY CHECKLIST: CHAPTER 3

Chapter validation. If you don't have 6 green ticks, the system is at risk.

- [ ] **AUDIT:** Have you done a 3D CBCT to rule out cavitations and silent infections?
- [ ] **METALS:** Have you removed amalgams and mixed metals (galvanic risk)?
- [ ] **RISK:** Do your gums bleed? (If yes = open barrier).
- [ ] **MONITOR:** Is your hs-CRP below 1.0 mg/L?
- [ ] **MATERIALS:** Have you chosen zirconia instead of titanium for any implants?
- [ ] **CHEMISTRY:** Do you use hydroxyapatite and xylitol?
- [ ] **STRUCTURE:** Do you assume the "Square" (D3/K2/Mg) and practice Mewing/Bite?
- [ ] **BIO-ECONOMICS:** Have you scheduled professional hygiene every 4-6 months?

Safety Status:

🔴 **RED:** Amalgam fillings, inflamed gums, high hs-CRP, sleep apnea.

🟢 **GREEN:** Metal-free, zirconia, hydroxyapatite, xylitol, negative CBCT.

CHAPTER 4

THE INTESTINAL BARRIER: DEFENSIVE PERIMETER AND NUTRITIONAL BIOECONOMY

"Are you what you eat? No. You are what you absorb and, above all, what you don't let in."

Imagine your intestine not as a simple digestive tube, but as **GALT (Gut-Associated Lymphoid Tissue)**: your body's military headquarters.

This is where 70-80% of your immune system resides.

It has a paradoxical task: it must be permeable to nutrients (friends) but impermeable to toxins and pathogens (enemies).

The problem is that the barrier separating these two worlds is composed of a single layer of cells (enterocytes). Thickness: **30 microns** (less than a hair).

I see a very thin line of defense under constant siege.

When this barrier falls (**Leaky Gut**), you don't have a "stomach ache," you have a security breach that allows hostile biological material to enter your bloodstream, triggering an inflammatory war that burns through your longevity reserves.

In this chapter, we will analyze the architecture of the barrier, advanced microbiology, and the economic strategy for feeding the biological elite.

PART 1: THE ARCHITECTURE OF THE FIREWALL (Microscopic Anatomy)

1.1 Tight Junctions

Enterocytes are "sewn" together by protein complexes called **tight junctions**, which are the customs gates.

In a healthy system, they are sealed, opening selectively only to allow micronutrients to pass through.

- **Zonulin Sabotage:** When gluten (gliadin) touches the intestine, or when bacteria detect glyphosate, enterocytes release a signaling protein called **zonulin**.
- **The Effect:** Zonulin acts as an "emergency open" command. The tight junctions break down, and the gates swing wide open.

  Now, viruses, bacteria, and undigested proteins enter the bloodstream unchecked.

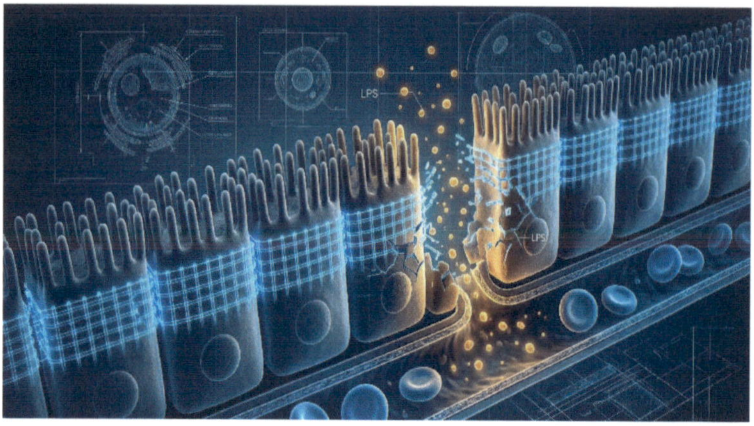

1.2 The Front Line: Mucus and Secretory IgA

Before reaching the cells, pathogens must overcome the "moat": the layer of **mucin**.

Secretory IgA (sIgA) patrols the mucus, special antibodies that "tag" and neutralize invaders before they touch the wall.

- **Audit Apex:** If your stool tests show low sIgA levels, your castle has no guards on the walls. You are vulnerable to any infection. Chronic stress (cortisol) is the primary destroyer of sIgA.

STEALTH SABOTEURS: EMULSIFIERS AND SWEETENERS

In addition to gluten, there are invisible enemies in processed foods (even "healthy" ones).

- **Emulsifiers:** (Carboxymethylcellulose, Polysorbate 80).

They act like **detergents**. They literally dissolve the protective mucus layer, allowing bacteria to directly touch the cells and inflame them.

- **Artificial sweeteners:** (sucralose, aspartame).

  They induce dysbiosis even in minimal doses, altering bacterial communication.

Apex Action: Without the "moat" of mucus, even the best defense system is overwhelmed. Avoid foods with long ingredient lists.

PART 2: THE TOXIC BREACH AND CYBER-SECURITY

2.1 Metabolic Endotoxemia: Fire in the Blood

What happens when the barrier falls? Fragments of the cell wall of Gram-negative bacteria, called **LPS (lipopolysaccharides)** or endotoxins.

- **The TLR4 Receptor:** When LPS enters the bloodstream, it binds to **TLR4** (Toll-Like Receptor 4) receptors on immune cells.
- **The Nuclear Reaction:** This binding activates the **NF-kB** pathway, the "master switch" of inflammation, and the body releases a storm of cytokines (IL-6, TNF-alpha).
- **The Result:** Low-grade systemic inflammation (*inflammaging*). You don't feel local pain, but you have

insulin resistance, depression, brain fog, and joint pain. You are literally poisoning your blood with every meal.

2.2 Molecular Mimicry and Autoimmunity

When whole food proteins (e.g., casein or gluten) pass into the bloodstream through a permeable barrier, the immune system attacks them by creating antibodies.

- **The Tragic Mistake:** Often these proteins resemble your tissues structurally (e.g., casein resembles thyroid cells). The antibodies, confused, attack both the cheese and your thyroid (Hashimoto's thyroiditis). This is the genesis of many autoimmune diseases.

2.3 Nervous Cyber-Security: The Gut-Brain Axis

The gut is not isolated. It is connected to the "Central Server" (Brain) via a biological fiber optic cable: the **Vagus Nerve**.

- **Neurotransmitters:** The gut produces 95% of the body's serotonin and 50% of its dopamine.
- **Cognitive Crash:** If the gut is inflamed (LPS), it sends constant "Danger" signals to the brain via the Vagus Nerve.

  This activates the brain's microglia (Neuro-Inflammation), causing drug-resistant anxiety and depression. If the perimeter is breached, the server crashes.

THE MIRROR BARRIER PRINCIPLE (LEAKY GUT = LEAKY BRAIN)

A Safety Officer must know that if there is a breach in the outer perimeter, the vault is at risk.

There is an almost total correlation between intestinal and cerebral permeability.

Zonulin not only opens the gates of the intestine; it travels in the blood and also loosens the junctions of **the Blood-Brain Barrier (BBB)**, exposing your neurons to toxins that should remain outside.

Apex Action: Repairing the gut is the only way to seal the brain vault.

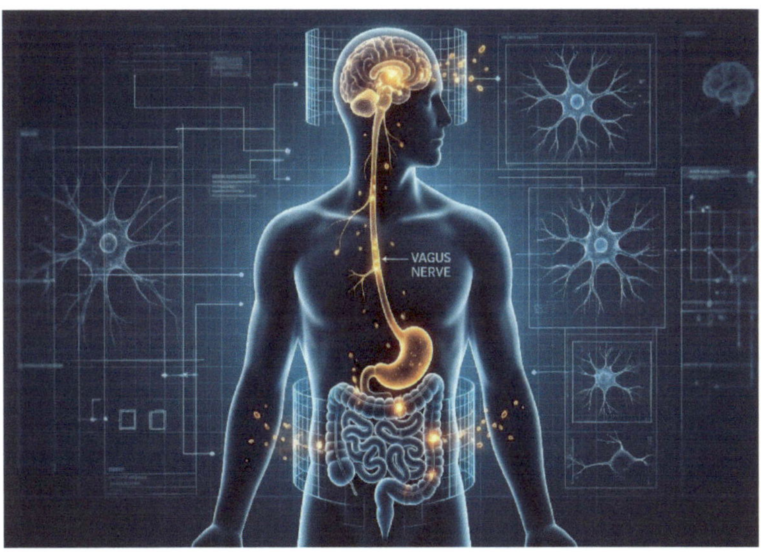

PART 3: ELITE MICROBIOLOGY (Not just "Lactic Ferments")

3.1 Key Species and Backup (Appendix)

Forget generic "Lactobacilli." A biohacker looks for "Ecosystem Engineer" species:

1. **Akkermansia muciniphila:** The "Guardian of Mucus."

   It eats old mucin and stimulates cells to produce new, thicker mucin.

2. **Faecalibacterium Prausnitzii:** The "Fuel Producer."

THE APPENDIX: THE BACKUP SERVER

The appendix is not a useless remnant of evolution. It is the microbiome's **safe house**. It is designed to store a "clean" copy of your original bacteria.

In the event of a serious infection or diarrhea that "resets" the gut, the appendix releases the backup to repopulate the system.

Apex Action: If yours has been removed, you don't have the offline backup. You need to be doubly rigorous with probiotics and nutrition after every illness.

EPIGENETIC FUEL: BUTYRATE

Butyrate (produced by bacteria from fiber) is not just food, it is a genetic signaling molecule that inhibits histone deacetylases

(**HDACs**), turns off inflammation genes, and turns on repair genes.

ZERO PRICE PROTOCOL: THE POTATO HACK

Here is the cheapest way in the world to produce butyrate. Cooking potatoes (or rice) and leaving them to cool in the refrigerator for 24 hours transforms normal starch into **Resistant Starch (Type 3)**.

This is not digested by us (it does not raise blood sugar) but arrives intact in the colon, becoming a royal feast for *Faecalibacterium*. Zero-cost food bioengineering.

APEX FRONTIER: Urolithin A (THE MITOCHONDRIAL LINK)

When specific bacteria process polyphenols (pomegranate), they produce **Urolithin A**.

This molecule activates **mitophagy**: the recycling of old mitochondria, which is the fuel for cellular longevity that originates in the intestine.

3.2 Photobiomics: Light as a Nutrient

Biohacking does not end on the plate.

- **The Concept:** The microbiome has photoreceptors.

  Red and near-infrared (NIR) light that touches the skin of the abdomen penetrates the tissues and sends a safety signal to the bacteria, improving butyrate production.

3.3 Glyphosate and the Shikimate Pathway

Why is the herbicide glyphosate so devastating?

- **The Mechanism:** It blocks the **Shikimate Pathway**, a process used by bacteria to synthesize amino acids.
- **The Impact:** It acts as a selective chronic antibiotic, killing beneficial bacteria and allowing resistant pathogens (Clostridia) to proliferate.

3.4 The Mechanics of Cleaning: The Migratory Motor Complex (MMC)

The intestine is not just chemistry, it is hydraulics.

Every 90-120 minutes, *only on an empty stomach*, a wave starts that "sweeps" away bacteria and residues: the **Migratory Motor Complex (MMC)**.

- **The Snack Mistake:** If you eat constantly, the MMC stops, food stagnates, bacteria rise from the colon to the small intestine and create **SIBO** (Small Intestinal Bacterial Overgrowth).

HYDRAULIC SAFETY: THE ROLE OF BILE

Bile acids (from the liver) are not only used to digest fats, they are also powerful **natural antibiotic cleansers**.

The Risk: If bile flow is poor (thick bile, see Chapter 2), colon bacteria can rise into the small intestine because there is not enough "disinfectant" to keep them at bay. Poor bile management is an open invitation to SIBO.

PART 4: NUTRITIONAL BIOECONOMICS (ROI & Anti-Nutrients)

4.1 Plant Defense: Lectins and Oxalates

Not all vegetables are harmless.

- **Lectins:** Proteins that open tight junctions (Gundry Protocol).
- **Oxalates:** Microcrystals that can accumulate in the kidneys.
- **Safety Action:** Soaking, fermentation, and pressure cooking destroy these toxins.

THE SILENT SABOTAGE: HISTAMINE

The Cause: **Histamine Intolerance** (DAO enzyme deficiency).

If your gut is inflamed, you don't produce enough DAO enzyme to break down histamine in fermented foods.

4.2 ROI (Return on Investment) of Spending

Healthy eating does not have to be elitist. Let's calculate the cost per nutrient.

"Poor" Food (Apex)	Cost/kg	Key Nutrients	"Rich" Food	Comparison
Beef Liver	€5-8	Vitamin A, B12, Copper, CoQ10	Beef tenderloin	Liver has 100 times more nutrients.
Sardines/Mackerel	€8-12	Omega-3, selenium	Salmon (Farmed)	Fewer metals, more real omega-3.
Organic Eggs	€0.50/egg	Choline, High-quality proteins	Protein bars	Eggs win on bioavailability.
Cabbage/Savoy cabbage	€1-2	Sulforaphane, Fiber	Bagged salad	Fermented cabbage is a superfood.

PART 5: THE REPAIR PROTOCOL (5R PROGRAM)

If you have symptoms of Leaky Gut, follow the **5R** protocol:

PHASE 0: AUDIT (Measure the Breach)

- **Fecal Zonulin:** The marker of the gates.
- **Lactulose/Mannitol Test:** The Gold Standard for Permeability.

PHASE 1: REMOVE

Eliminate triggers for 30 days. Gluten, A1 casein, alcohol, seed oils, emulsifiers, sweeteners.

PHASE 2: REPLACE

The Gastric Customs.

- **Stomach Audit:** If your gastric pH is not close to **1.5**, customs are open.
- ***Action:*** Apple cider vinegar or Betaine HCL.

PHASE 3: REINOCULATE

- ***Probiotics:*** Spore-based strains.
- ***Prebiotics:*** Resistant starch (potato hack), inulin.

SAFETY ALERT: THE PARADOX OF FIBER

Warning: If you have **SIBO**, fiber is fuel to the fire; bacteria in the wrong place ferment the fiber, causing explosive gas.

Safety Protocol: First repair gastric customs, bile, and motility (MMC), *then* introduce prebiotics.

PHASE 4: REPAIR

- **L-Glutamine:** Enterocyte fuel.
- **Bovine Colostrum:** Growth factors.
- **Bone Broth:** Liquid collagen.

PHASE 5: REBALANCE (Lifestyle)

The vagus nerve and circadian rhythms.

THE HIDDEN CENTRAL: INTESTINAL MELATONIN

The intestine produces **400 times more** melatonin than the pineal gland, making it the most powerful local antioxidant.

Apex Action: Production is regulated by darkness, so dim the lights when the sun goes down to avoid leaving the barrier unprotected.

PART 6: CHRONONUTRITION: THE RHYTHM OF EATING

We are not designed for continuous grazing.

Your metabolism is not an ON/OFF switch. It is a sine wave. The efficiency of insulin, digestion, and repair changes dramatically over a 24-hour period.

1. TACTICAL FASTING (TRF - Time Restricted Feeding)

It's not a diet, it's a maintenance window.

- **The Concept:** Intestinal stem cells and cleansing processes (autophagy) are only activated after 12-14 hours without calories.
- **Apex Protocol (16:8):** Eat within an 8-hour window (e.g., 11:00 a.m. to 7:00 p.m.). Fast for 16 hours.
- **Safety Warning:** Don't become a fanatic. If you are under extreme stress (high cortisol), prolonged fasting can worsen catabolism. In that case, reduce to 12:12.

2. CIRCADIAN LOAD (Early vs. Late)

Not all calories are created equal.

- **The Science:** Insulin sensitivity is highest in the morning and drops in the evening (melatonin inhibits insulin).
- **The Mistake:** Skipping breakfast and eating a huge dinner at 10 p.m. This is a metabolic disaster.
- **Apex Action:** Shift your calorie load. Eat breakfast/lunch like a king and dinner like a pauper.
    - **Golden Rule:** The last bite should be eaten at least **3-4 hours before bedtime**. If you digest while you sleep, you don't recover (low HRV, suppressed deep sleep).

PART 7: MATERIAL SELECTION: FORENSIC MACRONUTRIENTS

Quality beats quantity. Always.

1. PROTEINS: THE STRUCTURAL BUILDING BLOCKS

Without protein, you lose structure (sarcopenia). But not all proteins build lean muscle.

- **Amino Acid Profile:** Look for high-quality proteins with a high **leucine** content (the trigger for anabolism).
- **Sourcing (Bio-Security):**
    - **Meat:** Only *grass-fed*. Intensive farming meat (grain-fed) is inflammatory (too much omega-6) and full of antibiotics.
    - **Fish:** Only small fish (mackerel, sardines, anchovies) or wild-caught fish. Avoid predators (tuna/swordfish) due to mercury and farmed salmon (dyes and toxic feed).
    - **Eggs:** Only organic/free-range. The yolk is a multivitamin, don't throw it away.

2. FATS: CHANGING YOUR OIL

Your cell membranes are made of the fat you eat. Do you want flexible or rusty membranes?

- **The Enemies (Industrial Seed Oils):** Soybean, corn, sunflower, rapeseed. They are rich in unstable omega-6s that oxidize in the body. They are "biological paint" that inflames the arteries. **Eliminate them completely.**
- **Allies (Stable Fats):**

    - **Saturated:** Ghee butter, coconut oil, animal fat (if grass-fed). Stable when heated, essential for hormones.
    - **Monounsaturated:** Extra Virgin Olive Oil (EVOO), Avocado.
    - **Omega-3:** Fatty fish. Essential for reducing inflammation.

3. CARBOHYDRATES: TACTICAL FUEL

Don't demonize them, manage them. They are high-octane fuel for intense efforts (Zone 5) and for lowering cortisol in the evening.

- **The Choice:** Eliminate white flour (glue for the intestines). Choose tubers, roots, basmati rice, low glycemic index fruits (berries).
- **Timing:** Eat them **after** physical exertion or at dinner (to promote serotonin/sleep), never at breakfast if you want to stay awake and burn fat.

PART 8: CULINARY THERMODYNAMICS: COOKING WITHOUT KILLING

How do you turn healthy food into poison? By getting the temperature wrong.

This is where applied chemistry comes into play. Incorrect cooking generates **Neo-Formed Contaminants (NFC)**: toxins that were not present in the raw material.

1. THE MAILLARD REACTION AND AGEs

That brown, crispy crust on meat or bread is delicious, but it's toxic. It's **Advanced Glycation** End-products **(AGEs)**: sugars that fuse with proteins.

- **The Damage:** AGEs are "glue" that stiffens arteries, ages the skin, and inflames the kidneys.
- **Apex Action:** Avoid burning. If food is black or dark brown, it is damaged.

2. SMOKE POINT AND LIPID OXIDATION

Never cook with a fat above its smoke point.

- **The Mistake:** Frying or sautéing with vegetable oils or EVO at high temperatures. The double bonds in fats break down and form toxic aldehydes and free radicals.
- **Apex Action:**
  - For high temperatures: Use only **ghee** (clarified butter), coconut oil, or lard. These are stable saturated fats that do not oxidize.
  - EVO oil should **only** be used **raw** or for baking. Never let it smoke.

3. SAFE COOKING PROTOCOLS (Heat Hierarchy)

We rank the methods from safest to most toxic.

- **LEVEL 1 (Gold Standard - Safe):**
    - **Steaming:** Preserves nutrients, zero toxins, max temperature 100°C.
    - **Boiling/Poaching:** Excellent for meat and fish. No formation of AGEs.
    - **Sous-Vide (Vacuum-sealed):** Perfect temperature control. Tender meat without burning. (Use BPA-free bags).
- **LEVEL 2 (Acceptable with caution):**
    - **Oven (Low Temp):** Below 160-170°C. Use parchment paper, not aluminum foil in contact with food.
    - **Stew/Slow Cooker:** Long cooking times at low temperatures. Excellent for breaking down collagen in lean meats.
- **LEVEL 3 (Toxic - Avoid or mitigate):**
    - **Grill/Barbecue:** Fat dripping onto the fire creates carcinogenic fumes (Polycyclic Aromatic Hydrocarbons) that return to the meat. Charred meat contains Heterocyclic Amines (HCA).
    - **Frying:** Massive lipid oxidation.

    - **Mitigation:** If *you must* grill, marinate the meat first with lemon, vinegar, and rosemary/herbs. Antioxidants reduce HCA formation by 70-90%. And cut away the blackened parts.

4. CONTACT MATERIALS (Cookware Audit)

Do not cook healthy food in toxic cookware.

- **Eliminate:** Scratched Teflon (PFAS), bare aluminum (neurotoxic).
- **Use:** 18/10 stainless steel, cast iron, glass (Pyrex), 100% ceramic (not just coated).

PART 9: METABOLIC HACKING: GLYCEMIC CURVE MANAGEMENT

Keep the line flat.

Glucose spikes = Insulin spikes = Inflammation and fat accumulation. You don't have to be diabetic to suffer damage from high blood sugar.

1. THE ORDER OF ADDITIONS

The order in which you eat food changes your hormonal response.

- **Protocol:**

1. **Fiber (vegetables) first:** They create a network in the intestine that slows down absorption.
2. **Protein and fat second:** They satisfy hunger and do not raise insulin levels.
3. **Carbohydrates last:** If you eat them at the end, the glycemic peak is reduced by 30-50% compared to eating them at the beginning.

- **Action:** Never eat bread while waiting for the first course. Eat salad first.

2. VINEGAR AS MEDICINE

Acetic acid inhibits alpha-amylase (the enzyme that breaks down starches).

- **Hack:** One tablespoon of apple cider vinegar in a glass of water 10 minutes before a carbohydrate-rich meal reduces the glycemic and insulin response by up to 30%. It is the "poor man's metformin."

3. THE GOLDEN 10 MINUTES (Post-Prandial Walk)

Your muscles are sponges for glucose, but only if you contract them.

- **Hack:** After a meal, don't sit on the couch. Walk for 10 minutes.

- **Mechanism:** Muscle contraction activates GLUT4 transporters independently of insulin, immediately drawing sugar from the blood.

PART 10: THE ANTI-NUTRIENT MAP

Plants don't want to be eaten. They have chemical weapons.

Not all vegetables are harmless. Some contain **anti-nutrients** that steal minerals or puncture the intestine. The Safety Biohacker knows how to defuse them.

1. **Lectins (e.g., beans, nightshades):** They can damage the intestinal barrier.
    - ***Solution:*** Soak for a long time (24 hours) and cook in a pressure cooker (destroys lectins).

2. **Phytic acid (cereals, legumes, nuts):** Binds zinc, iron, and calcium, preventing their absorption.
    - ***Solution:*** Soak, sprout, or ferment (e.g., sourdough bread).

3. **Oxalates (spinach, Swiss chard, almonds):** Microscopic crystals that can cause kidney stones and joint pain.
    - *Solution:* Boil and discard the water (reduces oxalates). Do not eat raw spinach in industrial quantities in smoothies. Consume with a source

of calcium (dairy products/supplements) to bind them in the intestine and prevent absorption.

SAFETY OFFICER'S ADVICE

"Your intestinal barrier is the frontier between you and chaos. You can't build a security system on a foundation of sand. If you allow gluten, glyphosate, and emulsifiers to open the doors, you are inviting the enemy into your bloodstream. Repairing your gut is the highest ROI action you can take for your mental, physical, and immune health. And the good news? The repair materials (broth, eggs, fasting) are the cheapest on the market."

✅ SAFETY CHECKLIST: CHAPTER 4

Chapter validation. If you don't have 5 green check marks, the frontier is compromised.

- [ ] **SYMPTOMS:** Do you experience bloating, gas, or brain fog after meals (Mirror Barrier)?
- [ ] **ELIMINATION:** Have you eliminated gluten, seed oils, and emulsifiers (processed foods)?
- [ ] **CUSTOMS:** Do you use vinegar or betaine to ensure an acidic gastric pH (1.5)?
- [ ] **FLOW:** Do you have good bile flow and respect meal breaks for MMC?
- [ ] **ECONOMY:** Do you use the Potato Hack to produce butyrate at no cost?
- [ ] **LIGHT & TIMING:** Do you eat in natural light and avoid late-night eating?
- [ ] **MITOCHONDRIA:** Do you eat foods rich in polyphenols to produce Urolithin A?

Safety Status:

🔴 **RED:** Chronic bloating, antacids, sweeteners, midnight dinner.

🟢 **GREEN:** Quiet digestion, dense foods, active fasting, fluid bile.

PART 2: SYNCHRONIZATION & ENERGY (The Engine)

Operational Goal: Systemic Efficiency and Sustainable Power

The Concept:

In Part 1, we cleared the ground and built the walls. Now the system is secure, but it is **at a standstill**.

A Formula 1 car can be shiny and clean, but if the electronic control unit is out of phase (circadian rhythms out of whack) or if the cylinders don't burn fuel properly (mitochondrial dysfunction), it will remain stuck in the pits or blow its engine on the first lap.

Many people seek "energy" by abusing stimulants (coffee, pre-workout supplements).

That's not energy, it's **debt**. It's borrowing resources from the future with usurious interest rates. True biological energy (ATP) comes from synchronisation with the laws of physics: light, temperature and movement.

In this phase, we will move from **Safety** to **Performance**, we will start the engine, but we will do so while respecting the engine's revs.

The Battle Plan:

In this section, we will calibrate the biological machine for maximum energy yield:

- **Chapter 5:** We will reset the internal atomic clock.

  You will discover that sleep is not rest, but active maintenance, and that without **Chronobiology**, every other effort is out of time.

- **Chapter 6:** We will learn to "eat" light.

  Photobiomodulation (Solar Logic) will teach us how to use the sun and red light as essential nutrients for your cells.

- **Chapter 7:** We will build the **Metabolic Engine**.

  We will go beyond simple "gym" training for mitochondria (Zone 2) and maximum strength, creating an inexhaustible power reserve.

- **Chapter 8:** We will test resilience with **Thermodynamics**.

  We will use heat and cold not to "temper" ourselves, but to activate ancient survival genes (Hormesis) that make the system anti-fragile.

Don't start the engine until you've read the manual. Power without control is just an accident waiting to happen.

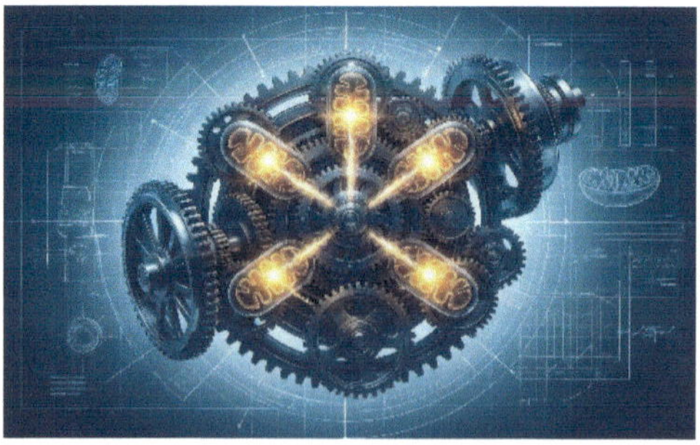

CHAPTER 5

CHRONOBIOLOGY AND SLEEP: SYSTEM MAINTENANCE

"Sleep is not a period of inactivity. It is the only time when your brain activates its cleaning crews to dispose of the toxic waste accumulated during the work shift. Skipping sleep is not heroism, it is accumulating hazardous waste."

In modern culture, sleep is seen as a "luxury" or a waste of time.

"I'll sleep when I'm dead," say burnout managers.

As **a Safety Officer**, I tell you that this is a very serious violation of safety protocols. Sleep deprivation is classified by the WHO as a probable carcinogen (shift work). Driving after 18 hours of wakefulness is equivalent to having a blood alcohol level of 0.05.

Sleep is the **Maintenance Shift**.

Imagine a chemical company that operates 24 hours a day without ever stopping the machines to clean the filters. Sooner or later, the plant will explode. Your body follows a precise rhythm (**circadian rhythm**) dictated by the Earth's rotation. If you ignore this rhythm, you are working against the laws of physics and biology.

In this chapter, we will not talk about "sleeping 8 hours," but about engineering rest: we will learn how to synchronize your

Master Clock, manage the chemical pressure of sleep, and activate the most advanced brain washing system that exists.

PART 1: THE MECHANICS OF THE TWO FORCES (Borbély Model)

You don't fall asleep "by chance." Sleep is the result of the mathematical collision of two opposing biological forces. Understanding this means being able to manipulate the system.

1.1 Process C: The Circadian Rhythm (The Clock)

Deep within your hypothalamus is a biological atomic clock: the **Suprachiasmatic Nucleus (SCN).** Regardless of how tired you are, it decides when to release cortisol (energy/alertness) and when to release melatonin (repair). It is a sine wave that lasts approximately 24 hours and 15 minutes.

- **The Signal (Zeitgeber):** The SCN has no eyes, but it is connected to the retina. The main signal that synchronizes it is **light**.
- **The System Error:** If you expose yourself to blue light (LEDs, smartphones) after sunset, you send a false signal to the SCN: "It's still noon." Melatonin release is blocked and the body remains in "Alert" mode instead of switching to "Maintenance" mode.

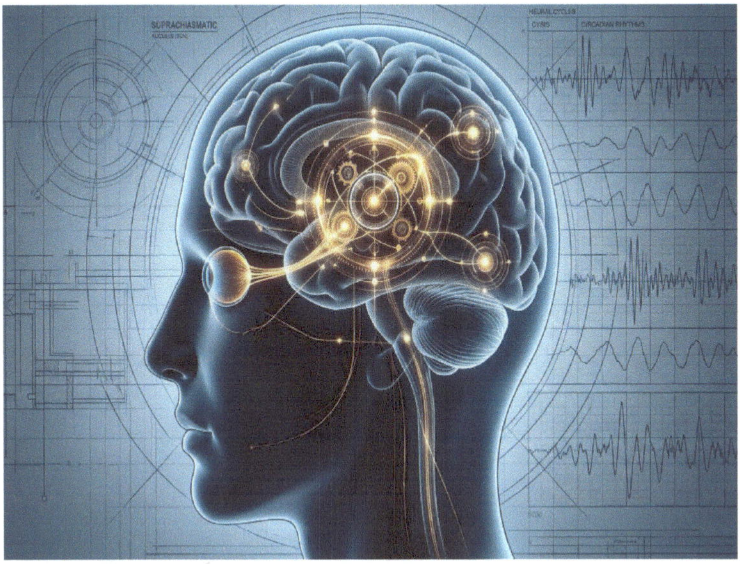

THE TRUTH ABOUT LIGHT: "DON'T LOOK OUT THE WINDOW"

Pay attention to a detail of optical physics: window glass (home, office, car) filters out most of the photons needed to reset the clock.

The Impact: Receiving light through glass takes **50 times longer** to achieve the same biological effect as direct light.

Apex Action: You need to go outside. No sunglasses, no windows. 10 minutes outside is worth more than 2 hours in front of a window.

THE DOUBLE SIGNAL: LIGHT + MOVEMENT

Don't just passively look at the sun. Move while you do it. Mechanical movement (e.g., a 5-minute brisk walk) increases the sensitivity of light receptors and accelerates the suppression of residual melatonin. It's the most powerful "Start" command for your operating system.

THE CORTISOL INJECTION: TAKE ADVANTAGE OF C.A.R.

Why is morning light so powerful? Because of the **Cortisol Awakening Response (CAR)**.

This is the physiological surge of cortisol that occurs in the first 30-45 minutes after waking up. Intense sunlight during this window "fixes" the peak.

The Timer: This not only gives you immediate energy, but also sets the timer for melatonin release **14-16 hours later**. If you miss the morning CAR, you will miss your evening sleep appointment.

VISION ENGINEERING: MELANOPSIN AND ipRGCs

It is not the cones and rods (vision) that synchronize the clock, but the intrinsically photosensitive retinal ganglion cells (**ipRGCs**). These contain a photopigment called **melanopsin**.

The Impact: This sensor is specifically calibrated to blue light at **480nm**. Even if you close your eyes or are visually impaired, if melanopsin is activated by bright light, your biological clock shifts. It is the safety sensor that decides whether to produce melatonin or cortisol. Protect it as you would a smoke detector.

BEYOND THE DARKNESS: THE LOGIC OF FIRE (THE SUNSET SIGNAL)

The absence of blue is not enough. The presence of **red** is needed. Melanopsin detects the absence of blue, but your mitochondria need the red/infrared signal typical of sunset to start cellular melatonin synthesis.

Apex Action: Switch to amber or red lights after dusk. For your ancient brain, this is the code for **"All Clear."**

THE CONFLICT OF SIGNALS: PERIPHERAL CLOCKS AND METABOLIC JET LAG

We've talked about the SCN (Master Clock), but every organ (liver, pancreas) has its own clock.

The Concept: Food is the Zeitgeber (synchronizer) of peripheral clocks. If the light says "Night" but you eat at 11 p.m., your liver receives the signal "Day."

The Impact: This temporal anarchy causes insulin resistance and blocks autophagy. For maximum safety, your "metabolic window" must close when the "light window" closes.

1.2 Process S: Sleep Pressure (Adenosine)

While you are awake and burning ATP to think and move, you accumulate a metabolic waste product: **adenosine**. Adenosine binds to receptors in the brain and creates "sleep pressure." The more hours you are awake, the more the pressure rises.

CAFFEINE HACKING (AND ITS COST)

Caffeine does not give you energy. Caffeine is structurally similar to adenosine and "parks" itself in its receptors, blocking them. You are tired, but your brain cannot "feel" the adenosine because the sensors are blocked by caffeine.

Safety Warning: The half-life of caffeine is 5-7 hours. The coffee you drank at 2:00 p.m. is still active in your blood at 9:00 p.m., preventing your brain from entering deep sleep.

PART 2: GENETICS AND CHRONOTYPES (The PER3 Gene)

We are not all the same.

Waking up at 5 a.m. ("The 5 Club") is good for some and destroys others. This is genetically determined by the length of **the PER3 gene**.

1. **Early Birds:** Long PER3 gene. They have an early melatonin peak. They are hyper-productive in the morning but crash at 9:00 p.m.
2. **Night Owls:** Short PER3 gene. Their cortisol peak comes later.
3. **The "Social Jet Lag" Risk:** Forcing an owl to get up at dawn creates a chronic misalignment between their biological clock and their social clock. This increases the risk of obesity, depression, and cardiovascular disease.

- *Apex Action:* Don't fight your genetics. Synchronize your most demanding activities with your natural peak.

PART 3: BRAINWASHING (Glymphatic System)

3.1 The Discovery of the Century

Until 2012, medicine thought that the brain did not have a lymphatic system to drain waste. This was a mistake. The **Glinphatic System** (Glia + Lymphatic) was discovered.

- **The Mechanics:** During deep sleep, the brain's glial cells physically "shrink" by 60%. This creates hydraulic channels between neurons.
- **Flushing:** Cerebrospinal fluid (CSF) floods these spaces at high pressure and washes away toxic proteins accumulated during the day: **Beta-Amyloid** and **Tau** (the plaques responsible for Alzheimer's).

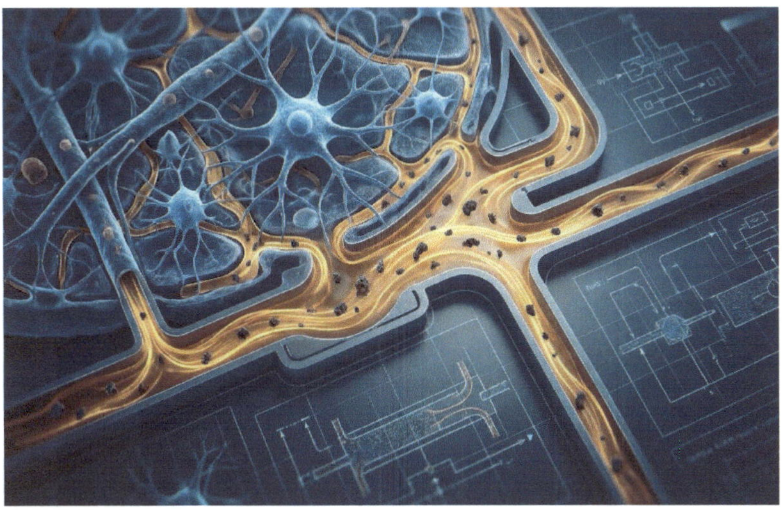

3.2 Applied Hydraulics: The Lateral Position

Glymphatic washing is a hydrodynamic process and is influenced by gravity.

- **Recent studies:** Sleeping in **the lateral position** (on your right or left side) is the most efficient configuration for toxin drainage compared to the supine (on your back) or prone (on your stomach) positions.
- **Safety Warning:** This flushing **ONLY** occurs during deep sleep. If you sleep 6 hours instead of 7.5, or if you wake up often, the flushing does not occur. Waking up with "brain fog" means starting the day with a toxic brain.

PART 4: SLEEP THERMODYNAMICS (Temperature Hacking)

To enter and remain in deep sleep, your core body temperature must drop by about **1°C**. If you stay warm, your brain will not shut down its alert systems.

4.1 The Warm Bath Effect Paradox

Many people think that a cold shower is necessary to cool down.

Wrong: Cold causes vasoconstriction (closes the pores) and traps heat inside.

- **The Apex Strategy:** Take a **hot** shower or bath (104°F) 90 minutes before bed.

- **The Physics:** Heat brings blood to the skin (massive vasodilation). When you get out of the bath, the "radiant" heat leaves the body quickly, causing the internal temperature to drop and inducing deep sleep.

4.2 The Thermal Accelerator: Glycine

We talked about the hot bath, but there is an internal metabolic hack.

- **The Concept:** The amino acid **glycine** (before bed).
- **The Impact:** Glycine acts as a metabolic coolant. It promotes peripheral vasodilation (, warm hands and feet), dissipating heat. This reduces sleep latency (you fall asleep faster) and improves the quality of deep sleep.

PART 5: PHASE ARCHITECTURE (Not all hours are equal)

Quality sleep is not a flat line, it is a 90-minute cyclical wave.

1. **Deep Sleep (NREM 3):** Occurs mainly in the first half of the night.
   - ***Function:*** Glinphatic cleansing, GH (growth hormone) release, muscle repair. This is the critical phase for the physical biohacker.
   - ***The Saboteur:*** Eating late (digestion = heat) kills Deep Sleep.

2. **REM (Rapid Eye Movement):** Occurs mainly in the second half of the night.
   - ***Function:*** Memory consolidation, emotional management, "software update." This is the critical phase for mental health.

SEASONAL AUDIT: ANNUAL CHRONOBIOLOGY

A biohacker knows that the protocol is not the same on June 21 and December 21. Don't force yourself to sleep 7 hours a day all year round.

Respect seasonal photobiology: your body is programmed for longer maintenance during the winter months (expansion of the repair phase).

METABOLIC SECURITY FAILURE: LEPTIN AND GRELINA

Poor sleep doesn't just make you tired, it makes you hungry. A single night of deprivation causes **leptin** (satiety hormone) to plummet and **ghrelin** (hunger hormone) to surge.

The impact: The next day, your "energy-starved" brain deactivates the prefrontal cortex (self-control). You are biologically programmed to seek out high-calorie foods (+25% calories). Resisting is almost impossible.

THE METABOLIC SABOTEUR: NOCTURNAL HYPOGLYCEMIA

If you regularly wake up between **2:00 and 4:00** a.m. with anxiety or tachycardia, your problem is not sleep, but metabolic stress.

The Mechanism: If dinner is poor or there is insulin instability, blood sugar crashes. The brain panics due to lack of fuel and orders a release of **adrenaline and cortisol** to raise sugar levels.

Apex Action: It's not insomnia, it's "chemical hunger." A small dose of healthy fats or a balanced dinner prevents the nighttime adrenaline spike.

THE ENEMY OF THE STAGES: ALCOHOL

Alcohol makes you "lose consciousness" (cortical sedation), but it is not sleep. Alcohol fragments rest and, above all, **suppresses the REM phase**.

The cost: You drink to relax, but you wake up emotionally unstable, anxious, and irritable because your brain didn't do its nighttime "emotional backup."

THE REST DASHBOARD: HRV AND TEMPERATURE

How does the Safety Officer know if the nightly "checkup" was successful?

1. **HRV (Heart Rate Variability):** The black box of recovery. A high value indicates that the parasympathetic nervous system has repaired the systems.

2. **THERMAL AUDIT (Skin Temp):** Modern wearables measure skin temperature deviation. If it is **higher than your baseline**, it is a system alarm signal: inflammation, late meal, or impending illness.

PART 6: THE NIGHT-TIME BIOENGINEERING PROTOCOL

PHASE 1: PREPARATION (10-3-2-1 Protocol)

A gradual shutdown procedure to ensure the system lands safely.

- **10 hours** before: Stop Caffeine (adenosine receptor cleansing).
- **3 hours** before: Stop Food (digestion stops, low T-core).
- **2 hours** before: Stop Work (low cortisol).
    - ***RAM emptying (Brain Dump):*** Before shutting down, write down everything that worries you or that you need to do tomorrow. This act moves data from your working memory (RAM) to an external "hard drive," allowing your brain to shut down active processes and slip into sleep without cognitive loops.
- **1 hour** before: Stop screens (or use blue blockers for melanopsin).

STEP 2: ENVIRONMENT (The Nighttime Clean Room)

Your bedroom should be a cave.

1. **Total Darkness:** Not even the TV light, your skin has photoreceptors. Use a mask if necessary.
2. **Cold:** Target environment 64-68°F.
3. **Silence:** Earplugs or white noise.
4. **EMF Audit:** Your room should be a virtual **Faraday Cage**. The pineal gland is sensitive to electromagnetic fields. Turn off Wi-Fi and put your smartphone in airplane mode. Melatonin is a photosensitive and electrosensitive hormone.
5. **Air audit:** Excess carbon dioxide in the room (>1000 ppm) activates the brain's alert sensors (amygdala), preventing access to deep sleep stages. Total darkness, but with guaranteed air circulation (door ajar or transom window).
6. **Light Geometry:** In the evening, place amber or red lights at **floor or table level**, never on the ceiling. Simulating the light of a low fire tricks the ancient brain much more effectively than a filtered ceiling light (which mimics the midday sun).

STEP 3: TACTICAL EQUIPMENT

- **Mouth Taping:** (See Chapter 1). Mandatory to prevent oxidation, apnea, and maintain CO_2/O_2 balance.
    - ***The Physics of Oxygenation (Bohr Effect):*** Taping is not only useful for preventing snoring. By maintaining physiological nasal levels, you

ensure that oxygen is effectively "released" from hemoglobin and delivered to neurons (**Bohr Effect**).

  - ***The Nasal Catalyst (Nitric Oxide):*** Breathing through the nose during sleep is the only way to inhale **the nitric oxide** produced in the paranasal sinuses. This gas acts as a powerful vasodilator, ensuring that the blood is "fluid" and oxygenated for glymphatic cleansing.
  - **SAFETY OVERRIDE:** Never practice mouth taping if you have acute nasal congestion or suffer from severe undiagnosed obstructive sleep apnea (OSAS) without consulting your doctor. For safety, always use an internal or external nasal dilator.

- **Weighted Blanket:** The weight (5-7 kg) stimulates proprioception, raises serotonin, and lowers cortisol (the "hug" effect).
- **Magnesium Bisglycinate & Glycine:** The ultimate muscle relaxant (Mg) combined with a thermal accelerator (Glycine).

THE PARADOX OF EXOGENOUS MELATONIN

Many biohackers abuse melatonin supplements. This can desensitize receptors and "turn off" endogenous production.

Apex Action: Melatonin is not a sleeping pill, it is a chronobiotic (rhythm regulator).

If you want to use it, "less is more": low doses are often more effective and safer for resetting your rhythm without creating biochemical dependence.

TECHNICAL BOX: THE STRATEGIC FOLD (Power Nap)

If you can't sleep at night, use a tactical nap to relieve adenosine pressure.

Rule: Either **20 minutes** (light rest only) or **90 minutes** (full cycle). Never 60 minutes.

Safety Window: Take your tactical nap preferably between **1:00 p.m. and 3:00 p.m**. Beyond this time, you will empty your adenosine "reservoir" too much, making it difficult to fall asleep at night.

The *"Nappuccino"* trick*:* Drink a coffee, then sleep for 20 minutes. You will wake up feeling energized as soon as the caffeine enters your bloodstream.

SAFETY OFFICER'S ADVICE

"Sleep is the foundation of the safety pyramid. You can eat keto, fast, and train like an Olympic athlete, but if you sleep 5 hours a night, your risk of mortality from all causes skyrockets. Don't 'steal' hours from sleep to be productive. It's like driving a car with the handbrake on: you consume more and go slower. Sleep is performance."

✅ SAFETY CHECKLIST: CHAPTER 5

Chapter validation. If you don't have 5 green ticks, the system is crashing.

- [ ] **LIGHT:** Do you expose yourself to direct sunlight (no glass) and move around within 30 minutes of waking up?
- [ ] **DARKNESS:** Do you use red/low lights after sunset (Twilight) and eliminate blue light?
- [ ] **CAFFEINE:** Do you respect the 10-hour curfew (Adenosine Management)?
- [ ] **METABOLISM:** Do you eat dinner 3 hours before bedtime and respect the light window (no Metabolic Jet Lag)?
- [ ] **THERMODYNAMICS:** Do you use a hot bath or supplement with glycine to lower your temperature?
- [ ] **AIRWAY:** Do you use mouth taping (if your nose is clear) to take advantage of the Bohr effect?
- [ ] **DASHBOARD:** HRV and Skin Temperature monitors to validate maintenance?

Safety Status:

🔴 **RED:** Lights on in the evening, late dinner, Wi-Fi active, alcohol, nocturnal hypoglycemia.

🟢 **GREEN:** Solar rhythm, dark/cold/screened room, energetic awakening.

CHAPTER 6

PHOTOBIO-MODULATION (SOLAR LOGIC): LIGHT AS A NUTRIENT

"We are bio-photon beings. Your mitochondria don't just eat glucose and oxygen; they eat light. Ignoring the solar spectrum and living under artificial lights is like trying to grow a forest in a neon-lit garage."

Until a few years ago, medicine considered the sun in only two ways: "Vitamin D" (good) and "Melanoma" (bad).

This is a two-dimensional and outdated view.

Light is electromagnetic radiation that acts as a variable-dose drug and, above all, as **an essential nutrient**.

Forty percent of sunlight is visible light. Fifty-four percent is infrared (which you cannot see but feel as heat). Only 6% is UV.

The modern problem is **spectral malnutrition**: we spend 93% of our time indoors (Indoor Generation), exposed to "junk light" (isolated blue LED) and lacking in regenerative frequencies (red and infrared).

In this chapter, we will explore advanced **Solar Logic**: from enzymatic activation to cellular water physics to pulsed technologies for the brain.

PART 1: APPLIED PHYSICS (The Mechanism of Action)

1.1 Cytochrome C Oxidase: The Cellular Solar Panel

Why does red light heal us? It's not magic, it's photo-chemistry.

In your mitochondria (the powerhouses of your cells), there is an enzyme called **Cytochrome C Oxidase** (CCO). It is the last step in the electron transport chain to produce ATP (energy).

- **The Blockage (Stress):** When you are stressed, sick, or inflamed, **Nitric Oxide (NO)** displaces oxygen and binds to CCO. Energy production stops. The cell suffocates.
- **The Unblocking (Light):** Red light (660nm) and Near Infrared light (850nm) penetrate the tissues and strike the CCO. The energy of the photons "displaces" the Nitric Oxide.
- **Result:** Oxygen returns, **ATP** production resumes at full capacity, and oxidative stress collapses. You are literally recharging the battery.

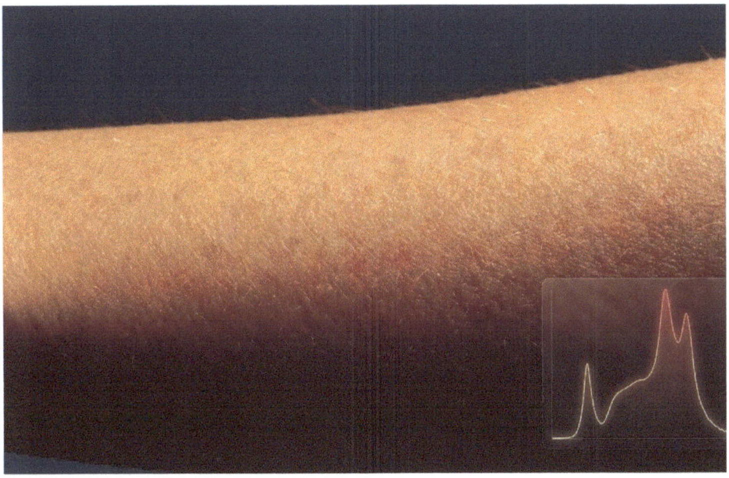

1.2 The Hydraulic Battery: EZ Water (Fourth Phase)

This is the most advanced concept in quantum biology (Gerald Pollack).

Your body is 99% water (in terms of molecules). But the water in your cells is not liquid like tap water.

- **The Concept:** When infrared light (3000nm+, present in the sun and saunas) hits intracellular water, the molecules reorganize. They go from a disordered state (H2O) to an orderly hexagonal crystalline structure: **H3O2** or **EZ Water (Exclusion Zone)**.
- **The Impact:** This water becomes a negatively charged gel, creating a veritable **liquid battery**. It expels toxins and facilitates protein folding.

- **Safety Insight:** Without infrared light, your cells are like dead batteries unable to conduct bioelectr r signals, no matter how much water you drink.

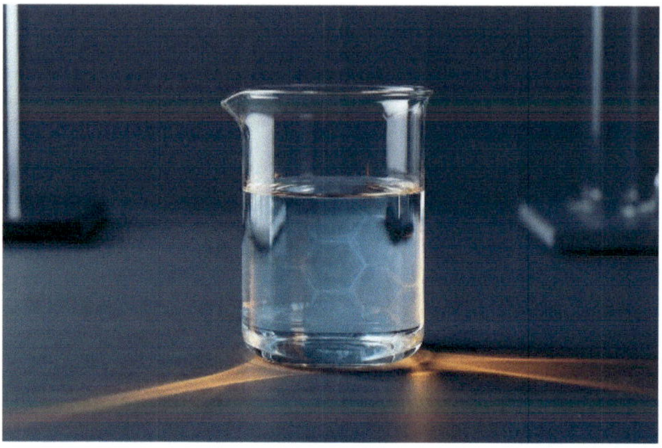

QUANTUM HEMODYNAMICS: THE EFFECT ON CAPILLARIES

Infrared light not only recharges cells; it acts as a **vascular lubricant**.

The Mechanism: By creating a layer of slippery EZ Water along the endothelium (the inner wall of blood vessels), it reduces blood flow friction.

The Impact: The heart works less hard to pump blood into the microcapillaries, improving peripheral oxygenation without increasing pressure.

THE SECRET OF MITOCHONDRIAL MELATONIN

This discovery rewrites biology.

The Concept: Only 5% of melatonin is produced by the pineal gland (for sleep). The remaining **95%** is produced within the mitochondria.

The Impact: Mitochondria produce melatonin as an "emergency antioxidant" when exposed to near-infrared (NIR) light.

Apex Action: It's not for sleep, it's for not burning. Exposing yourself to NIR (sun or panel) allows your mitochondria to produce the "internal shield" needed to neutralize free radicals. It's the engine's self-cleaning system.

1.3 The Biphasic Curve (Arndt-Schulz Law)

Light is a medicine.

- **Too little:** No effect.
- **Right:** Biological stimulation (Repair).
- **Too much:** Inhibition (Damage or shutdown of the system).

A Safety Officer knows that "more is not better." Spending 3 hours in front of a red lamp cancels out the benefits. Dosage is everything.

PART 2: SOLAR LOGIC (The Spectral Diet)

The sun changes its menu throughout the day. A Biohacker "feeds" on the right frequencies at the right time.

2.1 Dawn: The "Primer" (Red Light + IR)

As soon as the sun rises, there is no UV. There is an abundance of red and infrared light.

- **The Impact:** This light penetrates deeply and prepares the skin to receive UV later (**Pre-conditioning**). Exposing yourself at sunrise increases your resistance to midday sunburn. It is the evolutionary "sunscreen."

2.2 Midday: The Recharge (UVB)

When the sun is above 30° on the horizon (your shadow is shorter than you are).

- **The Impact:** This is when **Vitamin D** (steroid hormone) and **Beta-Endorphins** (well-being) are synthesized.
- **Safety Rule:** Direct exposure without glass. 10-20 minutes is enough. Never let your skin become erythematous (red).

PHOTOTYPE CALIBRATION (FITZPATRICK SCALE)

There is no universal dose. The "recharge time" depends on your hardware (your skin).

- **Fair skin (Phototype I-II):** 10-15 minutes is sufficient.
- **Dark skin (Phototype V-VI):** Melanin acts as a natural filter. It may take 5-10 times longer to synthesize the same amount of Vitamin D.

Apex Action: Know your skin type. The darker you are, the more "solar panels" (time) you need.

2.3 Beyond Vitamin D: Cholesterol Sulfate

We are told to avoid the sun to protect our skin, but we ignore the fact that avoiding the sun increases cardiovascular risk.

- **The Mechanism:** Skin exposed to UVB rays transforms cholesterol into **cholesterol sulfate**.
- **The Impact:** This molecule surrounds red blood cells, creating a negative charge (**Zeta Potential**) that causes them to repel each other.
- **Result:** Fluid blood, no clots, optimal pressure. Without sun, blood becomes "sticky." The sun is medicine for the heart.

BIO-REMOTE CONTROL: THE SKIN-GUT AXIS

This is the Elite frontier. New research shows that UVB exposure on the skin not only changes blood chemistry, but also diversifies the **gut microbiome**.

The Concept: Sunlight acts as a wireless signal for your bacteria. Proper exposure increases the richness of your microbiome, proving that the sun also "feeds" your internal symbionts without direct contact.

THE OMERA-LIGHT SYNERGY: DOPAMINE AND VISION

The eye is not just for seeing; it is an endocrine control center.

The Concept: Intense sunlight (over **10,000 lux**) strikes the retina and triggers the release of **dopamine**.

The Impact: Dopamine controls the axial growth of the eye (preventing myopia in children and adults) and stabilizes mood.

Apex Action: Without direct sunlight (without sunglasses), your dopamine production plummets, leading to brain fog, depression, and worsening vision.

2.4 Sunset: Repair (Red Light + IR)

The sun goes down, UV rays disappear, red light returns.

- **The Impact:** This light signals the end of the day and initiates the repair processes for DNA damage caused by midday UV rays.

PART 3: APEX TECHNOLOGY (Red Light Therapy - RLT)

If you can't live naked in nature, you have to bring the sun into your home. This is where technology comes in: red light panels (**Photobiomodulation**).

3.1 Critical Frequencies

Not all red lights work. Precise wavelengths are needed (Optical Window):

1. **RED (660nm):** Absorbed by the skin. Excellent for collagen, wrinkles, scars, acne.

2. **NIR (Near Infrared - 850nm):** Invisible to the eye. Penetrates 3-5 cm. Reaches muscles, joints, and **the brain**. Excellent for muscle recovery, deep inflammation, and neuroprotection.

3.2 Pulsation vs Continuous Wave (Advanced Tech)

Continuous light (CW) is excellent for the skin. But for the brain and deep tissues, **Pulsed Light** is superior because it speaks the electrical language of cells.

- **10 Hz (Alpha):** Resonance with brain Alpha waves. Promotes relaxation and physical recovery.
- **40 Hz (Gamma):** Resonance with Gamma waves. Studies (MIT) show that it activates microglia to clean amyloid plaques in the brain (Neuro-Cleanse).

3.3 Device Audit (What to Buy)

The market is full of useless toys. A Safety Officer checks 3 parameters:

1. **Irradiance:** Power. It must be >100 mW/cm^2 at a distance of 15 cm. If it is weak, it does not activate Cytochrome C.
2. **NNF (Non-Native EMF):** The panel must have electromagnetic emissions close to zero. There is no point in treating yourself with light if you are bombarded with dirty magnetic fields.

3. **Flicker:** Many cheap panels "flicker" imperceptibly. This stresses the nervous system. Look for "Flicker Free" devices.

PART 4: PROTECTION AND "DIGITAL AGING"

4.1 Nutritional "Sun Callus"

Chemical sunscreen is a last resort. The first line of defense is internal.

Industrial vegetable oils (oxidized Omega-6) insert themselves into the skin's membranes. When UV rays hit them, they react like burning plastic (**lipid peroxidation**) .

- **Anti-Sunburn Protocol:** Eliminate seed oils, increase Omega-3, and take **Astaxanthin** (the red pigment in crustaceans). It acts as an "internal sunscreen," protecting DNA.

SAFETY AUDIT: THE INTERNAL CHEMICAL FILTER (PHOTOSENSITIVITY)

A true Safety Officer monitors hidden variables.

The Risk: Some drugs (antibiotics such as tetracyclines, diuretics) or natural substances (St. John's wort) are **photosensitizing**.

The impact: In their presence, your tolerance threshold drops. Even a "normal" dose of light can cause phototoxic reactions. Always check the package insert before exposing yourself to the sun.

THE PARADOX OF SUNSCREEN (FILTER OR SABOTEUR?)

A Safety Officer must assess the risks of products.

The Risk: Chemical filters (oxybenzone, avobenzone) penetrate the bloodstream, act as endocrine disruptors (destroying testosterone), and kill the marine environment.

The Apex Solution: Use only **physical mineral filters** (zinc oxide or non-nano titanium dioxide). These act as mirrors that reflect light, not as chemical reagents that are absorbed by your skin.

4.2 Technical Box: Digital Aging

It's not just UV rays that age you. The blue light (**HEV - High Energy Visible**) from monitors penetrates the hypodermis, generating free radicals (ROS) that destroy the collagen and elastin matrix.

- **The Impact:** Spending 8 hours in front of a computer ages your skin as much as unprotected exposure to the sun ("Screen Face").
- ***Apex Action:*** If you work at a computer, use filtering software (f.lux, Night Shift) even during the day or apply a mineral sunscreen (zinc oxide) that reflects blue light.

THE LED DECEPTION: THE PARADOX OF ISOLATED LIGHT

We need to understand why white/blue LEDs in offices are toxic compared to the sun.

The Concept: In nature, blue light (high energy) never exists without its restorative counterpart (red and infrared).

The Impact: Modern LEDs emit "pure" blue without red. Delivering blue without red is like giving an engine **turbo** (oxidative stress) but removing its **cooling system** (mitochondrial melatonin). This causes cumulative damage that the sun balances, but LEDs do not.

PART 5: THE OPERATING PROTOCOL

PHASE 1: SYNCHRONIZATION (Morning)

- **Action:** Natural sun exposure (or red light panel if it is dark/winter) for 10 minutes on the face and chest.
- **Objective:** Mitochondrial activation and circadian signal.

OCULAR BIOHACKING: RESETTING THE RETINA

After the age of 40, the mitochondria in the retina lose efficiency (ATP decline), leading to vision decline.

Apex Protocol (UCL Study): **Three minutes** of exposure to deep red light (**670nm**) in the morning acts as a "defibrillator" for the mitochondria in the retina. It dramatically improves color sensitivity and night vision, slowing down ocular aging. (Do not look directly at the LEDs; use reflected light or close your eyes at a safe distance).

PHASE 2: ENHANCEMENT (Pre/Post Workout)

- **Pre-Workout:** RLT panel on muscles for 5 minutes. Increases ATP production and delays fatigue.
- **Post-Workout:** RLT panel for 10-15 minutes. Reduces lactic acid and inflammation, halving recovery times.

PHASE 3: DEEP THERAPY (Evening/Injury)

- **Target:** Joint pain, slow thyroid, or inflammation.
- **Distance:** 10-15 cm from the panel for 10 minutes. Use NIR (Infrared) mode.
- **Caution:** In the evening, use only red/NIR light. No blue screens after treatment.

TECHNICAL BOX: THE TESTICLES AND LIGHT

Studies show that direct exposure of the testicles to red/NIR light increases testosterone production (stimulation of Leydig cells) and sperm motility.

Protocol: 5-10 minutes of direct red light (no excessive heat, only light) per day. It is the most powerful and economical natural doping.

WINTER AUDIT: THE SOLAR DEBT STRATEGY

In winter, at our latitudes, the UV index is too low for vitamin D, but the need for light remains.

Apex Action: Manage your "Solar Debt" by doubling your use of RLT to keep mitochondrial melatonin production high and compensate for UVB deficiency with targeted **D3+K2** supplementation. Don't go into "photon hibernation."

SAFETY OFFICER'S WORD

"Light is the Wi-Fi of biology. It transmits data and energy. If you always live in 'Airplane Mode' (in the dark or under neon lights), your system drains its battery and loses signal. The EZ Water in your cells breaks down and your blood becomes thick. Don't be afraid of the sun, be afraid of artificial light. Go back to being a diurnal animal."

✅ SAFETY CHECKLIST: CHAPTER 6

Chapter Validation. If you don't have 5 green check marks, you are spectrally malnourished.

- [ ] **DAWN:** Do you expose yourself to natural light (or RLT) as soon as you wake up to pre-condition your skin?
- [ ] **WATER EZ:** Do you expose yourself to infrared light to charge your liquid battery and produce mitochondrial melatonin?
- [ ] **RETINA:** Do you use red light (670nm) in the morning for your eye audit?
- [ ] **TECHNOLOGY:** Do you own a low EMF RLT panel (660nm/850nm)?
- [ ] **DIGITAL AGING:** Do you protect your skin from blue light from screens (software filters or zinc)?
- [ ] **CREAMS & MEDS:** Do you check for photosensitizing medications and only use mineral filters?
- [ ] **PHOTOTYPE:** Have you calibrated your exposure time based on your melanin?

Safety Status:

🔴 **RED:** Indoor life, LED lights, "Screen Face," viscous blood, chemical creams.

🟢 **GREEN:** Sun callus, structured EZ water, mitochondrial energy, protected vision.

CHAPTER 7

THE METABOLIC ENGINE: BUILDING POWER (VO2 MAX, ZONE 2 & STRENGTH)

"Muscle is not just aesthetics, it is the organ of longevity. Frailty is not an accident, it is a choice of inactivity. If you don't build the engine today, tomorrow you won't have the power to get out of the disease curve."

Imagine your body as a high-performance safety vehicle.

- **VO2 Max** is the engine displacement (how many horsepower you have).
- **Zone 2** is fuel efficiency (how many miles you get per gallon).
- **Muscle strength** is the chassis and suspension (how much load you can carry without breaking).

Most people have a 50cc engine on a rusty chassis.

They get tired climbing stairs, are "short of breath," and have back pain. This is a **Structural Failure**.

According to the data, having a low VO2 Max is a greater risk factor for mortality than smoking, diabetes, and high blood pressure combined.

In this chapter, we will apply mechanical engineering to biology to build an indestructible hybrid engine.

PART 1: THE BASICS - ZONE 2 (Mitochondrial Efficiency)

Forget "No Pain, No Gain." For longevity, chronic "Pain" is often counterproductive.

Zone 2 is the magical metabolic state where you build the base of the pyramid.

1.1 The Biochemistry of Zone 2

When you train at low intensity (60-70% of your maximum heart rate), you force your mitochondria to burn **fat** (fatty acids) instead of sugar (glucose).

- **The Lactate Test:** In Zone 2, your blood lactate remains below **2.0 mmol/L**.
- **The Impact:** You create new mitochondria (**mitochondrial biogenesis**) and make them highly efficient.
- **Why it's safe:** If you have a poor aerobic base (bad Zone 2), at the slightest stress your body immediately

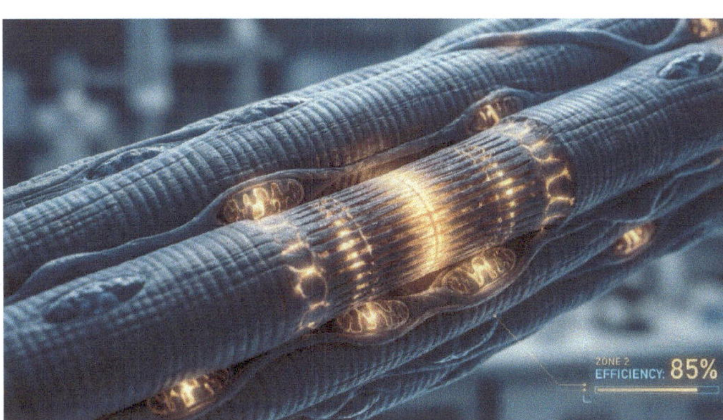

switches to burning sugars, producing acidic waste. You are a machine that revs up as soon as it is turned on.

THE MASTER REGULATOR: PGC-1\alpha

How does the body know it needs to build new mitochondria? Thanks to a signaling molecule: **PGC-1\alpha**.

It is the "General Manager" of the cell. It is activated by the volumetric stress of Zone 2 (and extreme cold).

Apex Action: The activation of PGC-1\alpha is the safety protocol to ensure that your power plants never go into blackout, increasing mitochondrial density per cell.

1.2 The Lactate Shuttle: From Waste to Super Fuel

We must correct the most common scientific error: "lactic acid burns muscles."

- **The Concept:** Lactate is not toxic waste. It is a high-octane fuel, preferred by the **heart** and **brain**.
- **The Mechanism:** When fast muscles work hard, they produce lactate. Slow muscles (trained in Zone 2) and mitochondria "suck it up" and use it to produce clean energy. This is the **Lactate Shuttle**.
- **Apex Action:** Training in Zone 2 increases the transporters (MCT-1) that enable this recycling. A biohacker does not want to "eliminate" lactate; they want to become a recycling machine to feed the brain under stress.

1.3 Zone 2 Audit: Talk Test and Maffetone

How do you know if you're in the right zone?

- **Quick Method (Talk Test):** You should be able to hold a conversation, but the other person should understand that you are exercising. If you have to pause for breath between words, you are going too fast.
- **Mathematical Method (Formula 180):** Subtract your age from 180. The result is the maximum heart rate you should not exceed to stay in pure aerobic Zone 2.
- **Elite Method (FatMax):** For the definitive audit, perform a metabolic test with gas analysis (calorimetry). This identifies your **FatMax**: the exact point at which your engine burns the maximum amount of fat per minute.

METABOLIC FLEXIBILITY (THE HYBRID ENGINE)

True security is the ability to switch from sugars to fats without disruption. An engine that can only use sugars has to stop at every gas station (hunger crisis).

Apex Action: Perform Zone 2 sessions in a state of **strategic fasting** (e.g., early in the morning). This teaches your cells not to "panic" when glucose is scarce, forcing the activation of the fat fuel line. It is the emergency procedure to avoid an energy blackout.

PART 2: THE ROOF - VO2 MAX (The Displacement)

If Zone 2 is the foundation, **VO2 Max** is the height of the skyscraper.

Definition: It is the maximum volume of oxygen that your body can absorb, transport, and use in one minute.

2.1 The Survival KPI

There is no biomarker with a stronger correlation to longevity.

- Moving from a "Low" VO2 Max to "Below Average" reduces the risk of death by **50**%.
- Moving to an "Elite" level reduces it by an additional **45**%.
- ***Safety Insight:*** VO2 Max declines by 10% every decade after age 30. If you are "average" at age 40, by age 70 you will not have enough "breath" to get up from a chair. You need to build a **Safety Margin** now.

FIELD AUDIT: ESTIMATE YOUR VO2 MAX (COOPER TEST)

How can you find out your VO2 max without a clinical laboratory?

The Protocol: Find a flat track. Run for **12 minutes** at the maximum constant speed you can maintain.

The Calculation: Measure the distance traveled in meters and apply this formula:

VO2 Max = [Distance (meters) - 504.9]/44.73

Benchmark example: A healthy 35-year-old man should exceed 40-45 ml/kg/min.

2.2 The Hidden Limiter: CO2 Tolerance

Many people "crash" during exercise not because they lack oxygen, but because their brain sensors panic due to the increase in carbon dioxide (**air hunger**).

- **BOLT Test:** Breathe out normally, pinch your nose. Time how long you can hold your breath before the first *involuntary urge* to breathe.
    - ***< 20 sec:*** System in constant alarm. Dysfunctional breathing.
    - ***> 40 sec:*** Elite. You have control of your autonomic nervous system.
- **Apex Action:** Train yourself to breathe less (nasally) during light exertion to raise your CO2 tolerance threshold. This improves brain oxygenation (Bohr Effect).

2.3 Training VO2 Max (Zone 5)

Intensity is needed here. You have to push your heart close to its limit.

- **Norwood Protocol (4x4):** 4 minutes at maximum sustainable intensity, 4 minutes of active recovery. Repeat 4 times.

It's brutal, but it's the fastest way to enlarge the engine cylinders.

SAFETY ALERT: FUEL FOR ZONE 5

While Zone 2 trains fat efficiency and loves fasting, Zone 5 (VO2 Max) is a combustion engine that requires **high octane fuel**.

Apex Action: Don't attempt VO2 Max on an empty sugar tank. To push your engine to 95-100%, you need available glycogen. Doing extreme intensity without carbohydrates is like trying to drive 300 km/h with half your cylinders shut off.

PART 3: THE FRAME - STRENGTH AND ANTI-FRAGILITY

Muscle is not just for flexing your biceps in the mirror.

Muscles are:

1. **Armor: They** protect bones and internal organs from impact.
2. **Glucose scavenger:** The more muscle you have, the more "tanks" you have to store carbohydrates (glycogen) without them turning into visceral fat.

THE MUSCLE PHARMACY: MYOKINES

Muscle is an immune and endocrine organ.

When it contracts intensely, it releases **myokines** (signal molecules).

- **IL-6 (Muscular):** Paradoxically anti-inflammatory, it tells visceral fat to melt away.
- **BDNF:** Tells the brain to create new neurons.

Apex Action: Every repetition in the gym is a "prescription" that your body writes for itself to fight chronic inflammation, cancer, and depression.

3.1 The Enemy: Sarcopenia and Raw Material

After age 30, you lose 3-8% of muscle mass per decade if you don't train it.

By age 60, sarcopenia (meat poverty) is the primary cause of falls and femur fractures.

- **Apex Action:** Lifting heavy weights is not "dangerous" for your joints. Being weak is dangerous.
- **Grip Strength:** Hand strength is not just muscle: it is a **biomarker of nervous system integrity**. A reduction in grip strength is related to accelerated aging of the brain and DNA.

THE RAW MATERIAL: THE LEUCINE THRESHOLD

You have the plan (training), but you don't have the building blocks?

To unlock protein synthesis and combat sarcopenia, it's not enough to eat "a little protein." You have to exceed the **Leucine Threshold**.

The Unlock Code: Anabolism is only activated if at least **2.5g of leucine** enters the bloodstream in a single meal (corresponding to about 30g of high-quality protein).

Safety Warning: If you only eat 10g of protein post-workout, the worker will not start building the structure.

SAFETY ALERT: TRANSMISSION (TENDONS)

Caution: Muscles adapt in weeks, but tendons and connective tissue take months.

The Risk: Many biohackers push the engine too hard too quickly and break the transmission.

Apex Action: Don't exceed the speed of your tendons. Use progressive loads and supplement with **collagen and vitamin C** 30 minutes before training to nourish the connective matrix.

3.2 Metabolic Deception: BFR (Blood Flow Restriction)

Want the muscles of a weightlifter without destroying your joints? Use **Blood Flow Restriction (BFR)** or the Kaatsu method.

- **The Concept:** Apply elastic bands (tourniquets) to the base of the limbs to occlude venous return but maintain arterial inflow.

- **The Impact:** Blood accumulates, oxygen levels drop (local hypoxia). The brain, in panic mode, recruits fast muscle fibers even with very light loads (20% of maximum).
- **Budget Hack:** You don't need $400 bands. Simple elastic physiotherapy bands work perfectly, if you know how to measure the pressure (7/10).

THE SUPER-CHARGE: CREATINE (THE EMERGENCY BACKUP)

It's not just for bodybuilders. It's a backup battery for ATP (cellular energy) in both muscles and the brain.

Apex Action: Think of it as "Capacitor Maintenance." It protects lean mass and dramatically improves brain resilience under stress and sleep deprivation.

3.3 The Operating and Braking System

A Ferrari with 800 horsepower and a steel chassis, but with wheels out of alignment, crashes at the first corner.

- **The Commander (Neuro-Muscular Connection):** Strength is not just fiber size, it's neural recruitment. Learn to "command" the muscle with your mind before loading it. The mind-muscle connection reduces the risk of structural injury by 40%.
- **The Anti-Collision Sensor (Proprioception):** It's not enough to be strong, you have to be connected. If your peripheral sensors are off (stiff shoes), power is blind.

Train your balance (standing on one leg while brushing your teeth) as you train your biceps. Integrate **DNS (Dynamic Neuromuscular Stabilization)** to stabilize your core.

- **The Braking System (Eccentric Strength):** In engineering, a powerful engine without brakes is a hazard. In biology, most injuries occur during the "braking" phase (e.g., going down stairs). Do not neglect the **eccentric phase** (descent) of weights: it is what protects your tendons and will allow you to walk down a mountain at 90 years old.

3.4 Coolant (Electrolytes)

If the muscle is the engine, electrolytes (sodium, potassium, magnesium) are the electrical fluid.

- **The Concept:** Without the right concentration of salts, the electrical signal from the brain to the muscle deteriorates (cramps, brain fog).
- **Apex Action:** Don't just drink water during training. Plain water dilutes sodium (hyponatremia), worsening performance. Use an electrolyte supplementation protocol to keep the system's conductivity high.

PART 4: REVERSE ENGINEERING (The Centennial Decathlon)

Why do you train? To have abs on the beach or to be independent at 90? The concept (by Peter Attia) is to design your life backwards.

4.1 The Mathematics of Decline

If you want to be able to lift your 15kg grandchild when you are 90, you can't wait until you are 89 to start training.

Knowing that you will lose about 10% of your strength per decade:

- To lift 15 kg at 90...
- You need to lift 25 kg at age 70...
- You need to be able to lift **40-50kg TODAY**.

Your gym membership isn't vanity, it's mathematical foresight.

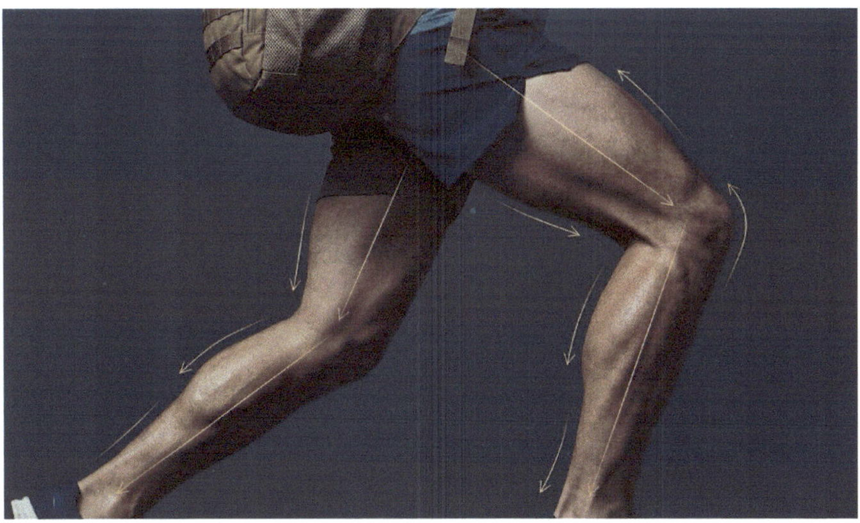

4.2 The 10 Events

Identify 10 physical tasks that are vital for your old age (e.g., getting up from the floor with one hand, carrying a suitcase into the overhead compartment on a plane, climbing three flights of stairs with groceries). Train today to master those movements tomorrow.

PART 5: THE OPERATING PROTOCOL (80/20)

How does the Biohacker with the eye of a Safety Officer put all this together?

With **Polarization**.

Most people make the mistake of training in the "Gray Zone": too hard to be Zone 2, too slow to be VO2 Max. Unnecessary effort and zero adaptation.

THE APEX WEEKLY PLAN (Example 4 hours/week)

1. **3 Hours (80%) - ZONE 2 (Aerobic Base):**
    - Slow running, exercise bike, rucking.
    - ***Rule:*** Breathe *exclusively* through your nose. If you open your mouth, slow down.
    - ***Safety Officer's advice:*** Perform one of the Zone 2 sessions on an empty stomach after fasting overnight. This "resets" your metabolic sensors and forces your body to test its fat fuel line.

2. **20-30 Minutes (10%) - ZONE 5 (VO2 Max):**
    - One session per week of high-intensity intervals (4x4 or hill sprints).
    - ***Goal:*** Lung and heart expansion.

3. **40-60 Minutes (10%) - STRENGTH:**
    - Free weights, weighted calisthenics, or BFR.
    - **Focus on the "Big 5":** Squats, Deadlifts, Pull-ups, Bench presses, Bench presses.
    - ***Goal:*** Myokine release and Centennial Decathlon.

THE DASHBOARD: BIOFEEDBACK & HRV

A safety officer doesn't just look at how fast the car is going, they look at the warning lights on the dashboard.

The Concept: How can you tell if you should do Zone 5 today or if you should rest? Look at **your HRV (Heart Rate Variability)**.

Apex Action: Use your **smartphone** or a wearable device. If your HRV is low compared to your average, the "Safety System" is on alert. Forcing the engine would lead to a short circuit (overtraining).

SCHEDULED MAINTENANCE: THE DELOAD WEEK

Even Formula 1 engines are dismantled and overhauled. If you always push yourself to the max (especially in Zone 5 and Strength), your **Central Nervous System (CNS)** will overheat before your muscles do.

Apex Action: Every 4-6 weeks, reduce your training volume by **30-50%**. This is not laziness, it is "preventive maintenance" to prevent your chassis from cracking due to chronic fatigue.

SAFETY CONNECTION: SLEEP (CHAPTER 5)

Warning: Metabolism is not built under weights, it is built in bed.

Apex Action: The engine repairs itself when the workshop is closed. If you train your VO2 Max but sleep 5 hours, you're trying to put a turbo on an engine that has no oil. Muscle and mitochondrial growth occurs thanks to the nighttime hormonal axis.

TECHNICAL BOX: RUCKING (THE SECRET WEAPON)

Want to do Zone 2 and Strength together without impacting your joints? Do **Rucking**.

Wear a backpack with 10-15kg and walk fast.

The Impact: It builds posture (pulls your shoulders back), strengthens your legs, burns 3x the calories of walking, but keeps your heart in Zone 2. It is the ultimate military training, adapted for longevity.

SAFETY OFFICER'S ADVICE

"Don't treat your body like a rental car, treat it like the only vehicle you'll have for your entire life. If the engine is smoking (poor VO2 Max) or the tires are flat (no muscles), you can't escape danger, whether it's a virus or a fall. Training is not a hobby, it's a mandatory maintenance procedure."

✅ SAFETY CHECKLIST: CHAPTER 7

Chapter validation. If you don't have 6 green check marks, your engine is at risk of melting down.

- [ ] **ZONE 2:** Do you do at least 150-180 minutes per week below 145 bpm (Formula 180)?
- [ ] **FATMAX:** Do you use the Talk Test to stay in the fat-burning range?
- [ ] **VO2 MAX:** Have you estimated your displacement with the Cooper Test?
- [ ] **STRENGTH:** Do you respect the Leucine Threshold (30g protein) after training?
- [ ] **BRAKES:** Do you train the eccentric phase (descent) to protect your tendons?
- [ ] **FLUIDS:** Do you use electrolytes during exercise to avoid diluting conductivity?
- [ ] **DASHBOARD:** Do you check your HRV on your smartphone before deciding on the intensity?
- [ ] **BALANCE:** Can you stand on one leg with your eyes closed for at least 20 seconds?

Safety Status:

🔴 **RED:** Sedentary, out of breath after climbing a flight of stairs, sarcopenia, low HRV.

🟢 **GREEN:** Hybrid engine, efficient lactate, structural strength, solid balance.

CHAPTER 8

THERMODYNAMICS AND SAFETY: HORMETIC SCALING (HEAT, COLD, AND MOLECULAR RESILIENCE)

"Comfort is a slow death. A body kept at 21°C is biologically 'asleep'. To activate genetic survival protocols, you must expose the system to extremes. We are not looking for suffering, we are looking for the adaptive response. The Safety Officer knows that a system that is never stressed is a system that will fail at the first emergency."

Modern humans live in an air-conditioned "thermal prison."

Summer and winter, the office and the home are always between 19°C and 24°C. From a biological safety point of view, this is a disaster.

Without temperature variation, thermoregulatory mechanisms atrophy and, with them, immune, vascular, and metabolic defenses.

In this chapter, we will discuss **hormesis**: the principle that "the dose makes the poison."

We will learn how to use the **sauna** not for relaxation, but as a mimic of cardiovascular exercise and a hormonal stimulator, and **ice** as a metabolic and neurochemical reset.

PART 1: THE THEORY - THE SAFETY CURVE (Hormetic Curve)

Before entering the ice bath, you need to understand the physics.

Hormesis follows an inverted "U" curve (Biphasic).

1. **Comfort Zone (Thermal Sedentariness):** No adaptation. Slow degradation, atrophy of blood vessels.
2. **Hormetic Zone (Safety Zone):** Acute but brief stress. The body responds by overcompensating (becoming stronger). This is where the Biohacker operates.
3. **Toxic Zone (Damage):** Too long or extreme exposure. Hypothermia, frostbite, or heatstroke. Structural damage to proteins.

The Safety Officer's job is to keep you right in the middle of the Safety Zone: enough stress to trigger the alarm, not enough to burn out the power plant.

PART 2: THE FURNACE - THE HEAT (Hyperthermic Conditioning)

The sauna is a **passive workout**.

Sitting in a sauna at 80-100°C raises your heart rate to 120-150 bpm, mimicking a Zone 2 cardio session, but with unique benefits at the molecular level.

2.1 Proteostasis: The Neural Defragmenter (HSP)

When the core temperature rises, DNA responds by activating **Heat Shock Proteins (HSP)**, particularly HSP70.

- **Function:** These are the "molecular paramedics." They scan cells, find damaged or misfolded proteins, and repair them (refolding).

  If they cannot repair them, they mark them for disposal (**autophagy**).

- **Neurodegenerative Prevention:** Diseases such as Alzheimer's and Parkinson's are caused by "protein folding errors" (plaques).

  HSPs act like defragmentation software for the protein hard drive.

- **Elite Data:** Finnish studies (Kuopio Ischaemic Heart Disease Risk Factor Study) show that taking a sauna 4-7 times a week reduces the risk of dementia and Alzheimer's by **65**%.

This is an immense safety margin.

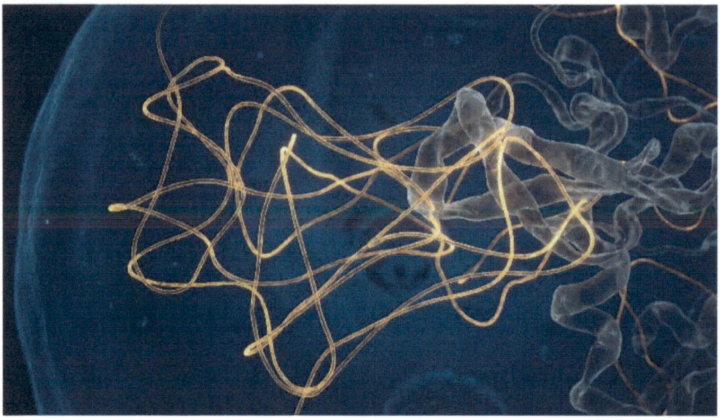

2.2 Hypervolemia: Legal Doping

Why do endurance athletes use saunas? For plasma expansion.

- **The Mechanism:** To cool itself down, the body sends blood to the skin. This reduces the amount of blood available to the organs. The kidneys sense the drop in pressure and order the body to retain water and sodium.
- **The Impact:** After a few sessions, your plasma volume increases by **7-10%**. More blood means more hemoglobin, more oxygen to the muscles, and superior thermoregulation. It's like doing natural EPO, but safe.

2.3 The GH (Growth Hormone) Protocol

Want to use heat for hypertrophy and anti-aging? Just "taking a sauna" is not enough.

A specific protocol is required.

- **The Concept:** Multiple sessions interspersed with cooling periods create a massive GH spike.
- **Elite Protocol:**
    1. 20 minutes in the sauna (80-100°C).
    2. 30-minute break (cooling down to room temperature).
    3. 20 minutes in the sauna.
        - ***Result (Studies):*** Growth hormone peaks up to **+1600%** compared to baseline. To be done once a week.

TECHNICAL BOX: Smartphone & BIO-MONITORING

Use your smartphone and wearable device to monitor your **Recovery Heart Rate (RHR)**. After leaving the sauna, your heart rate should drop by at least **20-30 bpm** in the first minute.

Safety Check: If recovery is slower, your autonomic nervous system is *overloaded*. Stop the protocol and rest.

2.4 Technology: Finnish vs Infrared (Extrapineal Melatonin)

- **Finnish Sauna (Convection):** Heats the air to 80-100°C. Great for HSP and cardio.
- **Infrared Sauna (Radiation):** Lower temperatures (100-120°F). But here's the secret.

- ***Mitochondrial Melatonin:*** Many associate melatonin only with sleep. But in elite biohacking, we know that infrared (NIR) light stimulates melatonin production directly **within the mitochondria**.
- ***Apex Action:*** The IR sauna is not just for sweating; it is an antioxidant recharge session that protects mitochondrial DNA from oxidative stress (ROS) produced during metabolism.

The best choice is a Finnish sauna equipped with IR lamps, killing two birds with one stone.

SELECTIVE SWEATING: DETOX PROTOCOL

Sweat is not just water. It is the preferred route for expelling **POPs (Persistent Organic Pollutants)** such as phthalates, bisphenol A, and heavy metals (cadmium, lead), which the kidneys struggle to filter.

Safety Procedure:

1. **Pre-Sauna: Take a** hot shower to open your pores and remove any creams/chlorine.
2. **Post-Sauna:** Shower *immediately* with natural soap. If you cool down without washing, the toxins expelled will settle on your skin and be reabsorbed. Wash away the poison.

PART 3: THE FREEZER - THE COLD (Cold Shock & Metabolism)

If heat repairs, cold transforms.

3.1 Biochemistry: Noradrenaline and Dopamine

Exposure to cold water (<15°C) is a systemic shock that the brain interprets as an imminent threat of death.

- **The Response:** Massive release of **Noradrenaline** (+530%) and **Dopamine** (+250%).
- **Difference from Drugs:** Unlike cocaine, cold raises dopamine levels steadily for 3-4 hours. Laser focus, stable mood, zero crash.

3.2 The Alchemy of Fat: UCP1 and "Beiging"

Everyone talks about brown fat (BAT), but the real hack is **beiging** (turning white fat into brown fat).

- **Apex Biochemistry (Uncoupling):** Thermogenesis in BAT occurs because the **UCP1** protein creates a "short circuit" in the electron transport chain. Instead of producing chemical energy, protons flow through the mitochondrial membrane, releasing energy in the form of dissipated heat.

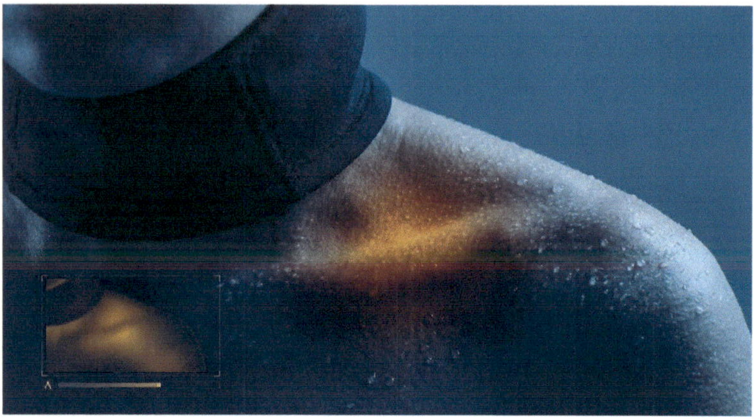

ADAPTATION KPI: BAT THERMOGRAPHY

How do we know if brown fat (BAT) is really activating? Here's an example.

The Signal: An efficient thermal system autonomously heats the supraclavicular area (where BAT resides) after exposure to cold.

Apex Action: Use an inexpensive thermal camera or infrared thermometer on the neck/clavicle area after icing. If that area remains warm while the rest of the body is cold, you have successfully activated your mitochondrial furnaces.

3.3 The Protocol: Thermal Randomization

Have you learned to tolerate the cold? Bad.

Predictability is the enemy of adaptation.

- **Murphy's Law of Cold:** If you always do 3 minutes at 10°C, the body becomes "too efficient" and stops producing the massive hormetic response.
- **Apex Action:** Surprise the nervous system. One time do 1 minute at 2°C (extreme shock), the next time 5 minutes at 15°C. Variability keeps the system alert and maximizes hormesis.

SAFETY DIAGNOSTIC: THE NEURO-HORMONAL BRIDGE (THYROID)

Thermal exposure is an audit of metabolic health.

The Concept: If you absolutely cannot tolerate cold (even moderate), the problem may not be "willpower," but thyroid inefficiency (inability to convert T4 to T3 to generate heat).

Safety Check: Measure your basal temperature in the morning. If it is consistently below **97.2°F**, your internal "thermostat" is off. Use cold gradually (alternating showers) to reactivate the axis, but do not force extreme ice until the thyroid engine is calibrated.

BREATHING TECHNIQUE: THE VAGAL BRAKE

Ice activates the sympathetic nervous system (fight/flight). Biohackers must know how to activate the parasympathetic nervous system to manage stress.

Apex Action: As you enter the cold water, do not hyperventilate. Use **Box Breathing (4-4-4-4)** or exhale twice as long as you inhale. You are telling your brain, *"There is a thermal emergency, but I am in control."* This is true psychological resilience training.

BOX: THE DNA TEST

We are not all the same in the cold.

If you have the **ACTN3** gene polymorphism or specific variants of the **UCP1** gene, your ability to produce heat or withstand the cold changes dramatically.

Apex Action: An Elite Biohacker tests his genetic predisposition before attempting diving records, to calibrate the " hormetic dose" to his genetic hardware.

PART 4: VASCULAR GYMNASTICS AND PERFORMANCE

4.1 Contrast Therapy (The Mechanical Pump)

Alternating hot and cold is like "weight training" with your blood vessels.

- **Nordic Cycle:** 15' Sauna -> 2' Ice -> 15' Sauna.

- *Safety Rule:* Finish with **cold** for energy/work. Finish with **heat** for relaxation/sleep.

4.2 The Stanford Hack: Palm Cooling

- **The Concept:** The palms of the hands, soles of the feet, and face (glabrous skin) are natural radiators.
- **The Action:** Between sets at the gym, cool your palms (cold water or gel packs at 10-15°C) for 2 minutes.
- **Result:** Lowers the temperature of returning blood, allowing you to increase your training volume by **40-60**%.

PART 5: SAFETY PROCEDURES (Safety Officer Override)

As Safety Officer, I must warn you of the real risks.

5.1 Afterdrop

When you get out of ice or very cold water, your temperature continues to drop for 10-20 minutes.

- **Apex Action:** Warm up with active movement (horse stance, squats). Do not take a hot shower *immediately* (risk of fainting).

5.2 Mammalian Dive Reflex

If you immerse your face in ice-cold water, your heart slows down (bradycardia) while your body speeds up (tachycardia).

- **Safety Protocol:** Enter the water slowly. Exhale as you enter. Never hyperventilate before diving (risk of blackout).

5.3 Timing and Hypertrophy

Cold blocks the acute inflammation necessary for muscle growth.

- **Rule: NEVER** take an ice bath within 4 hours of strength training (weights).

5.4 Male Fertility

Heat kills sperm.

- **Action:** Protect your testicles with a cold wet towel in the sauna and use local cooling after your session.

5.5 Mineral Audit (Supplementation with Module 2)

Profuse sweating expels heavy metals but also essential trace minerals.

- **The Risk:** Drinking only water after the sauna further dilutes electrolytes, risking cardiac fatigue.

- **Apex Action:** Replenish immediately with **magnesium bisglycinate** and potassium. The engine doesn't run on water alone; it needs the right coolant.

5.6 The Intestinal Connection (Thermal Gut Barrier)

A true expert knows that thermal stress impacts the intestinal barrier.

- **The Mechanism:** Extreme heat causes temporary intestinal ischemia (all the blood goes to the skin to cool it down), increasing permeability (**Leaky Gut**).
- **Apex Action:** If you suffer from intestinal permeability or inflammation, do not exceed 15 minutes in the sauna without massive hydration. Post-sauna cooling is essential for "sealing" the barrier, reducing systemic inflammation resulting from heat.

PART 6: THE INTEGRATED WEEKLY PROTOCOL

- **Monday (After Work):** 20-minute sauna (Recovery + HSP).
- **Wednesday (Morning):** Ice Shower (Randomized: 1 minute freezing cold or 5 minutes cool).
- **Thursday (During Workout):** Palmer Cooling between sets (Performance).
- **Friday (Evening):** Contrast Therapy (Sauna/Cold/Sauna) for "vascular flushing."

- **Sunday (GH Protocol):** "20-30-20" Sauna Protocol for hormonal peak.

SAFETY OFFICER'S WORD

"Fire tempers steel, but melts it if the temperature is wrong. The goal is not to prove how tough you are by staying in the ice for 20 minutes (that's ego). The goal is to administer the minimum effective dose to achieve the maximum hormetic response. If you shiver violently after the ice for hours, you have failed. Respect the curve."

✅ SAFETY CHECKLIST: CHAPTER 8

Chapter validation. If you don't have 5 green check marks, the system is thermally unstable.

- [ ] **HEAT:** Do you have at least 2-3 sauna sessions per week?
- [ ] **PROTEOSTASIS:** Do you use the sauna as a preventive tool for cleaning brain proteins?
- [ ] **SELECTIVE SWEATING:** Do you wash immediately after the sauna to remove POPs and metals?
- [ ] **COLD:** Do you reach a total of 11 minutes of exposure per week?
- [ ] **RANDOMIZATION:** Do you vary temperatures and times to avoid chronic adaptation?
- [ ] **CONTRAST:** Do you use hot/cold alternation for vascular gymnastics?
- [ ] **MINERAL RECOVERY:** Do you replenish trace minerals lost through sweat (not just sodium)?

Safety Status:

🔴 **RED:** Always at 21°C, lukewarm showers, heat intolerance, stubborn white fat.

🟢 **GREEN:** Efficient thermoregulation, active brown fat, active neuroprotection.

PART 3: THE INVISIBLE HARDWARE, BEYOND BIOCHEMISTRY

If you ask a traditional doctor what the human body is made of, they will respond with a list of chemical ingredients: proteins, fats, water, hormones.

He will talk to you about enzymatic reactions and receptors.

But if you ask a physicist, the answer will be different: the human body is an **agglomeration of electromagnetic fields and charged particles**.

For centuries, biology ignored physics.

We have treated humans as a "chemical soup," forgetting that every chemical reaction is, at its core, an exchange of electrons.

The heart does not pump without an electrical impulse, the brain does not think without membrane depolarization, muscles do not move without a voltage signal.

As **a Safety Officer**, I know that in a complex industrial plant, before checking the fluids in the pipes (blood/lymph), I must check that the **electrical system** and **sensors** are not short-circuited.

If the voltage drops, the machines stop; if there is too much interference (background noise), the sensors give incorrect readings and the automatic safety system does not trigger or triggers incorrectly (autoimmunity).

Today we live in a lethal paradox:

1. **We are drained:** We have isolated ourselves from our original "battery" (the Earth) with rubber shoes and synthetic flooring, losing access to the negative charge that shuts down inflammation.
2. **We are Overcharged:** We are immersed in an ocean of artificial radiation (nnEMF) that our DNA has never encountered in 200,000 years.

In this module, we will stop thinking like chemists and start thinking like **electrical engineers**.

We will learn that health is measurable in millivolts, we will learn that disease is, essentially, a loss of voltage.

We will learn how to shield human hardware from the interference of the modern world in order to restore its original conductivity.

Welcome to the world of Bio-Electromagnetism.

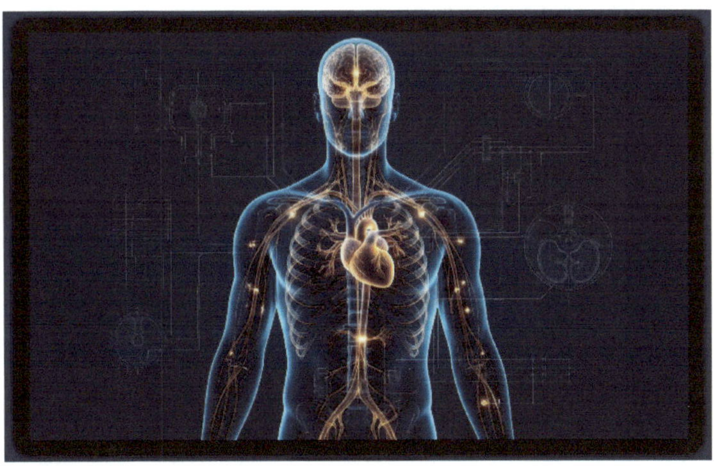

CHAPTER 9

BIO-ELECTROMAGNETISM AND GROUNDING: CELLULAR VOLTAGE AND EMF DEFENSE

"Cells are designed to function at a specific voltage. Chronic disease always occurs when we lose the ability to maintain that voltage. We are rechargeable batteries that have forgotten where the outlet is." — Dr. Jerry Tennant

The human body is a liquid crystal semiconductor. Each cell functions as a capacitor that stores energy.

Modern medicine focuses on "replacement parts" (organs), but the Elite Biohacker focuses on **Power Supply**.

In this chapter, we will explore the deep physics of life: from the Zeta potential of blood to the invisible threat of VGCCs, to the ancient solution of Grounding.

PART 1: THE PHYSICS OF LIFE (Voltage is Health)

You cannot have "energy" (feel good) if you don't have "energy" (electrons).

1.1 The Tennant Scale (pH and Voltage)

Dr. Jerry Tennant has shown that pH (acidity/alkalinity) is actually a measurement of voltage in a solution.

The formula is as follows:

Voltage (mV) = -59.1 x (pH - 7)

Cellular State	Voltage (mV)	Equivalent pH	Description
Healing/Growth	**-50 mV**	**~7.85**	Necessary for creating new cells (anabolism).
Standard Health	**-25 mV**	**7.45**	Optimal operating state for adults.
Fatigue / Onset of Illness	**-15 mV / -10 mV**	**7.25 - 7.15**	Lack of electrons, chronic pain.
Neutral Point	**0**	**7.0**	No energy flow.
Reversal (Cancer)	**+30 mV**	**~6.48**	Acidic, hypoxic (oxygen-depleted) environment.

1.2 The Electron Bank

The human body needs a constant flow of electrons (negative charge) to neutralize free radicals (positive charge/electron thieves).

- **Donors (Chargers):** Grounding, EZ Water, UV Sunlight, Raw Foods.

- **Thieves (Dischargers):** Heavy metals, Dental toxins, Scar tissue (which acts as a switch off), Blue light, Wi-Fi.

BLUE LIGHT AS AN ELECTRON THIEF (LINK CHAPTER 8)

We need to close the circle. Artificial blue light (LEDs/screens) is not just a sleep problem.

The Concept: It destroys the coherence of EZ Water in the mitochondria, leading to electron loss (oxidation).

Apex Action: Blue light is a **cellular battery drainer**. Protecting your eyes with blue-blocker glasses is an integral part of the voltage maintenance described in this chapter.

1.3 The Living Matrix: The Fascia as a Semiconductor

Do you have the hardware to generate your own energy? Yes. It's the **Fascia**.

- **The Concept (James Oschman):** Fascia (connective tissue) is a matrix of hydrated collagen that acts as "optical fiber" for electrons. It is called **the Living Matrix**.
- **Apex Action:** Movement is not only for muscles, but also serves to generate electricity through **the piezoelectric effect**. Every time you move, you compress the collagen crystals in the fascia, generating a voltage that recharges your cellular capacitors. Standing still literally means draining your battery.

THE BIOLOGICAL ANTENNA: WATER AND STRUCTURE (LINK MODULE 2)

Electromagnetic waves don't just affect receptors; they affect the water we are made of.

The Concept: Water molecules are electric dipoles. Artificial fields (nnEMF) create a chaotic "vibration" that destroys the coherence **of EZ** (Exclusion Zone) **Water** around proteins.

Apex Action: EMFs not only flood the cell with calcium, but they electrically "dehydrate" your proteins, making your blood and cytoplasm less structured. Grounding not only brings electrons, but it helps re-stabilize the crystalline structure of biological water.

PART 2: THE INVISIBLE ENEMY - nnEMF (Non-Native Electromagnetic Fields)

The telecommunications industry claims that radiation (Wi-Fi, 4G, 5G) is safe because it does not "heat tissue" (Thermal Effect).

As a Safety Officer, I tell you that this is a lie based on 1950s physics. The damage is not thermal, it is **Biological and Informational**.

2.1 The Mechanism: VGCC (Voltage-Gated Calcium Channels)

Research by Prof. Martin Pall has revealed the exact mechanism.

Our cells have voltage sensors on their membranes called **VGCCs**. They are designed to sense micro-electrical signals.

1. **The Interference:** Artificial electromagnetic fields (nnEMF) are millions of times stronger than natural signals. They activate VGCCs improperly.
2. **The Flood:** The channels open and calcium (Ca^{2+}) floods the cell.
3. **The Damage:** Excess calcium is toxic. It leads to massive oxidative stress.

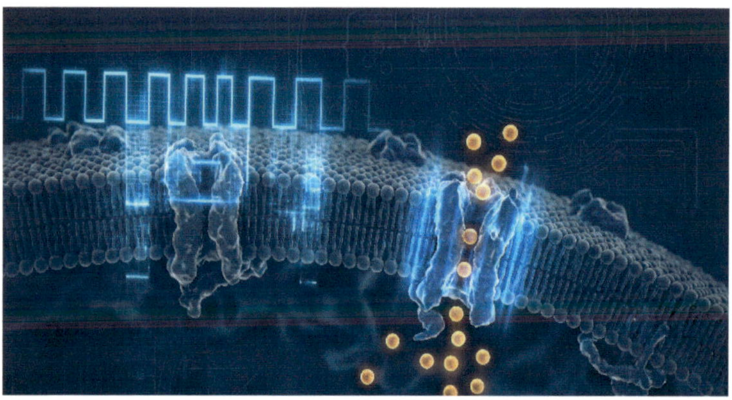

THE BIOLOGICAL TRANSDUCER: MAGNETITE IN THE BRAIN

The Concept: The human brain contains millions of biosynthesized **magnetite** crystals. These crystals act as transducers that couple external magnetic fields to cell membranes.

Apex Action: It is not just an electrical disturbance; it is a mechanical disturbance at the molecular level. Magnetite crystals vibrate in response to artificial frequencies, creating **mechanical micro-stress** that can alter the opening of ion channels regardless of voltage.

BIOCHEMISTRY OF DISASTER: PEROXYNITRITE

Here is the formula for damage that the industry ignores.

When VGCCs open, excess calcium stimulates the production of superoxide and nitric oxide. Their combination creates **peroxynitrite**, an oxidant that has no natural enzymatic defenses in the body:

Superoxide + Nitric Oxide = Peroxynitrite

The result: DNA strand breaks, lipid peroxidation of mitochondrial membranes, and destruction of energy production.

2.2 Symptoms of Electromagnetic Hypersensitivity (EHS)

You don't feel a "burning" sensation, but the system gradually crashes:

- **Neurological:** Insomnia, anxiety, brain fog (the brain is the organ with the most VGCCs).
- **Cardiac:** Palpitations, arrhythmias (the heart is an electrical organ).

- **Reproductive:** Infertility (sperm cells have no DNA repair mechanisms and are exposed).

PART 3: THE SOLUTION - GROUNDING

The Earth is not an inert rock. It is a giant, negatively charged electric generator. It is an unlimited supply of "Vitamin G" (Ground).

3.1 Physics of Grounding: The Umbrella Effect

We are insulated by rubber shoes. This causes our body to act like an antenna, accumulating positive static charge (inflammation).

When you touch the ground with bare feet:

1. **Equalization:** Your body voltage (often 2-5 volts AC in a modern home) instantly drops to zero (0 volts). Your body comes under the Earth's "electrical umbrella."
2. **Electron Flow:** Billions of free electrons flow up from the earth to the body, turning off inflammation.

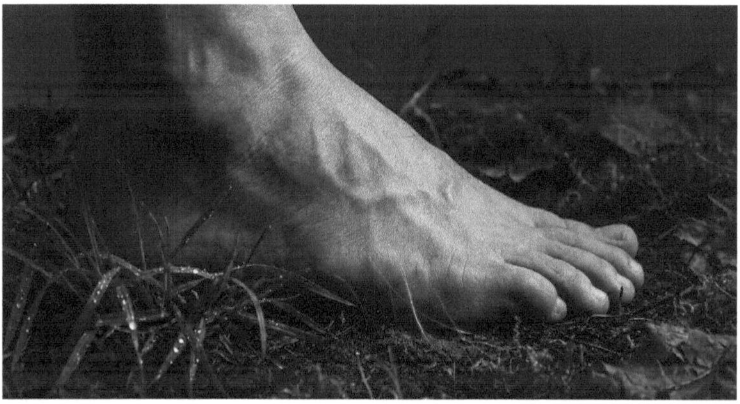

3.2 Hemorheology: Flow Safety (Zeta Potential)

Red blood cells have a negative surface charge (Zeta Potential) that causes them to repel each other.

- **The Risk (Rouleaux Effect):** Without the Earth, the charge is lost and the cells stick together. Thick blood forces the heart to pump harder and increases the risk of micro-thrombi.
- **Apex Action:** Grounding is not a spiritual hobby, it is a **blood thinning protocol**. Measuring Zeta Potential means drastically reducing blood viscosity, lowering stress on artery walls and preventing endothelial wear.

VISUAL EVIDENCE: DARK FIELD MICROSCOPY (LIVE BLOOD ANALYSIS)

Need proof? Zeta Potential is not a theory.

Visual Audit: Through dark field microscopy, you can see in real time red blood cells go from "piles of coins" (inflamed and hypoxic) to single, vibrant cells after just **20 minutes** of grounding. It is the optical validation of your voltage.

3.3 Schumann Resonance (7.83 Hz)

The Earth pulses at a specific frequency: **7.83 Hz**. Our brains evolved in this field (Alpha/Theta waves resonate here).

Living in isolation and immersed in Wi-Fi (2.4 GHz or 5 GHz) creates a desynchronization of the Master Clock.

BRAIN TRAINING: PEMF & SCHUMANN

The brain needs a "beat" to remain in homeostasis.

Apex Action: When you cannot ground yourself outdoors, use **PEMF (Pulsed Electromagnetic Fields)** devices calibrated to the Schumann Resonance. You are providing the body with the original terrestrial synchronization signal, counteracting the digital "noise" of artificial frequencies.

PART 4: REMEDIATION AND SHIELDING (Building Biology)

4.1 Dirty Electricity

In addition to Wi-Fi, there is an enemy in the walls: Dirty Electricity (voltage spikes caused by dimmers, power supplies, etc.).

- **Apex Action:** Use specific filters (e.g., Stetzer filters) in outlets to "clean" the current from these spikes that your body absorbs through capacitive coupling.

THE SILENT SABOTEUR: SMART METERS & PLC

New electronic meters use **Power Line Communication (PLC)** to transmit data.

The Concept: They constantly inject frequencies of 10-100 kHz into all the cables in your home, turning every wall into a radiating plate.

Apex Action: Check where your meter is located. If it is near the bedroom, shielding is a priority. Consider using elite capacitive filters at the entrance to the electrical panel to isolate the entire home from the "noise" of the public grid.

SAFETY ALERT: METAL-ELECTRICAL INTERFERENCE (THE LENS EFFECT)

Be aware of internal and external metals.

1. Implants: If you have plates or amalgams, they act as passive antennas.

2. Accessories (Lens Effect): Glasses with metal frames can act as local resonators, concentrating radio frequencies right next to the optic nerves and pituitary gland.

Apex Action: If you work in an office, you will undoubtedly have dense Wi-Fi, so choose acetate frames or non-conductive materials. Eliminate any unnecessary metal elements from the "perimeter" of your skull.

SAFETY ALERT: THE PARADOX OF INDOOR GROUNDING (GROUND LOOP)

Many people use grounding mats connected to their home's grounding outlet.

The Risk: If the building's ground is "dirty," the mat acts as an antenna that brings those frequencies **directly into your body**.

Apex Action: Before connecting, use a **Socket Tester** to check the ground connection and an **EMI Meter** to make sure the line is not carrying "noise." If the ground is dirty, indoor grounding is worse than isolation. A dedicated ground stake in the garden is better.

4.2 "Faraday" Night Protocol

1. **Kill Switch:** Physically turn off your Wi-Fi router at night (Timer).
2. **Distance:** No cell phones or "smart" devices on the nightstand.

CONTAINMENT PROCEDURE (LEVEL 3): THE FARADAY CAGE

We have talked about remediation, but for the Safety Officer there is a last line of defense when the external environment is "out of control" (e.g., 5G repeater 50 meters away).

Apex Action: If RF measurements remain above target despite the kill switch, the only "Zero-Stress" solution is a **Faraday Tent, preferably made of silver fiber,** over the bed. Creating an electromagnetic sanctuary where the signal is literally absent allows the glymphatic system to operate at 100% without interference.

TECHNICAL BOX: SMARTPHONE CALIBRATION

Use technology to protect yourself from technology.

Apex Action: On your smartphone, use **Modes and Routines if available**.

Set a rule:

"IF: Location is Home (or Time is 10:00 p.m.) -> THEN: Turn on Airplane Mode, Turn off 5G, Turn off Fast Charging."

SIGNAL MODULATION: DIGITAL "NOISE"

Many people think that only signal strength matters. This is not the case.

The Concept: The problem is not the frequency (Hz), but the **pulsed digital modulation**. The natural signal (Schumann) is a harmonious sine wave; Wi-Fi and 5G are violent square pulse trains that VGCCs perceive as a constant alarm.

Apex Action: Always choose 4G over millimeter wave 5G unless you need to download large files. The pulse density of 5G is biologically more difficult for your membrane sensors to ignore.

4.3 The Chemical and Circadian Shield

There is an even more subtle effect on the Master Clock.

- **Circadian Confusion (Phase Shift):** Electromagnetic fields are perceived by the suprachiasmatic nucleus as a "pseudo-light" signal. Even if the room is dark, if it is electrically "noisy," your Master Clock receives conflicting signals. Result: **chronic indoor jet lag**.
- **The Shield (Melatonin):** EMFs suppress melatonin, which is the only antioxidant capable of neutralizing peroxynitrite. Supplementing with melatonin and

magnesium (calcium antagonist) is vital for those who cannot clean up their environment.

4.4 The Textile Saboteur (Electrostatic Charge)

We have talked about rubber shoes, but not about "plastic clothing."

- **The Concept:** Synthetic fabrics (polyester, nylon, acrylic) generate enormous electrostatic charges through friction. These charges create a surface electric field that can exceed 2,000V, interfering with membrane voltage.
- **Apex Action:** Wardrobe Audit. Electrical safety comes from natural fibers (cotton, linen, wool, silk). Eliminating synthetics, especially in bed, drastically reduces the accumulation of positive static charge that "steals" electrons from the system.

4.5 Geopathies: Natural Electromagnetic Stress

An elite Safety Officer knows that the Earth does not only emit Schumann Resonance.

- **The Concept:** There are geopathogenic disturbance zones (Hartmann and Curry nodes, faults). These zones emit frequencies which, although natural, can act as chronic stressors if the bed is positioned above them.
- **Apex Action:** If HRV remains low after clearing artificial EMFs, perform a **geobiological audit**. Moving the bed just 50 cm can make the difference between

regenerative sleep and a state of constant systemic alarm.

PART 5: DIAGNOSTICS (The Safety Officer's Audit)

Don't guess. Measure.

1. **EMF meter (e.g., TriField TF2):** Target sleeping area: RF < 0.1 μW/m^2.
2. **Body Multimeter (Body Voltage Test):**
   - Connect the black probe to the ground. Red in hand.
   - Apex target: **< 100 mV** (0.1 V). If you read > 1 Volt or 1000 mV, you are under stress.

SAFETY OFFICER'S WORD

"We are the only species on the planet that lives electrically isolated from the surface on which it walks. We put on plastic shoes and surround ourselves with towers that pulse radiation. Modern diseases are often 'electrical inflammation'. Take off your shoes, turn off your router, check your grounding. Reconnect to the original electrical network."

✅ SAFETY CHECKLIST: CHAPTER 9

Chapter validation. If you don't have 5 green check marks, the circuit is unstable.

- [ ] **WI-FI:** Does your router turn off automatically at night (mechanical timer)?
- [ ] **ZETA POTENTIAL:** Do you do at least 20 minutes of grounding (outdoors) after training?
- [ ] **SMART METER:** Have you checked the meter location and considered PLC filters?
- [ ] **AUDIT:** Have you measured the Body Voltage in your bed? Is it below 100mV?
- [ ] **ACCESSORIES:** Do you use non-metallic glasses when working on your PC to avoid the lens effect?

  [ ] **DIRTY ELECTRICITY:** Have you removed dimmers and fluorescent light bulbs from your bedroom?
- [ ] **FABRICS:** Do you sleep in natural fibers (cotton/silk) to avoid electrostatic charges?

Safety Status:

🔴 **RED:** Wi-Fi 24/7, phone under your pillow, body voltage > 2V, brain fog.

🟢 **GREEN:** "Faraday" night, fluid blood, negative cell voltage (-25mV), clean ground.

CHAPTER 10

STRUCTURAL ENGINEERING: BAND, POSTURE, AND TENSEGRITY

"Structure dictates function. If your frame is misaligned, every movement generates micro-trauma. Pain is not the problem; pain is the red light on the dashboard telling you that the geometry of the system is compromised."

Most people (and doctors) think of the skeleton as the scaffolding of a skyscraper: bones stacked on top of each other that support the weight under compression.

This view is false.

If you removed all the soft tissue, your bones would collapse to the ground in a messy pile.

The human body does not function like a brick wall, but according to the principle of **Tensegrity** (Tension + Integrity).

We are like a camping tent or a suspension bridge: the rigid parts (bones) float in a sea of continuous tension (fascia). If a tie rod is too tight (contracture) or too loose (weakness), the entire structure deforms.

In this chapter, we will audit your frame to prevent **Structural Failure** (hernias, osteoarthritis, ruptures).

PART 1: THE THEORY - TENSEGRITY (Floating in Tension)

The concept, formalized by architect and inventor **Buckminster Fuller**, is simple: **discontinuous compression in a sea of continuous tension**.

1.1 Bones vs. Fascia (Struts and Cables)

- **The Bones (Struts):** These are the spacers that resist compression. They prevent the body from collapsing in on itself.
- **The Fascia (Cables):** This is the continuous tension network that envelops everything.
- **Apex Action:** Do not try to "straighten" a bone, but rather to balance the tensions. If you pull a cable at the ankle, you affect the tension at the neck. Often, if you have back pain (posterior), the cause is the anterior "cable" (psoas/abdomen) being too short, which overloads the system.

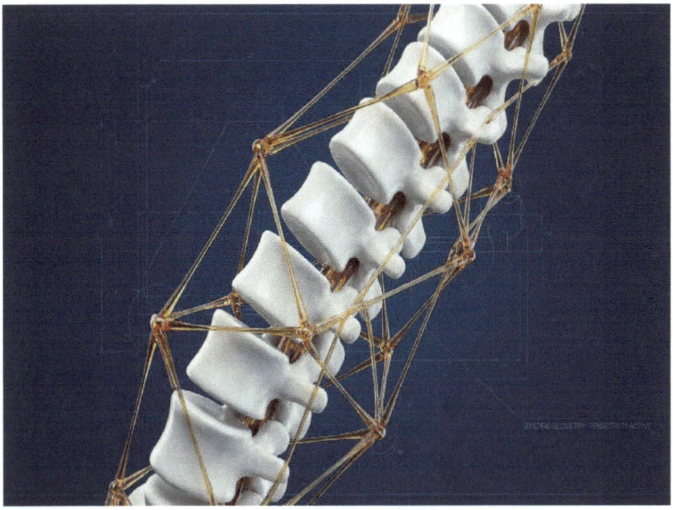

1.2 The Piezoelectric Matrix (Link Chapter 9)

The fascia is not inert. It is a piezoelectric liquid crystal.

- **The Mechanism:** Collagen fibers are crystals. When they are deformed by movement, they generate micro-electric currents.
- **Apex Action:** Fluid and varied movement is an electrical recharge. If your fascia is "stuck" (fibrosis) or there is scarring, it is an **electrical insult** because it interrupts this flow of charges to the cells. Structural rigidity leads to "electrical darkness."

PART 2: THE MATERIAL - THE FASCIA (Tissue Maintenance)

Healthy fascia is like a wet silk net: it glides without friction. Unhealthy fascia is like dry felt: it sticks and creates adhesions ("Fuzz").

2.1 Mechanical Hydration (Hyaluronic Acid)

Drinking water is not enough to hydrate the fascia. Water must be "pushed" into the tissues.

- **The Lubricant: Hyaluronic acid** is found between the layers of fascia. If you remain still for too long, it becomes thick and sticky (viscosity increases).
- **Apex Action:** Movement, especially elastic and multi-planar movement (not just linear movement such as running), makes hyaluronic acid fluid. You feel stiff in the morning because you have "dried out" during the night. Dynamic stretching is the "re-lubrication" of the engine.

2.2 SMR (Self Myofascial Release)

Foam rolling is not just for "loosening knots."

- **The Sponge Effect:** When you press on a muscle with the roller, you squeeze out old fluid and toxins. When you release, fresh, hydrated tissue is sucked in.
- **Protocol:** Don't roll fast. Find the sore spot, stop, and breathe for 30 seconds. Wait for the nervous system to "release" the tension.

PART 3: GEOMETRY - POSTURE AND ALIGNMENT

Posture is not "standing up straight for good manners." It is mechanical efficiency against gravity.

3.1 Tech Neck: The Weight of Modernity

The head weighs about 5 kg. For every centimeter you move it forward (looking at your smartphone), the perceived weight on your neck doubles (disadvantageous leverage).

- **The Damage:** At a 60° angle (texting on your phone), the weight on your neck is **27 kg**. It's like carrying an 8-year-old child sitting on your cervical spine for 4 hours a day.
- **Apex Action:** Bring the phone to your eyes, not your eyes to the phone. Train your deep neck muscles (Chin Tucks) to realign your cervical vertebrae.

SAFETY ALERT: VAGAL COMPRESSION (NEURO-POSTURE)

The cost of "Tech Neck" is not just physical pain.

The Concept: The vagus nerve and jugular vein pass through narrow spaces at the base of the skull. **Forward Head Posture** creates mechanical compression that reduces venous drainage from the brain and "strangles" vagal tone.

Neurological Audit: If your head is forward, your nervous system is in a constant state of alert because the vagal signal is disturbed. Correcting the neck is a prerequisite for mental calm.

3.2 The Fulcrum: The Psoas and Sitting

Sitting ("The New Smoking") dramatically shortens the Ileo-Psoas, the muscle that connects the legs to the spine.

- **The Consequence:** When you stand up, the short psoas pulls the lumbar spine forward, compressing the discs.
- **Counter-Move:** For every hour of sitting, perform 2 minutes of "Couch Stretch" or lunges to open the hip. Do not allow the psoas to calcify in a shortened position.

3.3 Spinal Decompression (Viscoelasticity)

We fight gravity 16 hours a day.

The intervertebral discs lose water and flatten (we are 1-2 cm shorter in the evening).

- **"Dead Hang" Protocol:** Hang from a bar for 1-2 minutes a day (active or passive shoulders).
- **The Impact:** Creates negative pressure in the discs, drawing in hydration and nutrients. It is the only preventive maintenance for herniated discs.

3.4 Disc Maintenance: Segmental "Pumping"

You've done the Dead Hang, but the intervertebral discs have no blood vessels, they only "eat" through pumping movement (**imbibition**).

- **The Concept:** If you only move "as a whole" (rigid spine), some areas of the disc do not receive nutrients and "starve."

- **Apex Action (CARs):** Insert **Controlled Articular Rotations** of the spine.

  Learn to move one vertebra at a time (segmental flexion/extension). This is the "contact cleaning" of your frame, which forces nutrients into the cartilage by diffusion.

3.5 The Internal Piston (Pressure Cylinder)

Tensegrity needs an internal pressure system to prevent collapse.

- **The Concept:** The core is not a set of abdominal muscles, it is a hydraulic piston composed of **the Diaphragm** (above) and **Pelvic Floor** (below) . If the two are not aligned, the pressure escapes.
- **Apex Action:** Aligns the two diaphragms. This creates **Intra-Abdominal Pressure (IAP)**.

CYLINDER BIOMECHANICS (LATEX INTEGRATION)

The stability of the lumbar spine is guaranteed by Laplace's law applied to the trunk.

Internal pressure acts on the walls of the abdominal cylinder, creating a stabilizing tension:

Where is the radius of the trunk and the thickness of the abdominal wall.

An aligned "piston" core maximizes support, reducing the compression load on the vertebrae by up to **40%**.

3.6 McGill's Triad (Spinal Safety Protocol)

Quoting **Dr. Stuart McGill**, the world's leading expert on spinal biomechanics: stability does not come from flexibility, but from **stiffness** (protective rigidity under load).

- **Apex Action:** Enter the **"McGill Big 3."**
    1. **Bird-Dog:** For extensor stability.
    2. **Side Bridge:** For lateral stability (square of the loins).
    3. **Modified Curl-up:** For anterior stability (without crushing the discs).
- ***Objective:*** To create a corset of muscles that protects the nerves like armor.

3.7 The Drainage System (G-Force & Lymph)

We talked about how gravity compresses the discs, but gravity is also the engine of your "waste disposal" system.

- **The Concept:** Unlike blood (pushed by the heart), lymph moves only through muscle movement and gravity. If your structure is rigid, the drainage of metabolic debris stops.
- **Apex Action (Postural Inversion):** You don't need a complex bench. Just 5 minutes of **"Legs up the Wall"**

(Viparita Karani) in the evening is enough. This reverses the pressure gradient, decongests the veins in the legs, and facilitates lymphatic return to the thoracic ducts, "washing" the hardware from the inside.

PART 4: TACTICAL ERGONOMICS

As Safety Officer, you must clean up the workstation.

4.1 The 50/50 Rule

Do not switch to a standing desk all day (it causes varicose veins and static back pain).

- **The ideal:** Alternate. 30 minutes sitting, 30 minutes standing.
- **Variability:** The best posture is "the next one." The body hates stagnation. Keep moving.

4.2 The Fundamentals: The Podalic Tripod

Modern shoes with narrow toes and raised soles destroy the structure. The foot is your interface with the Earth (grounding) and your stability sensor.

- **The Tripod:** The foot must rest on three points: **heel, base of the 1st metatarsal, base of the 5th metatarsal**.
- **Apex Action:** Wear barefoot shoes or shoes with a wide toe box. Practice the **Short Foot Maneuver**: learn to lift

the arch of your foot by contracting your intrinsic muscles, without curling your toes.

4.3 Unconscious Posture (The Ergonomics of Sleep)

We spend 8 hours in a static posture. If the setup is wrong, we undo the work of the day.

- **The Concept:** Pillows and mattresses are not furniture; they are passive alignment tools.
- **Apex Action:**
  - ***If you sleep on your side: Place*** a pillow between your knees to prevent your hip from rotating and pulling on your psoas.
  - ***If you sleep on your back: Place*** a small support under your knees to reduce lumbar disc tension. The spine must remain neutral.

PART 5: STRUCTURAL DIAGNOSTICS (Audit)

Do this test in front of a mirror:

1. **Thumb Test:** Relax your arms at your sides. Do your thumbs point forward or toward your thighs?
   - ***Towards your thighs: Your*** shoulders are rotated inward (desk/smartphone syndrome).

2. **Wall Test:** Lean your back, buttocks, and heels against the wall. Can you touch the wall with the back of your head while keeping your gaze horizontal?
    - ***No:*** Forward head posture (Tech Neck).

3. **Toe Spread:** Can you spread your toes voluntarily as you do with your hands?
    - ***No:*** Atrophy of the intrinsic muscles of the foot (Foundation Failure).

5.2 The KPI of Longevity: Gait Speed

We need to connect the structure to your longevity mission.

- **The Concept:** Walking speed is defined in scientific literature as the **"Sixth Vital Sign."** It is a more accurate predictor of mortality than blood pressure.
- **Apex Action:** Use your smartphone's sensors (accelerometer and gyroscope) to monitor your natural cruising speed.
- ***Safety Benchmark:*** If it falls below 1 m/s, your structural efficiency is declining. An elite biohacker walks with intention and symmetry.

TECH AUDIT: Use your hardware.

Apex Action: Use your smartphone's motion sensors with a posture analysis app (or record a slow-motion video of your profile while walking).

Artificial intelligence can detect asymmetries in the Podalic Tripod or pelvic rotation that the human eye ignores, and of course, if it detects abnormalities, contact your orthopedist for a clinical evaluation.

PART 6: THE CRANIAL ANCHOR - THE TONGUE AND JAW

Many people correct their shoulders but ignore the "rudder" of the spine: the tongue.

6.1 Postural Orthodontics (Mewing)

If your tongue rests on the floor of your mouth, your neck loses its internal support.

- **Apex Action:** The correct resting position is: lips closed, teeth in light contact, **tongue stuck to the palate** (the entire surface, not just the tip).
- **The Test:** Swallow. If you use your cheeks or lips to swallow, you have a dysfunction ("infantile swallowing").

6.2 Airway Health (The Structure of Breathing)

Posture is a slave to breathing. If the airways are narrow, the body will move the head forward to "open the tube."

- **Safety Protocol:** At night, use **mouth taping** (tape over the mouth).

- **Tech Audit:** Use your smartphone to record nighttime noises. If you snore, your "Airway Health" is compromised.

PART 7: STRUCTURAL CHEMISTRY AND PHYSICS

LOAD BIOENGINEERING: WOLFF'S LAW

Bone and connective tissue adapt to mechanical loads according to Wolff's Law. Remodeling is proportional to the stress applied: where is the force applied and the cross-sectional area. The Keith Baar Protocol optimizes the biological response to this mechanical stress.

7.1 The Keith Baar Protocol (Collagen Loading)

Researcher Keith Baar discovered that tendons absorb nutrients for only 10 minutes after being loaded.

- **The Apex Protocol:**
    1. **30-60 minutes BEFORE** training: Take Hydrolyzed Collagen (or Gelatin) + Vitamin C.
    2. **Workout:** Movement pushes these amino acids into the tendon matrix just when it is receptive.

7.2 The Catapult Effect (Elastic Storage)

The main function of fascia is missing: **elastic return**.

- **The Concept:** Fascia is a spring. In elite athletes, movement does not come from muscles, but from the release of stored elastic energy, i.e., the elastic constant of your fascia.
- **Apex Action:** Integrate small elastic bounces (pogos, light jumps barefoot) to maintain the "elastic youthfulness" of collagen ("Fascial Bounce").

PART 8: THE SENSORY AND NEUROMECHANICAL SYSTEM

The fascia is not just "packaging." It is the body's most extensive sense organ.

8.1 Interoception (The Sixth Sense)

Fascia communicates to the brain not only "where you are" (proprioception), but "how you feel" (interoception).

- **Apex Action:** Working on the fascia (SMR, stretching) not only helps you move better, but also calms anxiety at its root.

8.2 Neural Flossing: Freeing the Cables

If fascia is fiber optics and nerves are electrical cables, sometimes the cables "stick" to the sheath.

- **The Concept:** A nerve "trapped" by stiff fascia sends pain signals that no amount of muscle stretching will resolve.

- **Apex Action:** Enter **Neural Gliding.** Specific movements that slide the sciatic or median nerve through the fascial tunnels. It's the procedure for eliminating signal interference in your cables.

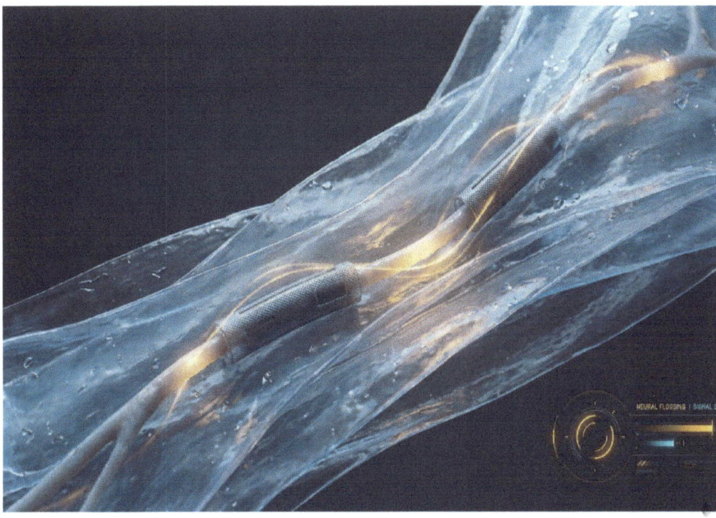

8.3 Scars: The Short Circuits of the Matrix

Every scar is a break in the fascial and piezoelectric network.

- **Neural Therapy:** Massage scars regularly with oil to break up adhesions and restore electrical conductivity to the area.

PART 9: VISION AND POSTURE (The Vestibular System)

The body follows the eyes. If your eyes are not functioning well, your neck will stiffen to stabilize your head.

9.1 The Horizon Line

The vestibular system and the eyes work together. If you spend 10 hours staring at a screen 40 cm away, your eye muscles lock up and your brain "freezes" your neck.

- **Apex Action:** Every 20 minutes, look into the distance (horizon). Do "Eye Yoga" exercises. Relaxing your eyes instantly relaxes your neck.

9.2 Sensory Conflict (Thalamic Gate)

We've talked about the eyes, feet, and vestibular system. But what happens if they are not synchronized?

- **The Concept:** If the data does not match (e.g., eyes say "stay still on the screen," feet feel "micro-oscillations"), the thalamus goes into alarm mode and creates **Protective Tension** (stiffness) to "immobilize" the structure.
- **Apex Action: Sensory Stacking**. When doing balance exercises or walking, turn your head or close your eyes. Train your brain to manage conflicting data to eliminate stiffness from "sensory conflict."

PART 10: HORMONAL FEEDBACK (CYBERNETIC POSTURE)

Posture doesn't just follow mood, it creates it. It's a feedback loop.

- **The Concept:** A "closed" (hyper-kyphotic) posture not only constricts the vagus nerve, but also sends a biochemical signal of submission/fear to the brain, raising cortisol and lowering testosterone.

- **Apex Action (High Power Posing):** Before an important meeting or stressful event, maintain a posture of maximum expansion (arms open, chest out, gaze on the horizon) for 2 minutes. You are hacking your endocrine system through your structural geometry.

SAFETY OFFICER'S WORD

"You are not a collection of mechanical parts screwed together. You are a hydraulic, electrical, and sensory tensile structure. If your tongue does not support your skull, if scars block the signal, if your tendons are starved and your eyes are fixed, no amount of 'gym' will give you regal posture. True structural engineering starts with the invisible to build the visible."

✅ SAFETY CHECKLIST: CHAPTER 10

Chapter Validation. If you don't have 5 green check marks, the structure is compromised.

- [ ] **HANGING:** Do you hang from the bar to decompress your spine?
- [ ] **MEWING:** Is your tongue stuck to the roof of your mouth (not your teeth) when you are at rest?
- [ ] **SCARS:** Have you treated/massaged your old scars?
- [ ] **ERGONOMICS: Do you** alternate sitting/standing (50/50 rule)?
- [ ] **ELASTICITY:** Do you feel an elastic "bounce" when you walk?
- [ ] **PISTON:** Are your diaphragm and pelvic floor aligned?
- [ ] **INVERSION:** Do you do 5 minutes of "legs up the wall" in the evening for lymphatic drainage?

Safety Status:

🔴 **RED:** Mouth breathing, low tongue, fragile tendons, active scars, stuck nerves, stagnant lymph.

🟢 **GREEN:** Perfect tensegrity, tongue on palate, conductive fascia, steel tendons, piston core, active drainage system.

CHAPTER 11

OFFICE BIOHACKING: OCCUPATIONAL SAFETY (ERGONOMICS, LIGHT, AND ATMOSPHERE)

"The chair is the cigarette of the 21st century, but the modern office is the whole tobacco pack. Stale air, junk light, forced immobility, and electromagnetic stress. The Safety Officer does not sit at a desk to die slowly; he designs a command post that nourishes biology while producing value."

Working in an office (or remotely) is an extreme endurance sport.

You are asking a hunter-gatherer to sit motionless in an artificially lit box, staring at a source of blue light 40 cm away, while breathing the recycled air of 20 other people.

From a safety perspective, this is a **Multiple Incident**.

1. **Metabolic:** Fat-burning genes (LPL) "shut down" after 20 minutes of immobility.
2. **Structural:** The spine collapses under gravity (disc creep).
3. **Cognitive:** CO_2 buildup reduces IQ by 15-50%.

In this chapter, we will apply industrial safety protocols to your workspace.

PART 1: THE COCKPIT (Ergonomic Setup)

You don't have to "adapt" to your desk. Your desk should adapt to you.

1.1 The 90-90-90 Rule (Sitting Mechanics)

If you have to sit, do so like a pilot, not like a tired passenger.

- **Elbows:** At 90°, resting on the armrests or tabletop, shoulders relaxed (not raised toward your ears).
- **Hips:** At 90-100°, use lumbar support to maintain natural lordosis.
- **Knees:** At 90°, feet flat on the floor (or on a footrest). If your feet dangle, circulation is blocked.
- **Apex action:** The top edge of the monitor should be **at eye level**. If you look down, you add 27 kg of load to your neck (Tech Neck). Use articulated arms for monitors or risers (books are also fine).

1.2 Standing Desk & Variability

As mentioned in Chapter 10, the best posture is "the next one."

- **Standing Desk:** Don't stand still like a statue (causes varicose veins). Use a **Balance Board** or anti-fatigue mat (topographic) to force your feet into continuous micro-movements.
- **The 30/30 Rule:** 30 minutes sitting (deep focus), 30 minutes standing (active work/calls).

PART 2: TACTICAL LIGHTING (Junk Light Defense)

Offices use cheap neon or LED lights that flicker and emit peaks of blue light. This destroys dopamine and strains the visual cortex.

2.1 Eye Shielding

- **Monitor:** Install **f.lux** or use your monitor's Eye Comfort Shield feature to reduce blue light peaks at 450nm.
- **Glasses:** If you work under fluorescent lights, wear **clear** (or slightly yellow) **Blue-Blocker** glasses during the day. They filter out the harmful peak without making you sleepy.

2.2 Bias Lighting

Staring at a bright screen in a dark or nearly dark room creates extreme stress on the iris (excessive contrast).

- **Apex Action:** Attach an LED strip (warm white 2700K or red) behind the monitor. This creates a halo of light that reduces the perceived contrast and saves your eyesight.

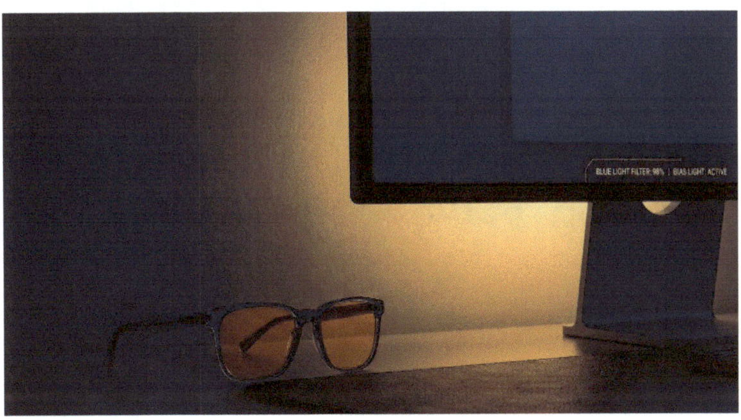

2.3 Flicker Management (Invisible Flicker)

Many LED lights pulse hundreds of times per second. You don't see it, but your brain does.

- **Solution:** If you can't change the bulbs, use a personal "Flicker-Free" desk lamp (incandescent or high-quality LED) and turn off the ceiling light above you if possible.

APEX INSTRUMENTATION: SMARTPHONE TECH AUDIT (ENVIRONMENTAL)

Your smartphone is a monitoring station. Use it.

- **Luxmeter:** Use the brightness sensor (via app) to check your desk.
    - ***Morning:*** Target **500-1000 lux** of cool light (to activate cortisol and wake up).
    - ***Afternoon:*** Target **< 500 lux** of warm light (to prepare melatonin).
- **Flicker Check:** Open the camera in **Slow Motion** mode and frame the office lights. If you see black bands scrolling, that light is stressing your optic nerve at 100Hz. It causes invisible brain fatigue.

PART 3: CONTROLLED ATMOSPHERE (Air Quality)

Indoor air is often 5 times more polluted than outdoor air (VOCs from printers, carpets, human CO_2), especially in offices.

3.1 The Silent Killer: CO_2 (The IQ Thief)

In modern offices, carbon dioxide levels quickly rise above 1000-1500 ppm.

- **The Fact:** A **Harvard** study showed that at 1400 ppm, cognitive performance (response and strategy) drops by **50%**. You are not tired from work, you are "intoxicated" by your own breathing.
- **Lucidity Audit:** Use a portable NDIR sensor. If it exceeds **1000 ppm**, the meeting should be interrupted or turned into a "walking meeting" outdoors or in the hallway.

BIOPHYSICS OF PERFORMANCE (CEREBRAL ACIDOSIS)

The rate of cerebral CO2 elimination is critical for maintaining the pH of cerebrospinal fluid. The accumulation of environmental CO2 shifts the chemical balance:

$$CO_2 + H_2O = H_2CO_3 = H^+ + HCO_3^-$$

The increase in H+ ions (local acidosis) alters neurotransmission, leading to what we call "office brain fog." Opening the window restores neuronal pH.

3.2 Biophilia (Plants as Filters)

They are not just for beauty.

- **Sansevieria (Mother-in-law's Tongue):** Produces oxygen at night and filters benzene/formaldehyde.

- **Pothos:** Extremely hardy, devours VOCs.
- **Action:** Place at least 2 plants within your field of vision. In addition to the air, looking at fractal greenery reduces visual cortisol.

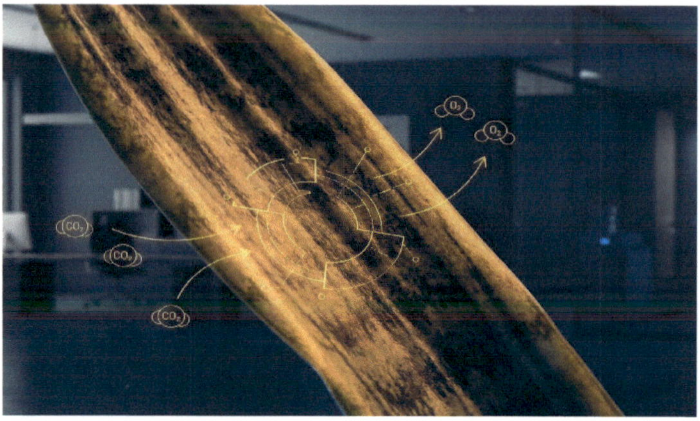

PART 4: INTEGRATED MOVEMENT (NEAT Engineering)

You cannot compensate for 8 hours of sitting with 1 hour at the gym. You must move *while* you work.

4.1 Exercise Snacks

Every hour, the timer goes off. You have 60 seconds.

- **Protocol:** 20 bodyweight squats or 10 push-ups against your desk.
- **The Impact:** Reactivates LPL (lipase), unlocks hip flexors, and pumps glucose to the brain.

4.2 Muscle Pump Syndrome (Venous Drainage)

Sitting not only destroys your back, it also stops the body's "second pump": the calf.

- **The Concept:** Blood stagnates in the legs, reducing venous return and, consequently, cerebral oxygenation.
- **Apex Action (Micro-Dosing of Movement):**
    1. **Seated Calf Raises:** Lift your heels rhythmically while typing.
    2. **The Ball:** Hold a tennis ball under the sole of your foot and massage it while you work. This keeps lymphatic and venous drainage active without having to leave your workstation.

4.3 Walking Pad

If you work from home or have a private office, the **Walking Pad** under your standing desk is the ultimate weapon.

- **Data:** Walking at 2-3 km/h does not interfere with typing, but burns 100 kcal/hour and keeps your metabolism active throughout the day.

PART 5: ELECTROMAGNETIC HYGIENE (Link to Chapter 9)

In the office, you are surrounded by the Wi-Fi of 20 routers.

1. **Cabling:** If possible, connect your PC via Ethernet cable and turn off your computer's Wi-Fi.

2. **Distance:** Do not keep the router on your desk 30 cm from your head. Move it at least 3 meters away.
3. **Headphones:** Use wired headphones (or Air Tube) for calls. Avoid keeping Bluetooth earphones in your ears for 4 hours straight.

PART 6: OPERATIONAL PSYCHOLOGY (Deep Work Safety)

Distractions are "cognitive accidents." Every time you are interrupted, it takes 23 minutes to return to deep focus.

6.1 Ultradian Rhythms

The brain cannot stay focused for 8 hours. It works in 90-minute cycles.

- **Protocol:** 90 minutes Focus (Deep Work) -> 20 minutes Decompression (No screens, look into the distance, walk).
- **Safety Tool:** Use noise-canceling headphones (ANC) with **Binaural Beats** (40Hz Gamma for focus, 10Hz Alpha for relaxation) to isolate yourself acoustically in open spaces.

PART 7: BIOLOGICAL AIR CONDITIONING (Humidity and Ions)

Office air is not only "stale" (CO_2), it is often electrically "dead" and biologically "dry."

7.1 The Hygrometric Audit (40-60%)

Air-conditioned offices often have a relative humidity of < 20% (like the desert).

- **The Damage:** Nasal mucous membranes dry out, losing their ability to trap viruses (the risk of airborne infection doubles). Eyes become dehydrated, increasing visual fatigue.
- **Apex Action:** Use an ultrasonic desktop humidifier. Maintain humidity between **40% and 60**%.

7.2 Negative Ionization (The Cascade Effect)

Computer screens and air conditioning generate an excess of **positive ions** (cations).

- **The Symptom:** Positive ions increase the production of serotonin (incorrectly) and histamine, causing irritability and headaches.
- **Apex Action:** Install a **negative ion generator** (ozone-free) on your desk. Negative ions (anions) neutralize the static charge of screens and purify the air of particulate matter.
-

PART 8: SENSORY NEURO-ERGONOMICS

8.1 Olfactory Hacking (The Olfactory Nerve)

Smell is the only sense directly connected to the limbic system.

- **Protocol:** Smell **rosemary** essential oil (1.8-cineole) *only* when you need to enter "Deep Work" mode. The brain will create a Pavlovian association:

  Smell of Rosemary = Extreme Focus

8.2 Soundscaping: Pink Noise vs. White Noise

- **Apex Action:** Use **Pink Noise** (similar to rain) or **Brown Noise**. It has a frequency that calms the nervous system and covers sudden disturbances better than White Noise.

PART 9: DYNAMIC VISION AND NEURO-PROTECTION

9.1 Panoramic Gaze (Peripheral Vision)

When you are stressed or stuck on a problem, your vision narrows ("Tunnel Vision").

- **Protocol:** Without moving your eyes from the screen, consciously try to widen your field of vision until you can perceive the side walls.
- **The Impact:** Instantly releases the stress response (sympathetic).

9.2 Zoom Fatigue Defense (Mirror Neurons)

Video calls are tiring because there is a micro-delay in the audio, and seeing your own face (self-view) keeps your brain in a state of "self-monitoring."

- **Apex Action: Hide your view (Hide Self-View)** and use **Audio Only** whenever possible.

PART 10: TACTICAL DESK NUTRITION

Eating at your desk is a metabolic disaster, but *what* you drink while working changes your performance.

The Polyphenol Diet (Brain Blood Flow)

Sitting reduces blood flow to the brain.

- **The Fuel:** Keep a jug of **green tea (Matcha)** or **raw cacao** on your desk.
- **The Mechanism:** Flavanols increase nitric oxide in the brain, partially compensating for the reduction in flow.

SAFETY OFFICER'S WORD

"Your desk is not a piece of furniture, it is a life support station. You have control over the air you breathe (ions/humidity), the light that hits your retina, the sounds that enter your ears, and the geometry of your skeleton. If you neglect these parameters, the office will consume you. If you master them, the office becomes the place where your biology performs at its highest level. Don't be an employee, be the architect of your habitat."

✅ SAFETY CHECKLIST: CHAPTER 11

Final Validation. If you don't have 5 green check marks, the habitat is hostile.

- [ ] **MONITOR:** Upper edge above eye level, arm's length away?
- [ ] **90-90-90:** Correct sitting posture with lumbar support?
- [ ] **STANDING:** Alternating sitting/standing (30/30 minutes)?
- [ ] **CO2 AUDIT:** Do you measure the air? If >1000 ppm, do you open the window or go outside?
- [ ] **FLICKER:** Have you checked for flickering with Slow Motion?
- [ ] **MICRO-DOSING:** Do you do calf raises or use a ball under your foot while working?
- [ ] **ANCHORING:** Do you use aromas (rosemary) to trigger the Flow State?

Safety Status:

🔴 **RED:** Dry, stale air (cerebral acidosis), strobe lights, chronic fatigue.

🟢 **GREEN:** Bio-optimized cockpit, laser focus, active metabolism 24/7.

CHAPTER 12

BIO-INTEGRATED DERMATOLOGY: THE SKIN AS AN ENDOCRINE ORGAN

"The skin is not a shell, it is an antenna and a chemical factory. What you put on your skin enters your bloodstream faster than what you eat, because it does not pass through the liver filter. The safety rule is brutal: if you wouldn't eat it, you shouldn't put it on your skin."

Classical dermatology often treats the skin as a tissue to be "plastered" with creams, steroids, and antibiotics. The **Elite Biohacker** knows that the skin is:

1. **An Endocrine Organ:** It produces vitamin D, cholesterol sulfate, and local sex hormones.
2. **An Ecosystem:** It hosts trillions of bacteria (Skin Microbiome) that are the true first line of immune defense.
3. **A Sensor:** It detects temperature, pressure, and light to calibrate the circadian rhythm.

The modern problem?

We bombard this organ with **endocrine disruptors** (in cosmetics), sterilize it with harsh soaps, and suffocate it with synthetic fabrics. The result is not only acne or wrinkles (which are just warning signs), but infertility, thyroid dysfunction, and systemic inflammation.

In this chapter, we will apply **Bio-Security** to skin care.

PART 1: THE SAFETY BARRIER (Acid Mantle & Microbiome)

Your skin is designed to be slightly acidic (pH 4.5 - 5.5).

This is the **Acid Cloak**. "Good" bacteria (e.g., *Staphylococcus epidermidis*) thrive in acid. Pathogens and fungi thrive in alkaline.

1.1 The Soap Mistake

Most commercial soaps and body washes have a pH of 9-10 (extremely alkaline).

- **The Damage:** Every time you wash with harsh soap, you destroy the acid mantle. It takes **14 hours** for the skin to restore the correct pH. If you wash twice a day, your skin is perpetually defenseless.
- **Apex Action:** Use pH-balanced cleansers (pH 5.5) or cleansing oils (which cleanse by lipid affinity without stripping away the hydrolipidic film).
- **Bio-Security:** Stop sterilizing yourself. A Biohacker doesn't smell, but doesn't "smell like chemicals" either.

1.2 The Physical Barrier (Stratum Corneum)

Imagine the skin as a brick wall. The bricks are the cells (corneocytes), the mortar is the lipids (ceramides, cholesterol, fatty acids).

- **Leaky Skin:** If you use water that is too hot or aggressive exfoliants, you dissolve the mortar. The skin becomes permeable ("Leaky Skin"). Toxins enter, water exits (TEWL).

- **Integration:** Nourish the barrier from within with **Omega-3** and **GLA** (Borage Oil) to produce high-quality ceramides.

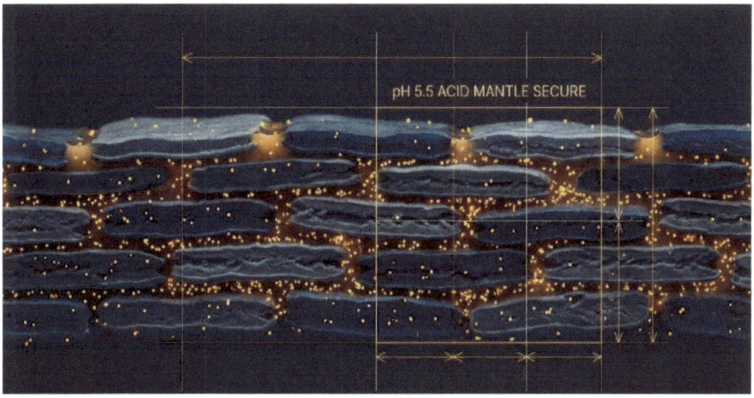

PART 2: TRANSDERMAL TOXICOLOGY (The Trojan Horse)

Why is the skin a critical safety point?

When you eat a toxin, the intestines and liver (first-pass metabolism) try to neutralize it. When **you apply** a toxin, it enters the capillaries and goes straight into the systemic bloodstream.

FICK'S LAW (BIOENGINEERING OF ABSORPTION)

The rate of transdermal absorption is described by Fick's law.

The Danger: Areas with thin skin (low) such as **the armpits, scrotum, neck, and eyelids** absorb toxins 100% faster than other areas.

BIOSAFETY: THE PERMEABILITY COEFFICIENT

Absorption is not only a matter of concentration, but also of lipid affinity. The permeability coefficient of a substance through the stratum corneum is predicted by its octanol-water partition coefficient.

Safety Insight: Small, highly lipophilic substances (such as many synthetic fragrances, phthalates, and preservatives) pass through the barrier as if it did not exist. Your skin is a selective sieve that lets the worst poisons through.

2.1 The "Dirty Dozen" (To be eliminated NOW)

Audit your bathroom. Eliminate anything that contains:

1. **Parabens:** Mimic estrogen.
2. **Phthalates:** Hidden under the heading "Parfum." They lower testosterone.
3. **Triclosan:** Destroys the thyroid.
4. **Aluminum:** Blocks sweat pores above the axillary lymph nodes.

2.2 Sunscreens: Protection or Poison?

Many chemical filters (oxybenzone) are endocrine disruptors.

- **Apex Action:** Use only physical mineral screens (**zinc oxide** or titanium "non-nano"). They reflect light instead of reacting chemically.

PART 3: THE SKIN AS A SOLAR PANEL (Endocrinology)

The skin is a biological photovoltaic panel.

3.1 Cholesterol Sulfate

When the skin is exposed to UV rays, it converts cholesterol into **cholesterol sulfate**.

- **Function:** Essential for heart and brain health.
- **Safety Alert:** If you always use sunscreen or wash with soap immediately after exposure, you block this synthesis.

3.2 Nitric Oxide (NO)

UVA rays stimulate the skin to release nitric oxide into the blood (vasodilation, low blood pressure).

- **Apex Action:** "Solar Callus." Gradually build up tolerance to the sun.

3.3 Skin Opsins and Non-Visual Photoreception

We must link this chapter to Light (Chapter 6).

- **The Concept:** The skin has **opsins** (like the rhodopsins in the eyes). These proteins "see" light and activate biological responses independently of the eyes.
- **Apex Action:** Blue light from smartphones not only affects the retina, but also activates skin opsins, inducing hyperpigmentation and mitochondrial degradation even at night. Protecting the skin from artificial blue light in the evening (covering up or using red lights) is as vital as protecting the eyes.

PART 4: GUT-SKIN AXIS (Internal Skincare)

Acne, rosacea, and eczema are not "skin diseases." They are smoke signals from the gut.

4.1 The Inflammation Map

The skin is the backup elimination organ.

- **Acne:** Often related to excess **insulin**.
- **Eczema/Psoriasis:** Related to intestinal permeability (leaky gut).
- **Apex Action:** Eliminate gluten, industrial dairy products, and seed oils for 30 days.

4.2 The "Skin-Gut-Brain" Loop: Biochemical Reflexology

The location of a skin rash is never random; it is a projection of the suffering of the internal organs.

- **Forensic Map of the Face (Apex Action):**
  - **Forehead:** Intestinal or bladder stress (dysbiosis).
  - **Chin/Jaw:** Hormonal imbalance (gonads/ovaries/testicles).
  - **Cheeks:** Pulmonary or metabolic stress (Smoking/Pollution/Sugar).
- **Safety Insight:** Do not cover up the symptom. If you have breakouts on your chin, the problem is endocrine, not soap.

PART 5: NEURO-DERMATOLOGY (The Skin as an Exposed Brain)

The skin is not just a barrier; it is embryologically linked to the nervous system (both derive from the ectoderm).

5.1 Skin-Brain Axis

The skin produces its own neurotransmitters (beta-endorphins, dopamine) and has receptors for cortisol.

- **The Concept:** Chronic psychological stress raises skin cortisol, which degrades collagen independently of sugar and inflames the sebaceous glands.

- **Apex Action:** The skin "feels" stress before the mind does. Practices such as meditation or grounding (Chapter 9) are direct dermatological treatments.

5.2 EDA (Electrodermal Activity): The Truth Sensor

The skin is the only organ that cannot lie about your stress level.

- **The Concept:** The electrical conductance of the skin (EDA) changes instantly based on the activity of the sympathetic nervous system. It is the **"voltage of fear."**
- **Apex Action (Bio-Feedback):** Use your wearable device to monitor your skin's galvanic response throughout the day. If your conductance rises without physical activity, your skin "hardware" is signaling an overload of the security system (stress).

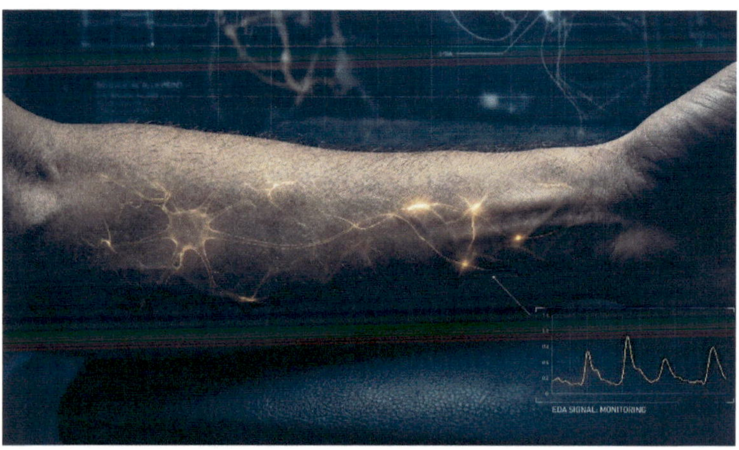

PART 6: REGENERATIVE BIO-AESTHETICS (Without Surgery)

6.1 Collagen Banking & GHK-Cu

- **Copper Peptides (GHK-Cu):** Stimulates skin regeneration and remodels scar tissue.
- **Microneedling:** Pure hormesis. Creates micro-holes to stimulate collagen production.

6.2 Skin Autophagy and Senolysis

Why do peptides and fasting work? Because they activate internal cleansing.

- **The Concept:** Old and damaged (senescent) cells remain in the skin, emitting inflammatory signals ("Zombie Cells").
- **Apex Action (Cleansing Protocol):** Intermittent fasting (Chapter 3) and molecules such as **spermidine** activate skin autophagy: the skin literally " " its damaged proteins to recycle them into new collagen.

6.3 Photobiomodulation (Red Light)

- **Action:** 10 minutes of red light (660 nm) and NIR (850 nm) increase ATP in fibroblasts.

PART 7: THE SECOND SKIN (Clothing)

7.1 Textile Toxins

Synthetic fabrics release microplastics and generate electrostatic charges.

- **Apex Action:** Return to natural fibers (cotton, linen, wool, silk). The skin must breathe and exchange electrons.

7.2 The Textile Saboteur: Washing Residues

We have talked about natural fibers, but an elite biohacker must look at what remains inside those fibers.

- **The Concept:** Conventional detergents and fabric softeners leave residues of phthalates and synthetic fragrances which, when in contact with the skin and body heat, are absorbed 24 hours a day through the skin (see Fick's Law).
- **Apex Action (Laundry Audit):** Use only eco-friendly, fragrance-free detergents or ceramic balls. Don't let your clothes become a **slow-release patch** of endocrine disruptors.

PART 8: THE GAS CHAMBER (The Danger of Showering)

8.1 Disinfection Byproducts (DBPs)

Under hot water, chlorine vaporizes to form chloroform.

- **Apex Action:** Install a **KDF-55 Shower Filter**. It converts free chlorine into chloride (harmless) before it touches your skin and lungs.

PART 9: GLYCATION AND BIOPHYSICS

Why does skin age? It's not just time. It's sugar (Maillard reaction).

9.1 Collagen Cross-Linking

Sugar binds to collagen, forming **AGEs** (Advanced Glycation End-products). The fibers "weld" together and become stiff.

BIOPHYSICS OF STRUCTURAL RIGIDITY

The collagen aging process is accelerated by the covalent binding of sugars to proteins.

The probability of AGEs formation is proportional to the exposure time and the average glucose concentration in the interstitial fluid.

Significance: Since we cannot change our internal temperature, the only safety variable we can act on is lowering the area under the glycemic curve. Carnosine and Benfotiamine are inhibitors of this reaction.

PART 10: HYDRAULICS, CHRONOBIOLOGY, AND DETOX

10.1 Dry Brushing

Dry brushing to activate the superficial lymphatic pump and drain toxins.

10.2 Skin Chronobiology

- **Morning:** Antioxidants (Vitamin C).
- **Evening:** Repair (retinoids).

10.3 Sweat as a Forensic Tool (Active Detox)

We have talked about toxins entering the body, but the skin is also your secondary "exhaust valve."

- **Apex Action (Sweat Audit):** Skin that smells acrid (ammonia-like) or has sudden rashes after a sauna is **dumping toxins**.

10.4 Phase III Detoxification (ABC Transporters)

- **The Concept:** The liver processes toxins, but the skin is **Phase III**. If membrane transporters (ABC proteins) are blocked, toxins remain trapped in the dermis.
- **Apex Action (Transporter Support):** The use of sulfur compounds (**MSM**) and cellular hydration ensure that the skin's cellular discharge pumps do not become blocked.

10.5 Skin Vascular Exercise (Cold Tightening)

Cold water is not just for waking up.

- **The Concept:** Exposure to cold causes vasoconstriction followed by reflex vasodilation, which "trains" the smooth muscle of the dermal capillaries.

- **Apex Action (Thermal Snap):** Ending your shower with **30 seconds of ice-cold water** tones the skin's elastic matrix, increasing firmness and reducing lymphatic stagnation that causes "dull skin."

PART 11: FRONTIER MOLECULES & DELIVERY

11.1 The Mitochondrial Secret (Methylene Blue)

It acts as a topical mitochondrial super-antioxidant, increasing ATP and collagen, which we will discuss later.

11.2 The Transdermal Portal: Selective Nutrition

The skin is an absorption organ. We can use this to our advantage.

- **Apex Action (Transdermal Magnesium):** Use magnesium oil (spray) on the skin, especially after the sauna.

PART 12: VISUAL DIAGNOSTICS

12.1 The Skin as a Mirror of Biological Age

The skin is not just an organ, it is a biomarker.

- **Facial Biological Age:** People whose skin looks visibly younger than their chronological age almost always have longer telomeres and a lower cardiovascular risk.
- **Safety Insight:** Deep wrinkles are a **visual audit** of your cellular efficiency.

TECHNICAL BOX: DIGITAL DERMATOLOGICAL AUDIT

Use your smartphone's sensors.

- **Pore Analysis:** Macro photography to monitor the "texture."

  Dilation = Inflammation.

- **UV Check:** UV lenses to see deep sun damage ("ghost spots").

PART 13: FACIAL ARCHITECTURE (LINK CHAPTER 10)

13.1 The Oral-Cutaneous Axis (Mewing & Microbiome)

The structure of the face and the oral microbiome directly influence skin aging.

- **Apex Action:** Tongue posture and nasal breathing act as a **natural facelift from within**.

SAFETY OFFICER'S WORD

"Your skin is the dashboard of your internal health. Inflamed skin is an alarm signal from the central security system. Covering it with foundation or bombarding it with cortisone is like removing the oil warning light from your car. Don't treat your skin; treat your body, and your skin will glow as an inevitable side effect."

✅ SAFETY CHECKLIST: CHAPTER 12

Final Validation. If you don't have 5 green check marks, your PPE is defective.

- [ ] **SHOWER FILTER:** Have you installed a KDF filter on your shower?
- [ ] **NO SUGAR:** Do you keep your blood sugar stable to avoid "caramelization" (AGEs)?
- [ ] **pH 5.5:** Do you only use acidic cleansers that respect the microbiome?
- [ ] **SOAP DETOX:** Have you eliminated Triclosan, Parabens, and Phthalates?
- [ ] **MICROPLASTICS AUDIT:** Is your detergent free of microplastics?
- [ ] **SUN:** Do you expose yourself to nitric oxide and cholesterol sulfate?
- [ ] **OPSIN SHIELD:** Do you protect your skin from artificial blue light in the evening?

Safety Status:

🔴 **RED:** Chlorinated showers, sugary diet, inflamed and glycated skin, chronic skin stress, toxic clothing.

🟢 **GREEN:** Intact acid barrier, elastic collagen, active skin mitochondria, zero toxic load, efficient detox.

PART 4: MOLECULAR OVERCLOCKING: THE SOFTWARE

Imagine you have the most powerful computer in the world (your body optimized in Parts 1-3), but you run it on Windows 95, full of bugs and viruses.

No matter how fast the hardware is, if the software is corrupted, the system will crash.

Human "software" consists of chemical signals: **hormones** (Chapter 13), **neurotransmitters** (Chapter 14), and **genetic signals** (Chapter 15).

These molecules are the lines of code that tell your cells what to do: "Burn fat," "Build muscle," "Sleep," "Focus," "Repair."

In traditional medicine, the software is only intervened upon when the system is already in "Blue Screen of Death" mode (diabetes, depression, hypothyroidism).

The **Safety Biohacker** acts differently.

We don't wait for the crash. We do **Safe Overclocking**.

In this section, you will learn how to:

1. **Modulate the Control Panel:** Optimize Testosterone, Thyroid, and Cycle for maximum efficiency (not to "pump up," but to perform).
2. **Rewrite the Mental Code:** Hack dopamine and cortisol for indestructible focus.

3. **Cheat Death:** Activate the pathways of longevity (autophagy, sirtuins) to slow down the biological clock.
4. **Read the Telemetry:** Use Elite Diagnostics (DNA and Blood) to guide decisions, don't guess.

Caution: Overclocking generates heat (oxidative stress).

If you haven't followed Parts 1-3 (Reclamation and Structure), pushing the accelerator now will blow up the engine.

But you've done your homework. Your engine is ready.

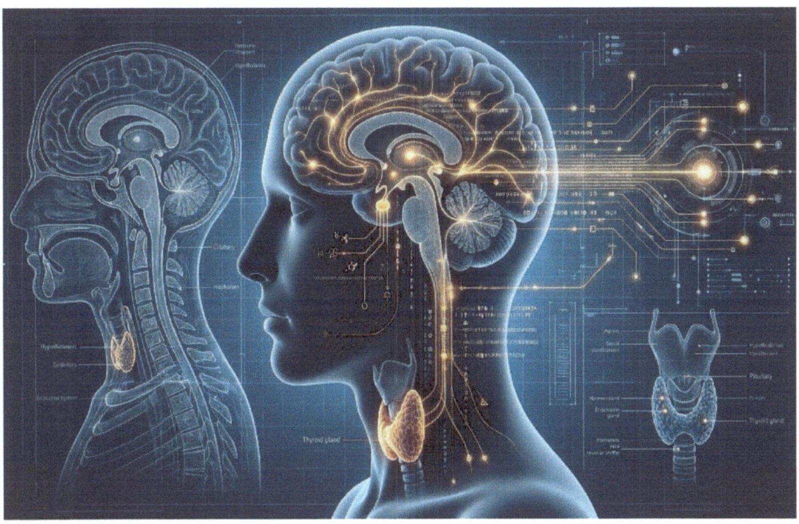

CHAPTER 13

THE ENDOCRINE SYSTEM: MEN & WOMEN (TESTOSTERONE, THYROID, AND CYCLE SYNCING)

"Hormones aren't just 'chemicals'. They're urgent emails that the brain sends to the organs. If the inbox is full of spam (endocrine disruptors) or the server is slow (sluggish thyroid), the company goes bankrupt. You can't have the will of a lion if you have the chemistry of a sloth."

The endocrine system is your body's Wi-Fi network.

Different glands (routers) send invisible signals (hormones) to specific receptors (antennas).

Today, we are living in a **Global Endocrine Crisis**.

- Male testosterone has declined by 1% per year since the 1980s. A 30-year-old man today has the hormone profile of a 60-year-old man in 1980.
- Thyroid disorders and female infertility are epidemic.

Why? Because our environment is hostile.

Plastic, blue light, chronic stress, and inflammatory foods are hacking the system for you.

In this chapter, we will regain control of **the Command Console**.

PART 1: LIGHT AS A HORMONE (The Optic-Gonadal Axis)

Many people think that testosterone is produced in the testicles/ovaries. False. The order comes from the eye.

The HPG (Hypothalamic-Pituitary-Gonadal) axis is activated by light.

1.1 Kisspeptin and GnRH

Morning sunlight (blue/UV spectrum) hits the retina, activates the suprachiasmatic nucleus (SCN), and stimulates the production of **kisspeptin** in the hypothalamus.

- **The Mechanism:** Kisspeptin is the "trigger" that starts GnRH (Gonadotropin-Releasing Hormone), which in turn instructs the pituitary gland to release LH and FSH (which tell the testicles/ovaries to work).
- **Apex Action (Solar Loading):** Don't just expose your skin. Expose your eyes (without sunglasses) to natural light within 30 minutes of waking up.

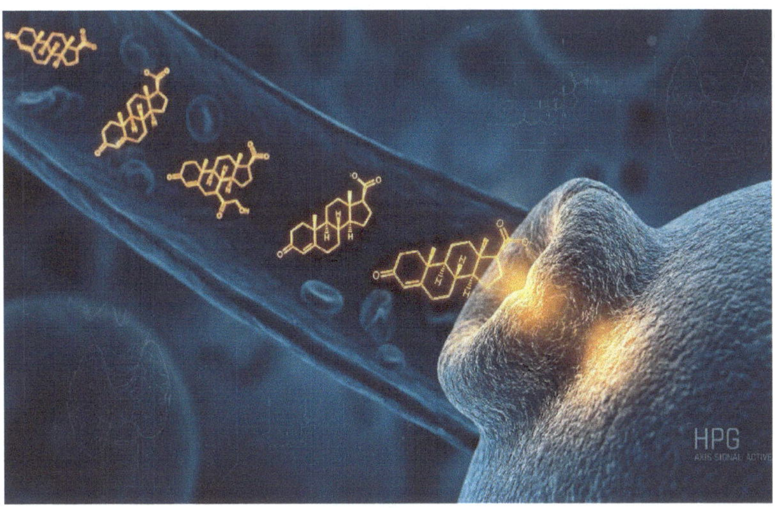

TECHNICAL BOX: (LIGHT MEASUREMENT)

Don't guess. Measure.

Apex Action: Use the brightness sensor (Luxmeter) on your smartphone when you wake up.

- **Target:** You need at least **10,000 lux** for 15-20 minutes to activate Kisspeptin.
- **Reality Check:** If it's cloudy, you need to stay outside longer.

1.2 Red Light Therapy (Photon Doping)

Red light (660nm) penetrates tissue and directly stimulates the mitochondria of Leydig cells (T production) and the thyroid.

- **Protocol:** 10 minutes per day, close distance on the neck (thyroid) or gonads.

PART 2: THE METABOLIC THERMOSTAT (THE THYROID)

Before talking about "muscles" or "libido," we need to talk about **energy**. The thyroid is the accelerator pedal.

2.1 T4 vs. T3 (The Conversion)

The thyroid produces T4 (inactive). It must be converted to T3 (active) by the liver and intestines.

- **The Block:** Stress (high cortisol), fatty liver, or intestinal dysbiosis block conversion. You have normal TSH, but you are tired, cold, and gaining weight ("functional hypothyroidism").
- **Apex Action:**
    - **Selenium & Zinc:** Essential cofactors. 2-3 Brazil nuts per day (selenium) are a must.
    - **Zero Gluten:** The gluten molecule resembles thyroid tissue. For a Safety Officer, gluten is an uncalculated autoimmune risk.

2.2 The "Handbrake": Reverse T3 (rT3)

In times of stress or famine, the body converts T4 into **Reverse T3** (a mirror image of inactive T3). It is the metabolic speed limiter.

APEX BIOCHEMISTRY: THYROID EFFICIENCY

Cellular hypothyroidism occurs when Reverse T3 (rT3) occupies the receptors intended for Free T3 (FT3). The safety formula for the Safety Officer is:

$$\mathbf{FT3\ (pg/mL)/[rT3\ (ng/dL) \times 10]}$$

- **Elite Target:** > 20
- **Safety Risk:** < 15 (The engine is in forced energy-saving mode).

Action: If the ratio is low, you must remove the stressor (toxins/inflammation), do not add caffeine.

2.3 The Hidden Thyroid (Barnes Thermometry)

Blood tests can lie. Body temperature cannot.

- **Protocol:** As soon as you wake up, measure your axillary temperature. Target: **98.5°F - 98.8°F.**

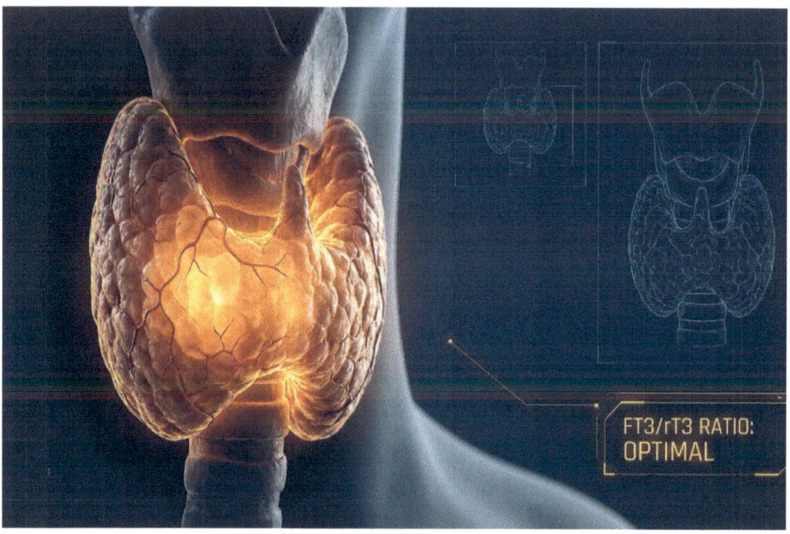

PART 3: THE CONDUCTOR (INSULIN)

You can't talk about sex hormones without mentioning insulin. It is the "master" hormone that determines metabolic priority.

- **The Concept:** Chronic hyperinsulinemia (caused by sugar and frequent snacking) is the number one cause of testosterone collapse in men (activates aromatase) and excess androgens in women (PCOS).

- **Apex Action (Insulin Shield):** Keep fasting insulin **< 5-7 uIU/mL**. If insulin is high, any attempt to optimize testosterone or progesterone will be sabotaged at the outset.

PART 4: MEN'S PROTOCOL (TESTOSTERONE OPTIMIZATION)

4.1 Enemies and aromatase

1. **Aromatase:** Converts testosterone into estrogen. Visceral fat is an aromatase factory.
2. **SHBG (Sex Hormone Binding Globulin):** Sequesters testosterone.

4.2 The Liver: The Distribution Center (SHBG)

We have referred to SHBG as a "sequestrant," but where is it produced?

- **The Concept:** SHBG is produced by the liver. If the liver is congested (steatosis, excess alcohol or fructose), SHBG production goes haywire. In an inflamed liver, SHBG can rise excessively, rendering even excellent testosterone production useless.
- **Apex Action (Liver Audit):** You cannot have elite hormones if your liver is not clean. Hormonal health is a byproduct of metabolic liver health.

4.3 Scrotal Hyperthermia (Occupational Hazard)

- **The Risk:** Sitting for 8 hours increases testicular temperature. A **1°C** increase reduces testosterone production by **40%**.
- **Apex Action (Cooling Protocol):** Get up every 30 minutes. Never keep a hot laptop on your lap (Wi-Fi + Heat = Sterilization).

4.4 The Winner Effect and the Mental "Firewall"

Testosterone is not stable. It fluctuates based on your perceived social status.

- **The Mental Firewall (Hypothalamic Feedback):** The hypothalamus is the security sensor. If it senses chronic defeat, it activates **somatostatin**, which blocks both GH and TSH.
- **Apex Action (Winner Effect):** Engineer your day to have 3-4 guaranteed "Micro-Wins." This tells your hypothalamus that the environment is safe, unlocking Somatostatin and raising Testosterone and Dopamine.

4.5 Tactical Supplementation

- **Zinc & Boron:** To optimize free T.

PART 5: WOMEN'S PROTOCOL (CYCLE SYNCING)

Women have a 28-day infradian rhythm.

1. **Follicular Phase (Spring):** High estrogen. Fasting and HIIT.

2. **Ovulation (Summer):** Hormonal peak. Maximum strength.
3. **Luteal Phase (Fall):** Progesterone. Metabolism accelerates. **Stop fasting.** Complex carbohydrates.
4. **Menstruation (Winter):** Reset. Magnesium and iron.

PART 6: ESTROGEN METABOLISM AND MICROBIOME (Safety Detox)

It's not just how much estrogen you produce that matters, but **how you dispose of it**.

6.1 The Estrogen Traffic Light (2-OH, 4-OH, 16-OH)

We want the **2-OH** (clean) pathway. The **4-OH** pathway damages DNA.

- **Apex Action:** Broccoli sprouts (sulforaphane) and **DIM** (diindolylmethane) to force the safe metabolic pathway and block aromatase.

6.2 The Estrobolome: The Intestinal Drain Valve

We've talked about the liver, but the last mile is missing.

- **The Concept:** There is a collection of gut bacteria called **the Estrobolome**. If these bacteria produce an enzyme called **Beta-Glucuronidase**, the estrogens that the liver has struggled to "package" are discarded in the gut, reactivated, and reabsorbed into the bloodstream.

- **Apex Action (Intestinal Audit):** If you have constipation or dysbiosis, your hormonal detox is at a standstill. **Calcium D-Glucarate** is the security key to blocking this enzyme and ensuring that the email (hormone) is actually deleted after use.

PART 7: DEFENSE AGAINST EDCs (Xenoestrogens)

Chemicals that "mimic" estrogen.

1. **BPA/Plastic:** Never put hot food in plastic.
2. **Receipts:** Do not touch thermal paper.
3. **Water:** Reverse osmosis is mandatory.
4. **Triclosan:** Get rid of antibacterial soaps that block the thyroid.

PART 8: PRO-HORMONE NUTRITION AND STRESS MANAGEMENT

8.1 The Raw Material: Cholesterol

- **Apex Action:** High-quality saturated and monounsaturated fats. Cholesterol is the precursor to sex hormones.

8.2 Vitamin D: The Steroid Pro-Hormone

We need to stop calling it a "vitamin." It is a steroid hormone that is essential for genetic transcription.

- **The Concept:** Without optimal levels (> 60 ng/mL), testosterone and thyroid receptors lose sensitivity. It's like having a Wi-Fi signal but a broken antenna.
- **Apex Action:** Don't accept the "normal" range (30 ng/mL). Aim for hunter-gatherer levels.

8.3 Pregnenolone Theft (Cortisol Steal)

- **The Concept:** Cholesterol produces pregnenolone. Under chronic stress, the body diverts all pregnenolone to **cortisol** (survival), leaving testosterone and progesterone depleted.
- **Apex Action:** You cannot optimize T unless you put out the Cortisol fire.

PART 9: THE NIGHT WATCH (SOMATOTROPIN AND MELATONIN)

Testosterone and the thyroid repair the engine, but Growth Hormone (GH) is the skilled worker that only works at night.

9.1 The GH Window (11:00 p.m. - 2:00 a.m.)

- **The Enemy:** Insulin. If insulin is high, it blocks GH release.
- **Apex Action:** If you eat sugar within **3 hours** of sleep, you sabotage your nighttime repair.

9.2 Melatonin as a Mitochondrial Protector

Melatonin is not just for sleeping.

- **The Concept:** Leydig cells (testicles) and theca cells (ovaries) are full of mitochondria that are vulnerable to oxidative stress. Melatonin is the most powerful mitochondrial antioxidant that protects the glands from cellular "rust."
- **Apex Action (Mitochondrial Shield):** Red light stimulates local melatonin. Protecting sleep means protecting the physical integrity of the hormone glands.

PART 10: OPERATIONAL SAFETY (EXOGENOUS RISK)

For a Safety Officer, it is essential to warn about the risks of "shortcuts."

10.1 Negative Feedback: The Danger of Replacement Therapies

- **The Concept:** The hormonal system is a negative feedback loop. If you introduce synthetic hormones from outside (TRT or other) without control, the brain perceives "full Wi-Fi" and **permanently shuts down** the routers (gonads/thyroid).
- **Apex Action:** Elite biohacking aims to reactivate endogenous production (via light, nutrients, and the Winner Effect), not replace it.

PART 11: ADVANCED ENDOCRINE DIAGNOSTICS

11.1 Free Androgen Index (FAI)

BIOHACKER FORMULA:

$$[\text{Total Testosterone (nmol/L)}/\text{SHBG (nmol/L)}] \times 100$$

Elite Male Target: FAI > 70%.

11.2 DHEA-S: The Adrenal Buffer

- **The Concept:** DHEA is the precursor to sex hormones and acts as a buffer against cortisol. It is the biomarker of "resilience."
- **Apex Action:** Check your cortisol/DHEA ratio. If it is skewed toward cortisol, you are in "catabolic" (destructive) mode.

11.3 Beyond Blood: The DUTCH Test

Measures urinary metabolites and the circadian rhythm of cortisol.

TECHNICAL BOX: HORMONE TRACKING

Use your hardware.

- **Men (HRV Tracking):** Monitor your HRV (Heart Rate Variability) in the morning. A drop in HRV is a predictive signal of a cortisol spike that will suppress testosterone over the next 24 hours.

- **Women (Cycle Tech):** Use cycle tracking apps (e.g., Clue or Stardust) integrated with smartphone temperature sensors to accurately identify the transition between the "Spring" and "Fall" phases of your cycle.

SAFETY OFFICER'S WORD

"Your hormones are not destiny, they are the result of your environmental inputs. If you live in a toxic environment, eat junk food, and don't sleep, your software will go into 'Survival' mode. Endocrine Biohacking is not about taking synthetic hormones; it's about removing interference so that the body can produce the chemical symphony it was designed to produce."

✅ SAFETY CHECKLIST: CHAPTER 13

Endocrine System Validation. If you don't have 5 check marks, your software is unstable.

- [ ] **VIT D:** Are your levels > 60 ng/mL?
- [ ] **rT3 AUDIT:** Is your FT3/rT3 ratio > 20?
- [ ] **RED LIGHT:** Do you use red light on the thyroid/gonads to stimulate the mitochondria?
- [ ] **GH WINDOW:** No food 3 hours before bedtime to maximize GH?
- [ ] **PLASTIC DETOX:** Do you only eat and drink from glass/steel?
- [ ] **RECEIPTS:** Do you avoid thermal paper (BPA)?
- [ ] **THYROID:** Do you eat Brazil nuts (selenium)?

Safety Status:

🔴 **RED:** High insulin, fatty liver (SHBG out of whack), belly fat, thyroid "handbrake" activated, toxic estrogen.

🟢 **GREEN:** Efficient metabolism, low insulin, dominant sex hormones, solid DHEA reserve, clean Estrobolome.

CHAPTER 14

NEURO-ENGINEERING: ARCHITECTURE OF THE SUPERIOR MIND

"Your brain isn't broken; your inputs are garbage. In a world that monetizes your distraction, the ability to focus deeply (Deep Work) is the ultimate superpower. The Biohacker doesn't seek motivation; he builds a neural architecture where focus is the only option."

The human brain consumes 20% of your metabolic energy while weighing only 2% of your body. It is the most expensive machine you own.

Today, this machine is under constant DDoS (Distributed Denial of Service) attack: email, social media, news, strobe lights.

The result?

1. **Dopamine Burnout:** The reward system is fried. Nothing satisfies you, everything bores you.
2. **Attention Residue:** Jumping from task to task leaves "residues" of attention that lower your IQ by 10 points.
3. **Cognitive Cortisol:** The background anxiety that prevents access to long-term memory.

In this chapter, we will "reboot" the mental operating system.

PART 1: THE PHYSICS OF DOPAMINE (Cheap vs. Expensive)

Dopamine is not the "pleasure" molecule. It is the molecule of "craving" and action.

1.1 Cheap Dopamine (The Toxic Peak)

Sugar, social media, pornography.

- **The Mechanism:** They create a very high and immediate peak without effort.
- **The Crash:** For homeostasis, the brain must compensate for the spike by lowering the baseline below zero (pain/boredom).

1.2 The "Dopamine Detox" Protocol (Safety Reset)

If you feel unmotivated, you don't need "more stimulation," you need "less noise."

- **Apex Action (24-hour Reset):** One Sunday per month. No screens, no music, no sugar. Just boredom.
- The **Effect:** "Boredom" is the receptor cleansing tool. It resets sensitivity.

1.3 The Desire Equation (Reward Prediction Error)

The brain releases dopamine when you get **more than you expected**.

$$RPE = R_{actual} - R_{predicted}$$

- **"Random Rewards" Protocol:** Use intermittent reinforcement. Flip a coin after a difficult task: Heads = Reward, Tails = Nothing.

  Uncertainty keeps dopamine sky-high (Motivation Hacking).

1.4 Hormetic Reset: Dynorphins and Sensitivity

There is a biochemical accelerator for resetting receptors: heat stress.

- **The Concept:** Extreme heat (sauna) releases **dynorphins**, peptides that initially make you feel uncomfortable. However, they force the brain to over-regulate (increase) the density of dopamine receptors.
- **Apex Action (The Heat Reset):** An intense post-work sauna session acts as a "chemical flush" that makes your next day's achievements much more rewarding.

PART 2: FLOW STATE ENGINEERING (The Art of Focus)

2.1 TPN vs DMN: The Focus Switch

The brain has two main networks that compete with each other.

1. **TPN (Task Positive Network):** Focus, Action, "Here and Now."
2. **DMN (Default Mode Network):** Daydreaming, Anxiety.

- **Apex Action (TPN Lockdown):** When you start a Deep Work session, the goal is to force the activation of the

TPN. If your brain "wanders," use **Visual Anchoring** to shut down the DMN.

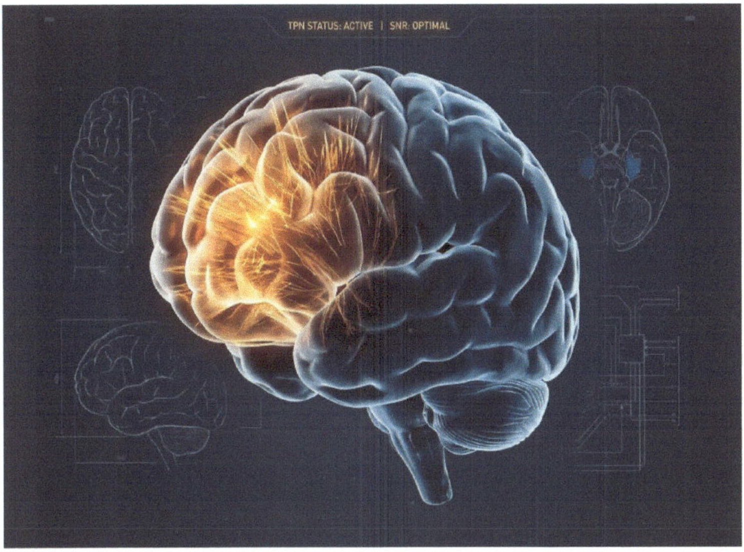

2.2 Visual Anchoring (The Brain Stem Switch)

Your eyes are an extension of your brain.

- **The Concept:** When your eyes converge on a fixed point, your brain enters "alert" mode (TPN).
- **Apex Action (Visual Focus Drills):** Before a Deep Work session, stare at a point on your desk or monitor frame for **60 seconds** without blinking. This muscular effort forces the release of acetylcholine exactly where it is needed.

2.3 Ultradian Rhythms (90 Minutes)

- **Safety Protocol:** Work in 90-minute blocks. After 90 minutes, the brain exhausts its neurotransmitters. Stop.

PART 3: OPERATIONAL NEUROCHEMISTRY (Safety Pharmacology)

The elite biohacker does not use "smart drugs" randomly. He uses chemistry to modulate his state.

3.1 The Adenosine Protocol (Caffeine Hacking)

- **The Concept:** Caffeine does not give you energy; it blocks adenosine receptors (fatigue). If you take it as soon as you wake up, the residual adenosine is not disposed of and hits you all at once when the effect wears off.
- **Apex Action (Caffeine Delay):** Delays caffeine for **90-120 minutes** after waking up.

3.2 Glutamate/GABA Balance (Accelerator vs. Brake)

The focus is not just on 'pushing' (Glutamate), but **on using the brake to eliminate background noise** (GABA). The goal is to maximize **Executive Precision**: there is no point in having a high-frequency processor if the signal is disturbed by cognitive 'static' or calculation errors. "

Signal Science:

- **Glutamate (The Accelerator):** Provides the computing power and excitement needed for action.
- **GABA (The Brake/Silencer):** Acts as a filter that turns off irrelevant neurons, allowing the main signal to stand out.
- **The Safety Risk (Excitotoxicity):** If glutamate dominates without GABA control, the system overheats ( ), causing anxiety, insomnia, and, in the long term, neuron death from electrical exhaustion.

BIOPHYSICS OF EXECUTIVE PRECISION

The stability of the central nervous system depends on the homeostatic balance between excitation and inhibition. The ratio between the main inhibitory neurotransmitter (GABA) and the excitatory neurotransmitter (glutamate) must tend towards stability to avoid **excitotoxicity**:

Action: Balance caffeine with **L-Theanine**.

3.3 Fuel for Dopamine (L-Tyrosine)

- **Protocol: L-Tyrosine** on an empty stomach. It is the direct precursor of dopamine.

PART 4: STRESS MANAGEMENT (The Handbrake)

4.1 The Prefrontal Brake (Top-Down Control)

- **The Concept:** The dorsolateral prefrontal cortex (dlPFC) is the brain's "safety officer."
- **Apex Action (Interceptive Audit):** When you feel the urge to check your smartphone, stop and observe the physical sensation in your body for **10 seconds**. This shifts the load from the limbic system (impulse) to the prefrontal cortex (control).

4.2 The Physiological Sigh

- **Technique:** Two quick breaths in through the nose, one very long breath out through the mouth. Immediate reset of anxiety.

4.3 Optic Flow (The Amygdala Silencer)

- **The Concept:** When you walk forward, objects pass sideways across your retina (**Optic Flow**). This mechanically suppresses amygdala activity.
- **Apex Action (Walking Reset):** If you are stuck, walk outdoors to activate your peripheral vision.

4.4 NSDR (Non-Sleep Deep Rest)

20 minutes of Yoga Nidra is equivalent to 3 hours of sleep for dopamine recovery.

PART 5: SYSTEM EFFICIENCY AND NEURO-SECURITY

5.1 The Signal-to-Noise Ratio (SNR Audit)

- **The Concept:** Too many stimuli (notifications, stress) create **neural "white noise."**
- **Apex Action:** Meditation and silence are protocols for increasing the SNR of Deep Work.

5.2 Decision Fatigue: Software Wear and Tear

Every choice consumes glucose in the prefrontal cortex.

THE DECISION LOAD EQUATION

Decision-making capacity declines exponentially with the number of choices made.

Apex Action (Load Elimination): Apply decision minimalism in the first 4 hours of the day.

5.3 Neuro-Security: Defense Against Cognitive Biases

If neurotransmitters are fuel, logic is code. An elite system must protect itself from system bugs.

- **The Concept:** The brain constantly seeks shortcuts (heuristics) that lead to wrong decisions under stress.

- **Apex Action (Logical Debugging/Pre-Mortem):** Before every critical decision, imagine that the project has already failed and ask yourself, "Why did this happen?" This forces the brain to bypass limbic optimism and activates the analytical circuits of the dorsolateral prefrontal cortex.

PART 6: BRAIN ENERGY AND LIGHT

6.1 Creatine Monohydrate (Brain Fuel)

- **Apex Action:** 5g per day to recycle neuronal ATP.

6.2 Ketones (MCT Oil C8): The Emergency Generator

"The human brain is an omnivorous consumer, but it often becomes 'blind' to glucose due to insulin resistance or postprandial glycemic drops."

- **Apex Action:** Add MCT oil (medium-chain triglycerides), specifically caprylic acid (C8), to your morning coffee or beverage.
- **The "Insulin Bypass" Mechanism:** Unlike long-chain fats, C8 is sent directly to the liver via the portal vein, where it is instantly converted into ketones. These ketone bodies cross the blood-brain barrier and provide energy to neurons without the need for insulin to enter the cells.
- **The Purpose:** To provide an **auxiliary power line**. While glucose fluctuates, ketones offer a steady stream of ATP,

eliminating brain fog and brain "chemical hunger" that follows sugar spikes.

6.3 Choline Loading: Broadband Enhancement

"If neurons are the hardware, acetylcholine is the data transmission protocol that enables computing speed. Without raw material, bandwidth narrows."

- **The Apex Action:** Strategic intake of elite choline sources, such as eggs (liquid yolk) or highly bioavailable supplements such as Alpha-GPC.
- **The Science of Raw Materials:** Acetylcholine is the primary neurotransmitter for working memory, executive focus, and muscle contraction. Choline loading saturates the system with the precursors necessary to avoid cognitive burnout during intense deep work sessions.
- **The Goal:** Increase **Processing Speed**. Alpha-GPC, in particular, is able to increase choline levels in the brain much more efficiently than standard choline, acting as an instant upgrade to the neural CPU.

6.4 Transcranial Photobiomodulation (tPBM)

We need to connect neuroengineering to light for direct hardware overclocking.

- **The Concept:** Near-infrared light (810 nm) passes through the skull and stimulates **cytochrome C oxidase** in the mitochondria of cortical neurons.
- **Apex Action (Cerebral Charging):** The use of an NIR device on the frontal lobe instantly increases oxygenation and cerebral ATP production, boosting TPN beyond standard biochemical limits.

PART 7: HARDWARE MAINTENANCE (DEFENSE AND CLEANING)

7.1 The Glinphatic System: Hardware "Flush"

- **Apex Action (Glymphatic Flush):** Head slightly elevated during sleep and last food intake at least **3 hours prior**. If you digest, you don't clean.

7.2 BDNF: The Fertilizer of Neurons

- **Apex Action (BDNF Trigger):** Intense aerobic exercise (Zone 4/5) and intermittent fasting for neurogenesis.

7.3 The Brain "Firewall": Microglia Reset

We have talked about energy, but not about defense against inflammation.

- **The Concept: Microglia** are the immune cells of the brain. If they perceive chronic stress, they go into "attack" mode (Microglia Priming), releasing cytokines that destroy the Signal-to-Noise ratio (Brain Fog).

- **Apex Action (Firewall Reset):** The integration of **luteolin** or **apigenin** acts as a fire extinguisher for microglia, returning them to a state of "maintenance" and extinguishing neural autoinflammation.

PART 8: LIMBIC FRICTION & TECH AUDIT

8.1 Cold Start: Overcoming "Limbic Friction"

- **Limbic Friction** is the biological resistance you feel when your prefrontal cortex (your will) wants to do something, but your limbic system (your instinctive side) resists because the action requires effort or causes discomfort.
- **The Mechanism:** Starting your day with a cold shower or a hyperventilation session isn't just about "waking up." These practices force an immediate and massive release of **norepinephrine** and **adrenaline**.
- **The Purpose:** This biochemical "shock" bypasses mental hesitation. By training yourself to enter the freezing water despite the urge to run away, you are literally strengthening the connection between the prefrontal cortex and the limbic system.

- **The Apex Action:** Use it as a "reset button" for inertia. The more you overcome Limbic Friction with hormetic stressors, the more capable you will become of tackling difficult tasks throughout the day without procrastinating.

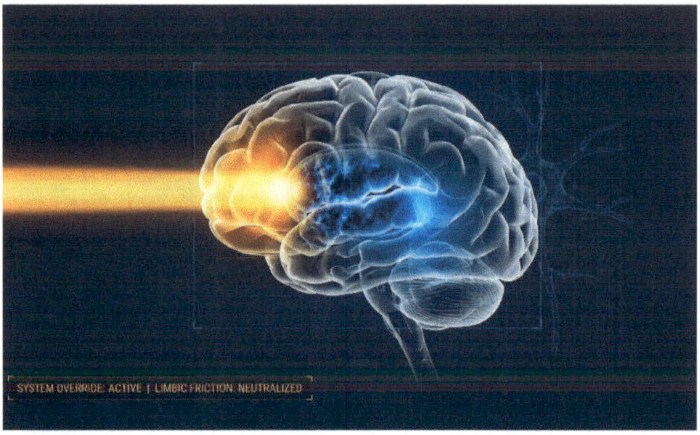

8.2 Apex Diagnostics: Pupillometry and SNR

- Your pupils are a direct window into your **Autonomic Nervous System (ANS)**. Their diameter responds not only to light, but also to your level of internal arousal.
- **The Science:** In a state of balance, your pupils constrict when you are relaxed (parasympathetic dominance). If they remain dilated even in normal light and at rest, it means you are in **Chronic Sympathetic Tone**: your body is stuck in a permanent "fight or flight" mode.
- **The SNR (Signal-to-Noise Ratio) Problem:** When you are chronically stressed, the neural "background noise" (cortisol and constant alertness) becomes so loud that it drowns out the "signal" (the important information you need to focus on).

- **The Apex Action:** If your "Pupil Audit" reveals constant mydriasis (dilatation), your cognitive efficiency is compromised. In this state, do not add stimulants (caffeine); instead, activate recovery protocols and the parasympathetic "brake."

8.3 Dual N-Back: Working Memory Enhancement

- **Working memory** is your brain's temporary storage space, the "RAM" you use to manipulate information in real time.
- **The Exercise:** Dual N-Back challenges you to track a visual and auditory sequence simultaneously, asking you to remember whether the current stimulus matches the one that appeared "N" steps earlier.
- **The Purpose:** It is the only scientifically validated *brain training* tool for increasing **intelligence fluency** and deep concentration skills.
- **Biological** ROI**:** 15 minutes of Dual N-Back per day expands your processing capacity. It's like weight training for your brain's CPU: the higher your working memory capacity, the more information you can manage simultaneously in your Master Plan without becoming cognitively overloaded.

SAFETY OFFICER'S WORD

"Your brain is a quantum processor trapped in a carnival environment. If you don't protect your inputs, the system will crash. Don't try to 'push' yourself harder. Stop drugging yourself with distractions, lower the background noise, and learn to hit the brakes when the curve picks up speed. The elite mind is a quiet mind, capable of exploding into action only when needed."

✅ SAFETY CHECKLIST: CHAPTER 14

Total Neural Validation. If you don't have 5 check marks, the pilot is ineffective.

- [ ] **CAFFEINE DELAY:** Do you wait 90-120 minutes after waking up before your first coffee?
- [ ] **ADENOSINE CLEARANCE:** Do you go out into natural light in the morning?
- [ ] **VISUAL ANCHORING:** Do you stare at a point for 60 seconds to activate TPN?
- [ ] **OPTIC FLOW:** Do you use the "Walking Reset" to shut down the amygdala?
- [ ] **GLYMPHATIC FLUSH: Do you** fast for 3 hours before sleeping?
- [ ] **BDNF TRIGGER:** Do you do intense cardio or fast for neurogenesis?
- [ ] **DOPAMINE DETOX:** Do you do a 24-hour reset every month?

Security Status:

🔴 **RED:** Afternoon crash, dominant DMN, inflamed brain (microglia), dilated pupils, emotional decisions.

🟢 **GREEN:** TPN on command, neuro-stability, clean hardware, high SNR, armored logic (Pre-Mortem).

CHAPTER 15

MOLECULAR LONGEVITY: GENOMIC MAINTENANCE PROTOCOLS

"Aging is the natural tendency of complex systems toward entropy. But in biology, entropy is caused by the loss of epigenetic information (the analog signal) that overshadows the genetic code (the digital signal). Aging is , like a scratched CD: the Safety Officer's job is to polish the disc and protect the original track to restore the software's readability."

Elite longevity is not about "living a long time in a house that is falling apart." It is about extending **Healthspan**. To do this, we must intervene in the mechanisms that govern cellular destiny: cleaning (Autophagy), repair (Sirtuins), structural protection (Telomeres), and energy efficiency (NAD+).

PART 1: THE BINARY SWITCH (mTOR vs. AMPK)

Every second, every cell must decide: "Do I grow or do I repair?" This decision is mediated by two protein sensors that function like a biochemical seesaw.

1.1 mTOR and Stem Cell Depletion

- **Function:** Stimulates protein synthesis and cell division. It is the accelerator of anabolism.

- **The Risk (Stem Cell Exhaustion):** If we stimulate mTOR 24/7, we force stem cells to divide continuously until they are exhausted.
- **Apex Action (IGF-1 Management):** Monitors **IGF-1**: if it is too high for too long, you are burning your biological "savings account" for immediate "interest."

1.2 AMPK: The Repair Sensor

- **Function:** Activates when energy drops. Orders the cell to stop growing and start repairing itself.
- **Apex Action:** Activate AMPK through Zone 2 exercise, intense cold, or **Berberine**.

PART 2: MITOCHONDRIAL ARCHITECTURE (CLEANING, BIOGENESIS, AND DYNAMICS)

It is not enough to clean old engines; we must increase the energy density and "quality control" of the network.

2.1 Mitochondrial Dynamics: Fusion and Fission

Mitochondria are not isolated entities, but a dynamic social network.

- **The Concept: Fusion** allows healthy mitochondria to compensate for damaged ones by sharing resources; **Fission** isolates diseased parts and sends them to mitophagy (disposal).

- **Apex Action:** Alternating between intense effort (**Zone 5**) and deep rest trains this mitochondrial "socialization" ability, ensuring that cellular voltage never suddenly

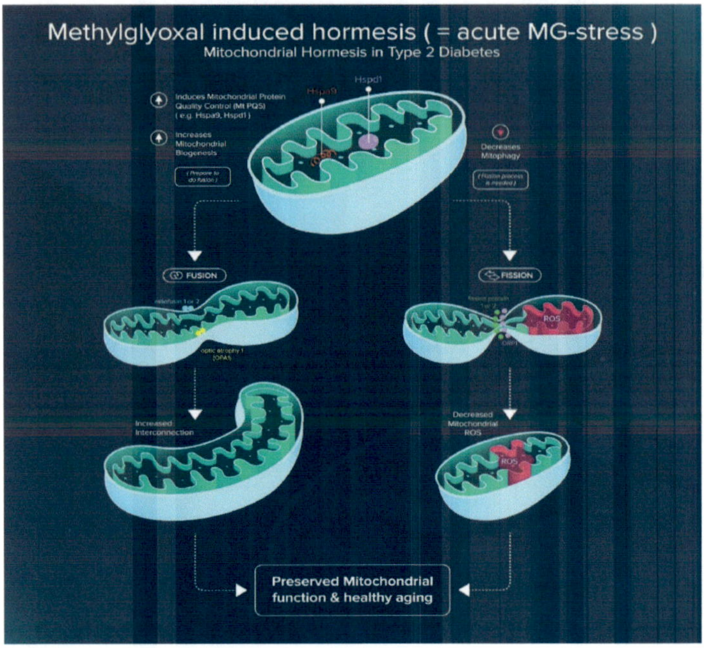

drops.

2.2 PQQ and Urolithin A (Construction and Cleaning)

- **PQQ (Pyrroloquinoline quinone):** Induces spontaneous **mitochondrial biogenesis**, creating new motors.
- **Urolithin A:** Induces **mitophagy**, eliminating motors that can no longer be repaired by fusion.

TECHNICAL BOX: (AGING AUDIT)

Apex Action (Digital Face Audit): Uses a high-resolution camera with polarized light filters to monitor the appearance of **lipofuscin** spots. This is a sign that your autophagy protocol needs to be intensified.

PART 3: THE NAD+ CYCLE AND REDOX POTENTIAL

NAD+ is the coenzyme essential for life. With age, silent inflammation (*inflammaging*) creates a "hole in the tank."

3.1 The Waste Rate and Apigenin

With age, inflamed macrophages produce **CD38**, an enzyme that destroys NAD+ before it can be used by sirtuins.

CELLULAR ENERGY BIOCHEMISTRY

The vitality of the system depends on the ratio between NAD+ and NADH. A "young" system maintains a high redox potential. Energy flow (ATP) is proportional to the availability of free NAD+.

Safety Insight: Investing in NMN without blocking CD38 (with **Apigenin**) is like trying to fill a bucket with holes in it.

PART 4: GENOMIC DEFENSE AND XENORMESIS

Sirtuins (SIRT1-7) are the firefighters of DNA. They are activated by the perception of environmental stress.

4.1 Xenohormesis: Stealing Resilience from Plants

- **The Concept:** Plants produce polyphenols when under stress (drought, pests). The body interprets these molecules as an alarm signal and activates repair genes.
- **Apex Action:** Choose organic or wild plants that have had to "struggle" to grow. They contain up to 10 times more Sirtuin activators.

PART 5: CODE BUFFERS (TELOMERES AND HBOT)

We talked about the "track length" of the biological CD. We need to protect telomeres.

5.1 HBOT & Telomerase (The Oxygen Effect)

Hyperbaric Oxygen Therapy (HBOT) is the most powerful longevity tool validated for telomere lengthening.

- **The Concept:** Elite studies have shown that specific HBOT protocols can lengthen telomeres by **20%** and reduce senescent cells by **37%** through the hyperoxic-hypoxic paradox.
- **Apex Action:** Incorporate **HBOT** as an "Extraordinary Maintenance Protocol." It is the only technology that measurably reverses the telomere clock in humans.

5.2 Telomerase and Methylation

- **Telomerase:** Also activated by Astragalus extract and heavy strength training.

- **Methyl Support:** Ensure **TMG, B12, and Folate** to keep the molecular "CD player" clean.

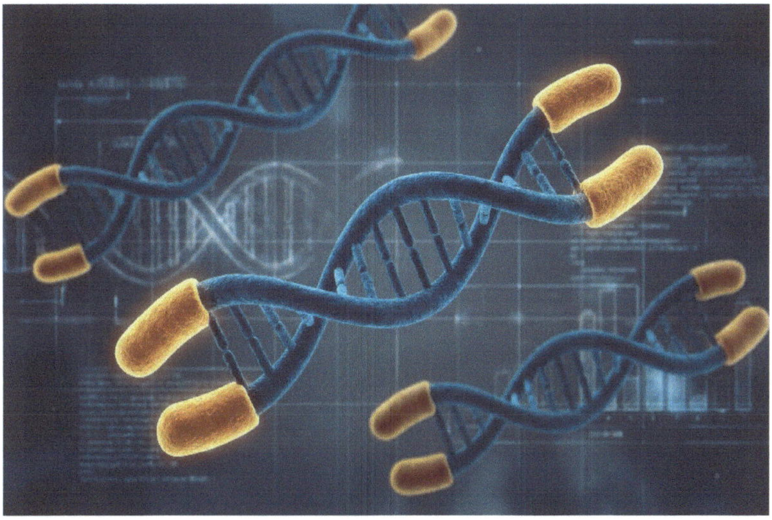

PART 6: GLYNAC (THE GLUTATHIONE SHIELD)

Aging is a collapse of endogenous antioxidant capacity.

- **GlyNAC Protocol:** The combination of Glycine and NAC removes the bottleneck for glutathione synthesis.
- **Apex Action:** Shuts down systemic inflammation and restores mitochondrial function to youthful levels.

PART 7: PROTEOSTASIS AND HEAT SHOCK PROTEINS (HSPs)

Aging is the accumulation of "protein garbage." **HSPs** straighten out misfolded proteins.

- **Apex Action:** The **Sauna** directly activates these proteins, preventing tissue degradation.

PART 8: SENOLYTICS (The Hunt for Zombie Cells)

- **The Concept:** Senescent (zombie) cells secrete inflammatory poisons (*SASP*).
- **Apex Action:** Use high doses of **fisetin** for 2 consecutive days, once a month, to "prune" these cells.

PART 9: THE MATHEMATICS OF RESILIENCE (HORMETIC CURVE)

We must define the "breaking point" to prevent biohacking from becoming a toxic stressor.

9.1 The Hormetic Safety Window

The law of hormesis follows an inverted U-shaped curve. Stress is only good if the system has the resources to respond.

THE RESILIENCE EQUATION

Resilience accumulated over time is the balance between hormetic insults and recovery capacity.

Safety Insight: If recovery is not greater than the stress applied (cold, fasting, sauna), the system enters accelerated entropy. Your job is to monitor that stress remains in the green window.

PART 10: ELITE DIAGNOSTICS (Biohacker Target)

Biomarker	Common Range	Elite Biohacker Target
C-Reactive Protein (hs-CRP)	< 3.0 mg/L	**< 0.5 mg/L**
Glycated Hemoglobin (HbA1c)	< 5.7	**4.8% - 5.2**
Homocysteine	< 15 µmol/L	**< 7 µmol/L**
Epigenetic age (GrimAge)	Chronological	**< Chronological (Delta -5/10 years)**

SAFETY OFFICER'S WORD

"Death is a technical failure. Aging is a communication error. Keep your NAD+ tank full, inhibit CD38, and train your mitochondrial dynamics with Zone 5. Don't be afraid of stress, but respect the mathematics of recovery. Time is a variable; your biology is the constant you can control."

✅ SAFETY CHECKLIST: CHAPTER 15

If you don't have 4 check marks, the software is unstable.

- [ ] **MITO-DYNAMICS:** Do you alternate Zone 5 sessions with deep rest (Fusion/Fission)?
- [ ] **MITOCHONDRIAL BIOGENESIS: Do you** supplement with PQQ and Urolithin A?
- [ ] **XENOHORMESIS:** Do you choose "stressed" vegetables for Sirtuins?
- [ ] **EPIGENETIC AUDIT:** Have you taken a GrimAge test to validate your methylation rate?
- [ ] **FACE AUDIT:** Do you use your smartphone to monitor lipofuscin spots?
- [ ] **SENOLYTIC FLUSH:** Do you follow the monthly fisetin protocol?

Security Status:

- 🔴 **RED:** Premature aging, loss of energy
- 🟢 **GREEN:** Slowed aging, more energy, and longer life

CHAPTER 16

ELITE DIAGNOSTICS & BIO-PRIVACY: THE HUMAN SYSTEM AUDIT

"Without data, you're just another person with an opinion. But beware: your DNA is the only password you can never change if it's hacked. Measurement is power, protecting the source code is survival."

In conventional ("curative") medicine, tests are only done when a symptom is felt or once a year for bureaucratic reasons. It's like waiting for black smoke to come out of the engine before checking the oil.

In **the Safety Officer's** view, this is a failed risk management strategy. We operate under a **Condition-Based Maintenance (CBM)** regime.

Your body leaves digital and biochemical traces every second. If you know how to read them, you can predict a critical failure years in advance.

But there is a *dark side*. Biological data is the new oil. Insurance companies, Big Pharma, and hackers don't want your money, they want your source code.

In this chapter, we will build an aerospace-grade **Control Dashboard**, shield your privacy, and create your **Digital Twin**.

PART 1: THE CYBER-BIOSECURITY PROTOCOL

Before taking a single drop of blood or saliva, we must secure the perimeter. Many "biohackers" send their DNA to foreign companies, unaware that they are giving away the most sensitive data they possess.

1.1 The Irreversibility Theorem

If your credit card is stolen, you block it. If your genome is stolen, **it is compromised forever**. You cannot change your DNA. You compromise your privacy and that of your descendants.

"GHOST" PROTOCOL: ANONYMOUS SEQUENCING

If you decide to sequence your DNA, strictly follow this procedure:

- **Burner Identity:** Never use your real name. Create a dedicated encrypted email account (e.g., ProtonMail) and use a pseudonym.
- **Ghost Payment:** Never use personal credit cards. Use anonymous prepaid cards or cryptocurrencies.
- **No Cloud Storage:** Request the *raw data*, download it to a local encrypted hard disk (cold storage), and request immediate deletion from the server.
- **Sample Destruction:** Flag the option for physical destruction of saliva after analysis.

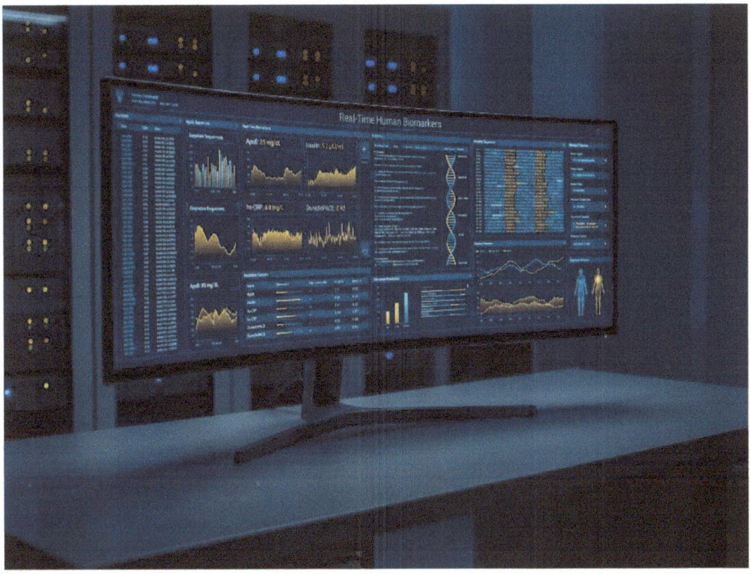

PART 2: BLOOD AUDIT DASHBOARD

The Safety Officer does not seek the average (mediocrity), but rather **the functional optimum**.

2.1 Cardiovascular Subsystem

- **ApoB (Apolipoprotein B):** Counts the *exact number* of atherogenic particles. Counting license plates is better than weighing cars (LDL). ***Safety Target:*** < 60 mg/dL.
- **Lp(a):** The "Silent Killer." Measure it **only once in your life**, because its levels in the blood are determined almost exclusively by your **genetics**.

Knowing this value allows the **Safety Officer** to immediately identify a genetic predisposition to cardiovascular events that would not respond to normal lifestyle changes, allowing the defense strategy to be customized from the outset.

2.2 Metabolic Subsystem

- **Fasting Insulin:** The true early warning sign. If your blood sugar is 90 but your insulin is >7 uIU/mL, you are in functional pre-diabetes.
- **HbA1c:** Average blood sugar over the last 3 months. ***Safety Target:*** < 5.0%.

2.3 Fire Alarm (Inflammation)

- **hs-CRP (High Sensitivity):** Detects low-grade inflammation burning the arteries. ***Target Safety:*** < 0.5 mg/L.

PART 3: HARDWARE vs SOFTWARE (GENETICS & EPIGENETICS)

3.1 Hardware: Fixed Bugs (SNPs)

- **MTHFR:** If you have the methylation bug, synthetic folic acid is toxic. Use only methylated folate.
- **APOE4:** Critical gene for Alzheimer's. If positive, avoid excess saturated fats.
- **COMT:** Neurotransmitter disposal speed. Defines stress resilience.

3.2 Software: The Aging Speedometer

- **DunedinPACE:** It doesn't tell you how old you are, but how fast you are aging *today*.
    - ***Value*** *< 0.8:* You are slowing down entropy.

3.3 Pharmacogenetics: Software Safety (ADR Prevention)

You cannot ignore individual variability in response to drugs.

- **The Concept (Cytochrome P450):** Over 50% of people have genetic variants in liver enzymes (CYP family). If you are a "Slow Metabolizer," a standard dose of a common statin or antidepressant can become toxic.
- **Apex Action:** Cytochrome P450 polymorphism testing. It is the final safety audit to avoid ADRs (Adverse Drug Reactions).

BIO-SAFETY: METABOLIC CLEARANCE

To add the final touch of scientific rigor, we define system clearance. The speed at which your system eliminates a substance (Cl) depends on your genetic profile. The safe dose (D safe) is a function of clearance and the administration interval (tau):

D safe = C target x Cl x tau

Without knowing your Cl coefficient (derived from the CYP450 test), any standard medical prescription is an unauthorized experiment on your biology.

C target (Target Concentration)

This value does not depend on you, but on the **molecule**.

- **Source:** It comes from pharmacological literature and "Gold Standard" clinical studies.
- **Meaning:** Represents the therapeutic window, i.e., the minimum concentration in the blood necessary to have the desired effect (e.g., DNA repair or mitochondrial activation) without exceeding the toxicity threshold.

Tau - Administration Interval

This is the variable of **chronobiology**.

- **Source:** It is determined by **the half-life (t1/2)** of the substance (how long it takes the body to halve its concentration).
- **The Meaning:** This is the time between doses (e.g., every 8 hours, every 24 hours, or once a week).
- **Apex Action:** For example, for Liposomal Vitamin C, tau is 24 hours thanks to Hydrogel technology, while for injectable BPC-157, tau is often 12 hours (twice a day) to keep the repair signal active.

PART 4: REAL-TIME TELEMETRY (CGM)

The **CGM (Continuous Glucose Monitor)** is a biomedical sensor that is applied to the arm for 14 days.

Bio-Individuality: Find out which "healthy" foods cause blood sugar spikes in *your* body. The goal is **Flat Glycemic Variability**.

PART 5: STRUCTURAL DIAGNOSTICS (IMAGING)

- **CAC SCAN (Calcium Score):** CT scan of the heart to see if there is calcium (plaque).

  Score 0 = Safe.

- **DEXA SCAN:** Maps visceral fat (VAT). Visceral fat is a toxic organ.

  Target: Zero.

PART 6: LIQUID BIOPSY (CANCER EARLY DETECTION)

Nowadays, waiting for a visible mass to diagnose a tumor is an engineering and medical failure.

The Concept: Cancer cells release fragments of DNA into the bloodstream (*cell-free DNA*) long before they form a mass. It's like finding a loose bolt on the track before the car breaks down.

Apex Action: Perform a **Multi-Cancer Early Detection** test every 12-24 months. It analyzes methylation patterns to detect over 50 types of cancer.

The probability of early detection increases dramatically.

PART 7: IMMUNO-BIOGRAPHY (THE AGE OF THE DEFENSE SYSTEM)

Methylation (DunedinPACE) tells us how much we run, but Immuno-Age tells us how much ammunition is left in the army.

The Concept (Naive vs. Memory T-Cells)

As we age, "naive" T cells (ready to fight new viruses) decline, and "memory" cells (specialized but old, senescent) increase.

Apex Action: Audit the **CD4/CD8** ratio and count **naive T cells**. This is the most accurate predictor of vulnerability to future pandemics or autoimmune diseases. A security system without a young army is a system destined to collapse.

PART 8: MICROBIOME FORENSICS (NON-HUMAN GENOME AUDIT)

You are only 43% human. The rest is bacteria.

The Test (Shotgun Sequencing)

Shotgun metagenomic sequencing is needed to map not only *who* lives in your gut, but *what metabolic functions* they perform.

Critical KPI: Akkermansia muciniphila

The guardian of the mucosal barrier. If it is low, you have *Leaky Gut* and toxins enter the bloodstream, triggering inflammation.

PART 9: ENVIRONMENTAL TOXICOLOGY (XENOBIOTIC AUDIT)

Heavy Metals: Mercury, Lead, Cadmium accumulate and block mitochondria.

Endocrine Disruptors: Measure phthalates and BPA. These compounds "hack" hormone receptors, rendering your testosterone useless.

Apex Action: If high, environmental remediation (air/water filters) is needed, not supplements.

PART 10: THE "DIGITAL TWIN" AND LOCAL AI

Your smartphone is not a phone, it is a biophysical laboratory and a neural computing center. It can help you see what may not be visible to the naked eye. Of course, you should then report your findings to your doctor.

10.1 Passive Sensors (Monitoring)

- **AI Pupillometry:** The camera monitors pupillary response (cognitive load and stress on the autonomic nervous system).
- **Voice Biomarkers:** AI analyzes voice jitter to detect neurological fatigue or pre-clinical depression.

10.2 The Digital Twin (Simulation)

Nowadays, uploading your data to an AI cloud is tactical suicide.

- **The Concept:** Smartphones have an NPU capable of running local language models (Local LLM).
- **Apex Action:** Do not send your raw data to external servers. Upload it to the local instance and create your **Digital Twin**: a simulation based on your historical data.
- **In Silico Testing:** Want to know what would happen to your ApoB if you switched to a carnivorous diet? Ask your Digital Twin. Crash test the simulation, not your skin.

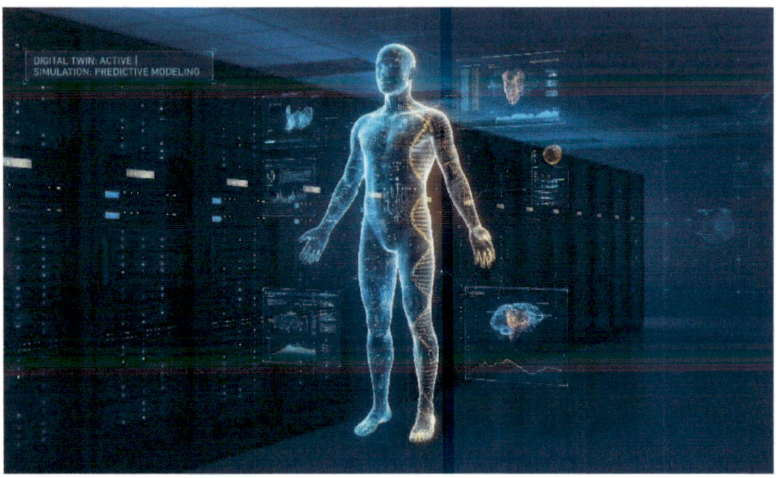

PART 11: BIO-ESTHESIA (DATA SYNCHRONIZATION)

Elite diagnostics fail if data remains isolated.

Safety Officer's Note: One isolated value is a point; three values are a trend. The power lies in the trend.

COMPARATIVE TABLE: STANDARD MEDICINE vs. ELITE BIOHACKING

Parameter	Standard Medicine	Elite Biohacking Implementation
Heart	Total Cholesterol	**ApoB** / Calcium Score (CAC)
Metabolism	Fasting Blood Sugar	**Insulin** / CGM / **Digital Twin Simulation**
Medications	Standard Dosage	**CYP450 Analysis** (Personalized Clearance)
Immunity	White Blood Cell Count	**Immuno-Biography** (Naive vs. Memory T-Cells)
Cancer	Diagnosis (Symptom)	**cfDNA Liquid Biopsy** (Prediction)
Intestine	"No pain"	**Shotgun sequencing** / Akkermansia

SAFETY OFFICER'S WORD

"The absence of evidence is not evidence of absence. Without data, you are just waiting for the impact. Hope is not a strategy. Measurement is the only way out."

✅ SAFETY CHECKLIST: CHAPTER 16

Total Neural Validation. If you don't have 4 check marks, the pilot is ineffective.

- [ ] **BIO-PRIVACY**: Have you encrypted the Raw Data in "Cold Storage" and are you using a Local LLM?
- [ ] **LIPIDS & HEART**: Do you know your ApoB value and have you scheduled a CAC scan?
- [ ] **PHARMACOGENETICS**: Have you mapped your CYP450 enzymes to avoid adverse reactions?
- [ ] **LIQUID BIOPSY**: Have you scheduled an MCED (cfDNA) test for early detection?
- [ ] **MICROBIOME**: Do you know your Akkermansia and bacterial diversity levels?
- [ ] **DIGITAL TWIN**: Have you integrated wearable and blood data into a local predictive model?

Security Status:

🔴 **RED:** Standard analysis, no genetic data, data in public cloud.

🟢 **GREEN:** Unified dashboard, active Digital Twin, protected DNA, known drug clearance.

CHAPTER 17

PEPTIDES AND BIOREGULATORS: SOURCE CODE INJECTION (SCRIPT INJECTION)

"Don't shout at the whole body with hormones. Whisper to the individual cell with peptides. The medicine of the future is not chemistry, it is information."

Until yesterday, if you wanted to repair an injury or improve your skin, you used systemic drugs that affected the *whole* body like a cluster bomb.

The **Safety Biohacker** rejects collateral damage. We seek **Molecular Surgical Precision**.

Welcome to the world of **Peptides**: short chains of amino acids (less than 50) that act as unlocking keys for specific functions. They add nothing foreign; they simply tell the body to do what it has stopped doing.

But be careful: we are manipulating growth factors and cellular metabolism. If you miss the target or get the dose wrong, the system crashes.

This chapter is a manual on **handling biological weapons**.

That's why, before taking peptides, it's essential to discuss it with and be monitored by a specialist doctor.

PART 1: HORMONES vs PEPTIDES (BROADCAST vs UNICAST)

To understand safety, you need to understand signal transmission.

- **Hormones (e.g., testosterone):** These are **broadcast** messages. You inject them, and they "shout" to all tissues (muscles, prostate, brain, heart). Powerful effects, but systemic risks.
- **Peptide (e.g., BPC-157):** This is a **unicast** message. It is an encrypted email sent only to the receptor responsible for repair.
  - ***Advantage:*** Zero impact on non-target organs.
  - ***Safety:*** Very short half-life (minutes/hours). It enters, delivers the message, and degrades into harmless amino acids.

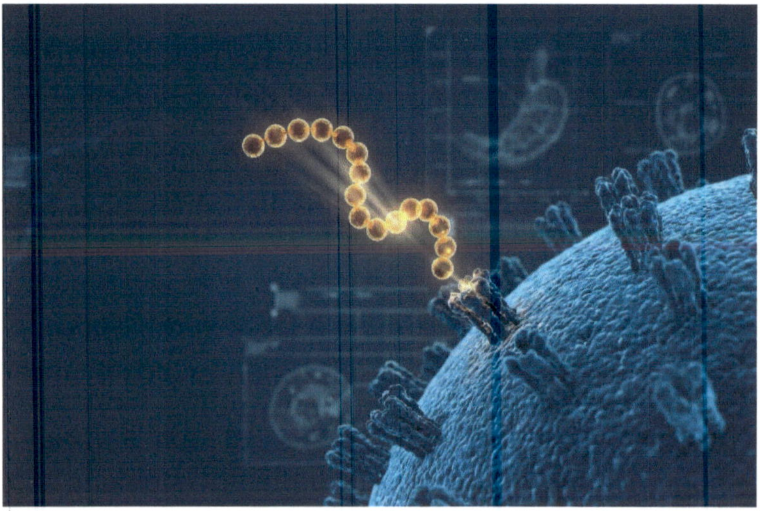

PART 2: THE REPAIR PROTOCOL (THE WOLVERINE STACK)

The first "Elite" use is accelerated recovery from structural damage.

2.1 BPC-157 (Body Protection Compound)

The "Master Builder." Signals angiogenesis (new blood vessels) and tendon repair.

- **Chemistry Matters: Arginate vs. Acetate.**

For a biohacker aiming for effectiveness, chemical form is everything. Many oral BPCs are destroyed by gastric juices if they are in "Acetate" form.

  - **Apex Action:** Specifies the use of **BPC-157 Arginate Salt**. It is the only form that is stable at room temperature and resistant to the acidic pH of the stomach, making oral absorption truly effective for treating the gut (Leaky Gut) and tissues.

2.2 TB-500 (Thymosin Beta-4)

The "Logistician." Regulates cellular actin, reduces inflammation, and prevents fibrous scarring.

- **Safety Warning (Oncology):** Because it stimulates angiogenesis and cell migration, it is **PROHIBITED** if you have a history of active cancer. You don't want to build highways for malignant cells.

PART 3: METABOLIC SYNERGIES & ORGAN SUPPORT

Peptides give the order, but the body must have the building blocks to execute it, the compass to navigate, and the energy to work.

3.1 The Builder Stack (Structure)

- **Order:** BPC-157 + TB-500.
- **Bricks:** Vitamin C + Hydrolyzed Collagen + Glycine.
- **The Compass (Mechanotransduction):** The master builder (BPC) needs to know *where* to go.
    - **Tactical Loading Protocol:** After injection, perform 10 minutes of **light isometric contractions** or mobility. This mechanical stress "calls" growth factors to the injury site via cellular biofeedback.

3.2 The Energy Stack (Mitochondria & Photons)

- **Order:** MOTS-c.
- **Activator:** Lactic Acid Exercise.
- **Photon Synergy (Module 8 Integration):** Peptides are the software, mitochondria are the energy. If the cell is depleted, the order is ignored.
    - **Apex Action (PBM Stacking):** Use **Red Light Therapy (660nm/850nm)** on the SubQ injection site or the area to be repaired 10 minutes after administration. The photons charge the

mitochondrial Cytochrome C Oxidase, providing the ATP needed to execute the repair script.

3.3 The Visceral "Security Patch" (Phase III Support)

Massive use of peptides puts pressure on disposal systems.

- **Apex Action:** Add **TUDCA** or **NAC** as a liver shield.
- **Monitoring:** Quarterly monitoring of **creatinine** and **eGFR** (renal filtration).

PART 4: RUSSIAN BIOREGULATORS (EPIGENETIC SWITCHES)

Prof. Khavinson discovered very short peptides (2-4 amino acids) that act on DNA.

- **Epitalon (Pineal):** Reactivates melatonin and telomeres.
- **Thymogen (Thymus):** Restores the immune army (T-cells).
- **Safety Action:** Used cyclically (e.g., 10 days every 6 months). Short and safe.

PART 5: MITOCHONDRIAL ENGINEERING & UPSTREAM HORMONES

5.1 MOTS-c & SS-31

- **MOTS-c:** Exercise mimetic. Increases insulin sensitivity.

- **SS-31:** Stabilizes mitochondrial cardiolipin. Repairs the powerhouse.

5.2 Kisspeptin-10 & PT-141

- **Kisspeptin:** Stimulates endogenous testosterone without atrophy.
- **PT-141:** Ignites central libido (brain). Beware of nausea.

PART 6: SENOLYTIC WARFARE (ZOMBIE CELL DETOX)

6.1 FOXO4-DRI

- **The Mechanism:** Breaks the FOXO4-p53 bond. The senescent "zombie" cell detects the damage and activates apoptosis.
- **Apex Action:** Short cycles for tissue "disinfestation."

PART 7: COSMETICS AND THE BRAIN (SKIN & BRAIN)

7.1 GHK-Cu (Copper)

Remodels the skin.

Safety: Supplement with zinc to balance.

7.2 Semax & Selank (Neuro)

- **Semax:** Focus and BDNF.

- **Selank:** Non-sedative anxiolytic.

PART 8: METABOLIC OVERCLOCK (GLP-1 SAFETY)

Semaglutide/Tirzepatide.

Sarcopenia risk: Muscle loss due to calorie deficit.

Safety rule: Double protein and weights.

PART 9: DOSAGE ARCHITECTURE AND HANDLING

Peptides are fragile. Incorrect handling turns them into expensive water.

The Cold Chain, Light, and Fibrillation

- **Temperature:** Refrigerator (43.2–46.4°F). Do not shake.
- **Light:** Peptides are sensitive to photolysis. Use **amber glass** and work away from direct light.
- **The Fibrillation Phenomenon (The Visual Audit):** In addition to photolysis, peptides are susceptible to aggregation. Vibration or temperature changes can transform the peptide into useless and immunogenic clumps.
    - **Apex Action:** Before each injection, check the vial with a flashlight. The solution should be crystal clear. If you notice a slight "fog effect" (**Tyndall Effect**) or filaments, the code is corrupted. Do not inject.

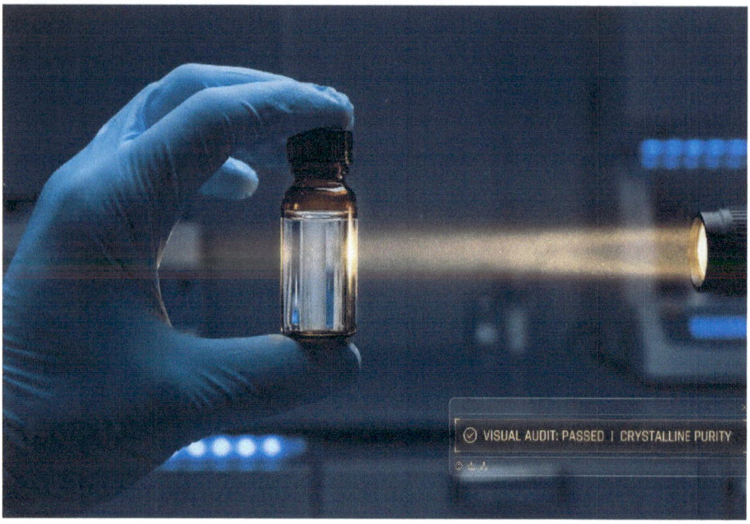

PART 10: BIOENGINEERING OF THE RECEPTOR RESPONSE (ARRESTIN)

The intensity of the biological response is proportional to the binding affinity and density of the receptors. Under chronic stimulation, the system activates **arrestin**, which internalizes the receptor, rendering the injection completely ineffective.

PART 11: RESCUE PROTOCOL (OFF-TARGET MANAGEMENT)

A Safety Officer must always have an emergency plan for adverse reactions.

Apex Action (Rescue Stack):

1. **H1/H2 Antihistamines:** Keep on hand for localized redness (common with GHK-Cu).

2. **Complex sugars:** If you use MOTS-c, monitor your blood sugar. A sudden drop can be managed with slow-release carbohydrates.
3. **BPC Anhedonia:** In rare cases, BPC-157 can "flatten" dopamine. If you feel emotionally detached, stop the cycle immediately: your **HRV Audit** will alert you before you consciously notice it.

PART 12: THE LEGAL AND ETHICAL FIREWALL

12.1 Forensic Sourcing (HPLC Audit)

Do not trust the PDF certificate. Use your smartphone and Local LLM to analyze HPLC peaks. Look for anomalies in the baseline.

- **Transparency:** Only use substances labeled for research. Take responsibility for the supply chain.

PART 13: INTRANASAL DELIVERY (THE BRAIN BYPASS)

Not all peptides need to be injected. The nasal route bypasses the blood-brain barrier.

13 Nasal Efficiency

- **High:** Semax, Selank, Oxytocin, PT-141.
- **Low:** BPC-157, TB-500.

SAFETY OFFICER'S WORD

"Peptides are not supplements, they are code. You are not giving bricks, you are giving orders to the foreman.

If the order is wrong, the site is empty, or the software is corrupt, you're going to build a disaster.

Respect the molecule. Respect sterility. Start with the minimum effective dose. We're not here to bulk up, we're here to last."

✅ SAFETY CHECKLIST: CHAPTER 17

Procedural Validation. Without sterility, there is no biohacking, there is infection. If you don't have 5 check marks, you are in danger.

- [ ] **VISUAL AUDIT:** Have you done the flashlight (Tyndall) test to rule out fibrillation?
- [ ] **STABILITY:** BPC-157 Arginate (oral) and Amber Glass (light)?
- [ ] **SYNERGY:** PBM (Red Light) post-injection and Mechanotransduction (Iso)?
- [ ] **VISCERAL SHIELD:** TUDCA/NAC active and creatinine monitored?
- [ ] **GEOMETRY:** 29-31G SubQ needles and calibrated MDNS spray?
- [ ] **SATURATION:** Active 5/2 Protocol (Arrestin Law)?
- [ ] **RESCUE READY:** Do you have antihistamines and sugars ready in case of a reaction?

Safety Status:

🔴 **RED:** Purchase from dubious sites, cloudy solution, exposure to light, reused needles.

🟢 **GREEN:** AI-validated sourcing, visual audit OK, PBM active, TUDCA present, rescue kit ready.

CHAPTER 18

BIO-HARMONY & SOCIAL EPIGENETICS: THE HUMAN NETWORK (THE HUMAN LAN)

"You can have the perfect diet and optimized sleep, but if you come home to a toxic environment, your cortisol will wipe out any progress. Bio-security doesn't end at your skin; it extends to your pack."

In the world of Safety Biohacking, we tend to view the body as a fortress to be defended. But evolutionary biology teaches us an uncomfortable truth: Homo sapiens is a compulsory herd animal.

Our autonomic nervous system not only regulates itself from within (**self-regulation**), but also constantly synchronizes with others (**co-regulation**).

If you live with an anxious partner, your heartbeats will synchronize upwards. If your work environment is hostile, your digestion will shut down (gut-brain axis) regardless of how many probiotics you take.

This chapter is not about "being nice." It's about **Shared Neural Network Engineering**. It's about how your biological state affects your family (Social Epigenetics) and how to protect yourself from "emotional contagion."

PART 1: THE PHYSICS OF CONNECTION (BIOLOGICAL WI-FI)

Your heart doesn't just pump blood; it generates a measurable electromagnetic field up to 1-2 meters away from your body.

According to studies by **the HeartMath Institute**, this field transmits information about your emotional state.

1.1 Neuroception (The Invisible Radar)

Dr. Stephen Porges (Polyvagal Theory) coined the term "neuroception."

It is the ability of your nervous system to scan the environment to detect "Safety" or "Danger" before your conscious brain notices it.

- **The Risk:** If you enter your home feeling stressed, your "field" transmits an alarm signal. Your wife, husband, and children will pick up on this and go into a state of alert (sympathetic tone).

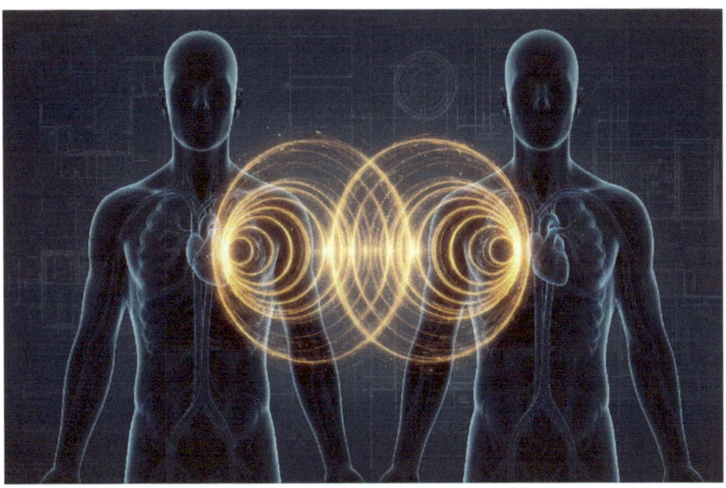

1.2 Bio-Safety: The Shared Coherence Coefficient (LaTeX)

The emotional stability of an environment (Sa) is proportional to the cardiac coherence of the dominant subject (Cleader) mediated by physical distance (d):

Sa = (Cleader x alpha)/d^2

Where alpha is the herd's receptivity coefficient.

- **Safety Action:** Safety is a function of distance and stability. Before crossing the threshold, perform a "Server Reset" to raise your Cleader and positively saturate the environment.

PART 2: THE PARADOX OF ORTHOREXIA (WHEN BIOHACKING BECOMES TOXIC)

As a Safety Officer, I see many Biohacker "colleagues" obsessed with avoiding toxins to the point of becoming toxic to those around them.

2.1 The Social Cost of Rigidity

The Mathematics of Damage:

Often, the inflammatory damage caused by relational stress exceeds the chemical damage of a pizza.

- **Apex Action:** The 80/20 rule. When you're alone, be a ruthless Safety Officer. When you're in a group, be a human being.

PART 3: CO-REGULATION (BEING THE STABLE SERVER)

Leadership in the family is not about giving orders. It is about modulating energy.

3.1 The Anchor Technique

You are the stable server that unstable clients connect to.

1. **Slow down your breathing:** < 6 breaths/min.
2. **Relax your jaw/shoulders:** Signal that the "all clear" has been given.
3. **Result:** Limbic resonance. The other person's heartbeat slows down to synchronize with yours.

3.2 Bio-Security: Entrainment Index

The speed at which an unstable system synchronizes with a stable one (Vsync) is a function of the strength of the coherence signal (Cl) and structural empathy (epsilon).

- **Safety Insight:** The deeper and more regular your breathing, the faster the "client" (child/partner) will download your state of calm. There is no need to speak; you need to emit coherence.

3.3 Bio-Mechanics of Listening (Vagus Nerve)

The muscles of the middle ear are innervated by the vagus nerve. Under stress, they relax to pick up predators (low frequency) and filter out the human voice.

- **Insight:** If you shout, the other person physically stops "hearing" the words and only hears a threat. Use low, melodic tones (prosody) to reactivate listening.

PART 4: MIRROR NEURONS AND NETWORK LATENCY

Your internal state is not private. It is open source.

4.1 Vocal Synchrony and Facial Feedback (The Soft Face Audit)

The facial muscles are connected to the cranial nerves that regulate the heart and lungs. If your face is "frozen," you convey a system error.

- **Apex Action:** Check the muscles around your eyes (orbicularis). Consciously relax them. This is the biometric signal for "Server Secure."

4.2 The Synchrony Signal: "Micro-Mimicry"

In relationships, synchrony occurs through involuntary micro-imitation (blinking, posture). If there is a delay (because you are distracted), the other person's nervous system detects a "lag" and activates danger neuroception.

- **Apex Action ("Zero Latency"):** During a critical conversation, subtly mimic the other person's posture. This is not manipulation; it is actively lowering the other person's defensive firewall to allow for an emotional software update.

PART 5: OXYTOCIN PROTOCOL & C-TACTILE FIBERS

Oxytocin isn't just cuddles. It's survival biochemistry.

5.1 C-Tactile Fibers (The Fiber Optics of the Nervous System)

There are receptors in the skin tuned to a specific speed (1-10 cm per second) that transmit the "social value" of touch.

- **Apex Action ("Care-Loading"):** Touch must not only be strong (hugging); it must be **slow**. Rubbing the back at this precise speed is the "root" command for resetting the amygdala.

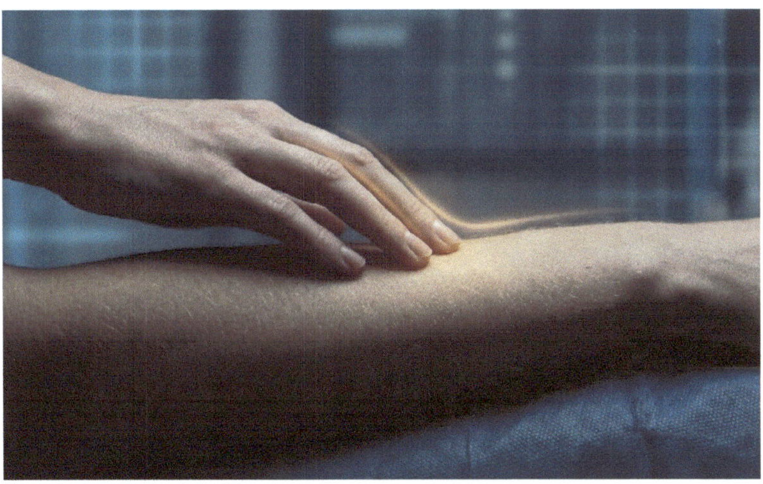

5.2 The 20-Second Rule

A hug lasting >20 seconds raises oxytocin and lowers blood pressure.

PART 6: BIOARCHITECTURE AND CIRCADIAN ENTRAINMENT

6.1 Circadian Synchronization (Entrainment)

If one family member uses blue lights at midnight, it resets everyone else's clock.

- **Apex Action ("Circadian Entrainment"):** The "Server" (you) must drag the "Clients" toward the same temporal efficiency (lights, meal times) to avoid domestic jet lag.

6.2 Lighting Design

At dinner, use only low, warm lighting (< 2700K). Avoid ceiling lights (skull/threat effect).

PART 7: SOCIAL EPIGENETICS (BIOLOGICAL INHERITANCE)

7.1 Intergenerational Trauma

Parental stress alters DNA methylation, predisposing children to anxiety.

- **Apex Action:** A calm father "programs" the stress receptors in his child's brain to be more efficient.

PART 8: CHEMOSIGNALS (THE OLFACTORY INTERNET)

8.1 Stress Sweat

Stress sweat contains alarm molecules. Avoid synthetic perfumes that mask the signal. Seek real cleanliness.

PART 9: CRISIS MANAGEMENT & SOCIAL BUFFER

9.1 The Social Pain Matrix (ACC Bypass)

Social pain activates the **Anterior Cingulate Cortex (ACC)**, the same area as physical pain. Treat verbal conflict as inflammation.

9.2 Bio-Security: The Flooding Index

When heart rate (HR) exceeds the critical threshold (HRcrit approximately 100 BPM), communication efficiency (Ec) declines according to an inverse logistic function.

- **Safety Insight:** Above this threshold, the prefrontal "processor" is isolated from the system. **Time-out** is not an option: it is a protocol necessity to avoid data corruption.

9.3 The "Social Buffer": The Gottman Ratio

Stability (Ks) = Positive Inputs / Negative Inputs.

- **Target Safety: 5:1** ratio.

- **Apex Action ("Positive Loading"):** Engineer 5 micro-moments of connection for every single negative feedback.

PART 10: SYSTEM MAINTENANCE & RESILIENCE

In every LAN, packets are lost. Resilience is not about avoiding error, but about repairing it quickly.

10.1 The System Restore Point Protocol

If a conflict is not repaired within 24 hours, the "Danger" signal is stored in long-term memory, creating a permanent "bug."

- **Apex Action (The Repair Script):** Apply the quick repair protocol. Recognizing the error is not submission, it is a command to clear the stress cache (Cortisol) before it becomes chronic.

10.2 The "Play" State: The Natural Antivirus

Dr. Porges identifies "Play" as the perfect combination of sympathetic activation (energy) and ventral vagal (safety).

- **Apex Action:** Engineer moments of unstructured "Social Play." Laughing together or playfully wrestling is how the pack performs a **Stress Test** on the network, increasing emotional bandwidth.

PART 11: FAMILY OPERATING SYSTEM (FamOS)

11.1 Sync Meeting & Phubbing Audit

- **Meeting:** Sunday evening (Retrospective + Logistics).
- **Digital Firewall:** Phubbing (ignoring someone to look at your phone) activates the other person's ACC.
    - **Apex Action (NPU Integration):** Use your smartphone's AI to monitor your screen time. If you look at the display while your heart rate indicates "sociality," the **"Network Intrusion"** alert should trigger.

PART 12: NVC - THE DATA TRANSMISSION PROTOCOL

If neurotransmitters are the signal, words are the packet format. Most conversations fail because data is sent as "Judgment" (Malware), which activates the firewall (Amygdala).

12.1 Action Apex (Data Packet Formatting)

Send data following the **OSRN** protocol:

1. Observation: Pure data, zero opinions ("I see socks on the floor," not "You're messy").
2. Sentiment: Internal state of the server ("I feel frustrated").
3. Requirement/Need: System requirement ("I need order").
4. Norm/Request: Specific, actionable command ("Can you put them in the hamper?").

- **Result:** The packet bypasses the defense and is processed by the other's prefrontal cortex.

PART 13: TOXICOLOGY AUDIT & MOAI

13.1 Energy Vampires & Moai Protocol

- **Identify/Isolate/Eliminate:** Remove toxic contacts.
- **Moai:** Create your external "Safety Team" (2-3 people). Share HRV data. Loneliness is inflammatory.

TECHNICAL BOX: (THE SOCIAL FIREWALL)

1. Voice Jitter Analysis

Analyze voice jitter to detect hidden stress. If out of range, do not negotiate; you can use your smartphone to do this.

2. Environmental Mirroring (Forensic Home Automation)

Use your smartphone's light sensors and microphone to map the "toxicity" of the room.

- **Apex Action:** If it detects excessive white noise or lights >6000K during dinner time, it activates an automatic routine that sets the lights to amber tones and lowers the volume of the devices. You are the architect, your phone is your environmental sensor.

SAFETY OFFICER'S WORD

"No man is a biological island. You can build the safest bunker in the world, but if you lock yourself inside, you will die sooner than those who live outside in community.

Bio-Harmony is the ultimate safety net. Build relationships that nourish your nervous system, not drain it. Be the pillar of calm for your family. Because in the end, longevity is useless if you have no one to share it with."

✅ SAFETY CHECKLIST: CHAPTER 18

Social Validation. Is your network safe or under attack? If you have less than 5 green check marks, you are not safe.

- [ ] **ENTRY RESET:** Do you perform a "Soft Face Audit" and breathe before entering?
- [ ] **RULE 80/20:** Do you avoid social orthorexic toxicity?
- [ ] **CARE-LOADING:** Do you use slow touch (1-10 cm/s) for C-Tactile Fibers?
- [ ] **FLOODING:** Do you apply Time-Out above 100 BPM (Flooding Equation)?
- [ ] **RESTORE POINT:** Do you resolve conflicts within 24 hours?
- [ ] **PLAY STATE:** Do you engineer moments of unstructured play for the pack?
- [ ] **MOAI:** Do you have an external support team?

Security Status:

🔴 **RED:** Shouting arguments, stiff face, phubbing, isolation, judgmental communication (malware).

🟢 **GREEN:** Soft Face active, Family OS installed, frequent Care-Loading, OSRN active, regular Play State.

PART 5: CLINICAL FRONTIERS (EXTRA-SAFETY)

Beyond Lifestyle: Heavy Engineering and Crisis Management.

THE BREAKING POINT OF DIY BIOHACKING

As **Safety Officer**, I must confront you with a brutal engineering reality: **Routine Maintenance cannot repair critical structural damage.**

- Eating blueberries will not rebuild knee cartilage that no longer exists ("bone on bone").
- Sleeping 8 hours will not remove the calcified plaque that has formed in your coronary arteries over the last 20 years.
- Meditating will not stop an arterial hemorrhage or a heart attack in progress.

WELCOME TO THE RED ZONE (CLINICAL GRADE)

This section, **Clinical Frontiers**, marks the transition from "Soft Biohacking" to "Hard Biohacking."

Here we stop whispering to cells and start operating on hardware with industrial tools.

In this part, we will explore two opposing but complementary concepts:

1. **Reconstruction (Chapter 19):** When a component is worn out, we don't polish it.

   We replace or regenerate it.

   We will talk about Stem Cells, Exosomes, and blood washing (Apheresis). It is the science of turning back the biological clock, not just slowing it down.

2. **Acute Resilience (Chapter 20):** The Safety Biohacker doesn't just plan for 100 years of longevity; he plans how to survive the next 10 minutes.

   We will talk about "Crisis Management": what to do (and what to have in your backpack) when the system suddenly crashes.

SAFETY WARNING

The strategies described in this section require:

- **High Budgets:** We are not talking about $20 supplements, but therapies costing thousands of dollars.
- **Mandatory Medical Supervision:** You cannot act alone here.

  Your role changes: from "Operator" you become "Project Manager" leading a team of medical specialists.

- **Risk Management:** Clinical intervention involves risks (infections, adverse reactions).

  Bio-security here means choosing the right clinic, the right protocol, and always having a backup plan.

Wear higher-level PPE. Let's enter the heavy laboratory.

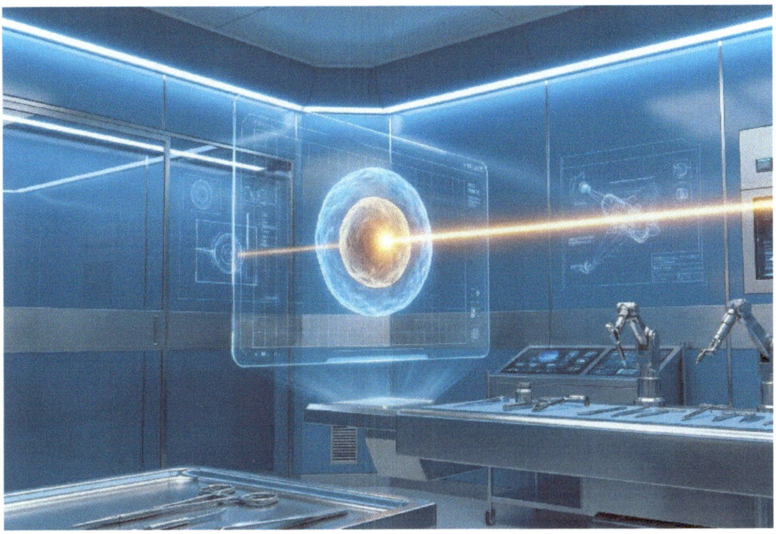

CHAPTER 19

REGENERATIVE MEDICINE: THE ENGINE OVERHAUL (HARDWARE OVERHAUL)

"Nutrition and sleep are routine maintenance. Regenerative medicine is when you take your car to the shop, take out the engine, and replace the worn parts. You can't repair structural damage just by eating blueberries."

There is an insurmountable biological limit: **Structural Damage**.

When cartilage is worn away ("bone on bone"), when neurons are dead, when the heart has scar tissue, lifestyle changes are no longer enough.

As a Safety Officer, I have to be brutal: biology has a point of no return.

Regenerative Medicine is the art of hacking that point, introducing "young" biological material or mechanically filtering the blood to turn back the clock.

We are not talking about science fiction, but about clinical therapies that require high budgets and, above all, a **Class 4 Bio-** . Here, the risk is not "it doesn't work," the risk is "infection," "rejection," or "tumor proliferation."

PART 1: REMEDIATION OF THE "NICHE" (PRE-REGEN AUDIT)

Before introducing new cells, you must remediate the terrain.

The Concept (SASP): Senescent cells (the "zombie cells" from Chapter 15) emit **SASP**, a toxic inflammatory fog. If you inject "master builders" (young stem cells) into a toxic construction site, the new cells die or become corrupted.

- **Apex Action ("Senolytic Clearing"):** A cycle of senolytics (**Fisetin** or **Dasatinib + Quercetin**) is mandatory 2 weeks before any regenerative procedure. You must make physical and chemical space in the stem cell "niche."

PART 2: KLOTHO (THE MANAGER OF YOUTH)

If stem cells are the workers, the **Klotho** protein is the project manager.

- **Apex Action:** Monitor soluble Klotho levels. If they are low, the effectiveness of stem cells will be halved. Optimize with intense exercise and precursors before therapy.

PART 3: STEM CELLS (THE GENERAL CONTRACTORS)

Stem cells act as paracrine signalers: they release growth factors that instruct *your* cells to repair themselves.

3.1 Autologous vs. Allogeneic

- **Autologous (Yours):** Safe, but limited by your age (short telomeres).
- **Allogeneic (Wharton's Jelly):** From the umbilical cord. They have "Day 0" age. They are turbo-charged and immune-privileged. **Elite Standard**.

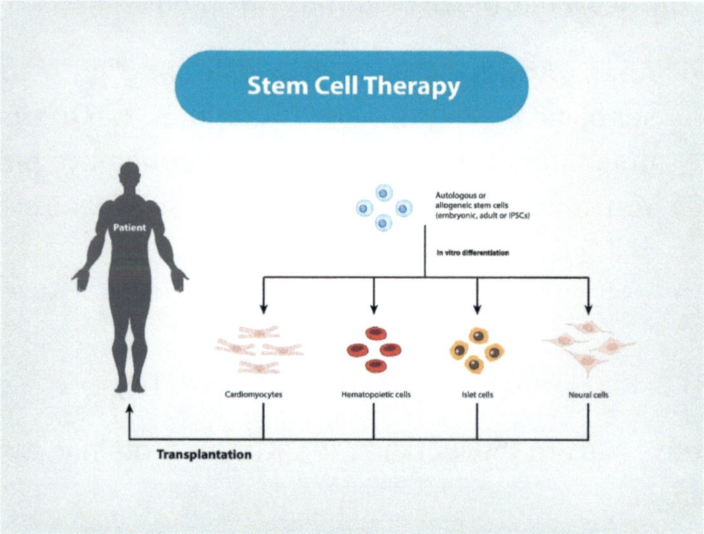

3.2 Laboratory Quality Audit (GMP Standard)

As a Safety Officer, I tell you that cell count is nothing without process purity.

- **Apex Action (GMP Standard):** Demand cells produced in **GMP (Good Manufacturing Practice)** certified laboratories.
- **Forensic Procedure:** Request the **Karyotype** report. This serves to confirm that the expanded cells have not developed chromosomal abnormalities (potentially carcinogenic) during duplication.

3.3 The Scaffold (Bio-Scaffolding & Hydrogels)

Stem cells in areas of high mechanical stress (knees) need a home.

- **Apex Action (Hydrogel Stacking):** The elite do not just inject cells, but cells suspended in **biocompatible hydrogels** or **fibrin glue**. These substances create a temporary 3D scaffold that protects the cells and keeps them *in place*, preventing them from being dispersed by the synovial fluid.

PART 4: VSELs (THE DORMANT RESERVE)

4.1 NIR Priming

VSELs (tiny stem cells in the blood) are dormant.

- **Apex Action:** Clinical protocols use **NIR lasers (810nm)** or thermal shocks to "wake them up" and provide the necessary ATP before re-infusion.

PART 5: EXOSOMES & SECRETOME (THE SIGNAL)

Stem cells are large. **Exosomes** are the stealth solution (nanoparticles of pure signal).

5.1 Technical Box: The Secret of the "Secretome"

The Secretome is the "broth" where stem cells are grown, rich in cytokines.

- **Apex Action:** In cases of rapid repair, infusion of the Secretome avoids the "lung trap."

5.2 Selection of the "Cargo" (Exosomal Tissue-Specificity)

Today, exosomes are no longer generic.

- **Apex Action:**
    - For **Structural Damage** (knee/shoulder): Require exosomes derived from **bone marrow MSCs**.
    - For **Cognitive Decline**: Look for **BDNF-loaded** exosomes derived from neural stem cells.

PART 6: MITOCHONDRIAL REFRESH (THE ULTIMATE UPGRADE)

If stem cells are the new workers, mitochondria are the batteries they carry with them.

6.1 The Concept (Mitochondrial Transfer)

An elite frontier of our times. It is not about injecting cells, but about injecting **young, healthy mitochondria** isolated from hyper-efficient donor cells.

- **Apex Action:** Insert the infusion of exogenous mitochondria as a final "Power-Up" for the tissues with the highest energy consumption (**Heart and Brain**), where damage is often mitochondrial before it is cellular.

PART 7: NAVIGATIONAL ENGINEERING (HOMING)

7.1 Lung Trap & SDF-1

70% of stem cells stop in the lungs.

- **Apex Action (The Beacon):** Before injection, use **PEMF** or **Shock Waves** on the target area. This releases **SDF-1**, which guides circulating cells where they are needed.

7.2 The Dynamics of Vascular "Gates" (NO-Stacking)

Stem cells travel in the blood. If the "highways" (capillaries) are blocked, your investment gets stuck in traffic. Bioavailability depends on Nitric Oxide (NO).

- **Apex Action:** 30 minutes before intravenous infusion, use nitric oxide precursors (**beet nitrates** or **L-citrulline**) and ensure hyper-electrolyte hydration. You must "open the vascular gates."

PART 8: APHERESIS & TPE (THE OIL CHANGE)

Therapeutic Plasma Exchange (TPE)

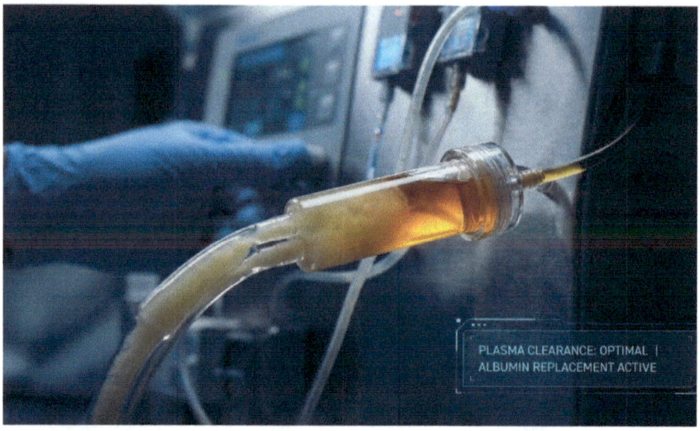

Remove old ("dirty") plasma and replace it with clean albumin. Dilute your biological age.

PART 9: PRP & PRF (BASIC CLINICAL BIOHACKING)

9.1 PRF > PRP

Use **Fibrin (PRF)** for slow release (7-10 days) instead of the immediate burst of plasma. Essential for joints.

PART 10: HYPERBARIC OXYGEN (HBOT)

10.1 Henry's Law

At **>2.0 ATA** (Hard Chamber), oxygen dissolves into plasma, regenerating hypoxic tissues.

PART 11: THE POST-OP PROTOCOL (THE NURSERY)

You have invested $15k. The next 7 days and the next 6 months will determine your ROI.

11.1 Absolute Prohibitions

- **NO NSAIDs:** Turning off acute inflammation means turning off the signal.
- **NO ALCOHOL:** Poison for newborn cells.

11.2 Peptide Synergy (Peptide Priming)

Use **BPC-157** and **TB-500** in the 15 days post-infusion to accelerate angiogenesis.

11.3 Technical Box: Clock Validation

Apex Action: Perform a **DunedinPACE** test 6 months after the regenerative procedure. If the protocol has worked, you will see not only a decline in static biological age (Horvath), but a drastic deceleration in the current rate of aging. This is the ultimate **KPI (Key Performance Indicator)** of your investment.

PART 12: THE ONCOLOGY SAFETY & BIO-PRIVACY CHECKLIST

Growth factors nourish everything, even tumors. And your data is sensitive.

12.1 Safety Protocol: The "Cancer Screen"

Before injecting growth factors:

1. **Complete Tumor Markers.**

2. **Liquid Biopsy (cfDNA):** Exclude circulating tumor DNA.
3. **Whole Body Resonance.**

12.2 Genomic Encryption (Karyotype Privacy)

Karyotype reports and sequencing generate the most sensitive data of your existence.

- **The Risk:** Many laboratories store your genetic profile on vulnerable clouds. If that data is hacked, your "biological password" is compromised forever.
- **Apex Action:** Demand that the laboratory destroy the physical samples after sequencing and deliver the raw data to you exclusively on **encrypted physical media** (offline hard drive). Your regeneration should not become a database for Big Pharma.

SAFETY OFFICER'S WORD

"Regenerative medicine is the last line of defense. It is expensive, invasive, and powerful.

These therapies only work if the 'terrain' is clean. If you inject young cells into an inflamed body, they will die.

First clean up (senolysis), open the gates (NO-stacking), then repair (stem cells + mitochondria), and finally protect the data (privacy). Respect the order of operations. Don't put the turbo on a seized engine."

CHAPTER 20

CRISIS MANAGEMENT & RESILIENCE: THE TACTICAL 'SAFETY KIT'

"Resilience is not how hard you can hit, but how quickly you can restart the system after taking a hit. In an emergency, you don't rise to the level of your expectations; you fall to the level of your training (and your equipment)."

The world is chaotic. Entropy constantly seeks to disrupt your biology.

While the previous chapters were devoted to long-term health, this chapter is devoted to managing the **next 10 minutes**.

When the ambulance is far away, or when you have to perform despite a physiological breakdown, you need tools that work immediately. Not supplements that work in 3 months. Medications and tech that work in 3 minutes.

PART 1: THE CONCEPT OF "BIO-EDC" (EVERYDAY CARRY)

EDC is what you carry in your pockets every day. Bio-EDC is what keeps you alive or functional when you are away from your "safe base."

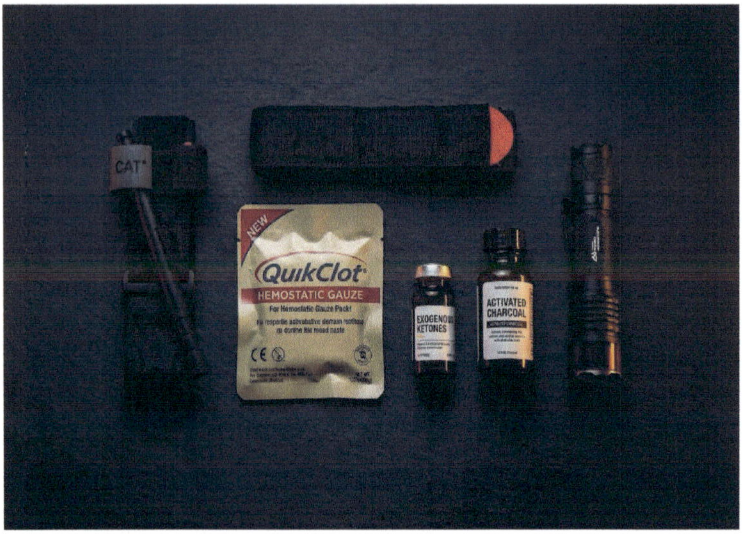

1.1 The "Digestive Rescue" Module

If you eat something toxic, you have about 30 minutes before it enters your bloodstream.

- **Activated Vegetable Charcoal:** The "Undo button." It binds to toxins, preventing their absorption.
- **High-Dose Proteolytic Enzymes:** To quickly "digest" inflammatory proteins (e.g., accidental gluten).

1.2 The "Energy Crash" & Cognitive Fuel Module

A sudden hypoglycemic drop can cause fainting, but adrenaline burns glycogen so quickly that sugar is sometimes not enough.

- **Dextrose/Liquid Glucose:** Simple sublingual sugar for immediate hypoglycemic shock.

- **Cognitive Emergency Fuel (Exogenous Ketones):** Adrenaline depletes sugar reserves. When they run out, the brain shuts down ("bonking").
    - *Apex Action:* Insert a bottle of **Ketone Esters or Salts**. They are the only fuel that bypasses the metabolic block caused by stress, providing energy to the brain in 15 minutes regardless of glucose. It is the emergency "Battery Pack" for your CPU.
- **Electrolyte Sticks (LMNT):** For rapid rehydration.

1.3 Forensic Bio-Hydration (Purification Module)

In the survival equation, water is the universal solvent. In a crisis, "clear" water is not "safe" water.

- **The Risk:** Metals, PFAS, or pathogens (Cholera/Giardia) can corrupt hardware in hours.
- **Apex Action (Purification Kit):**
    1. **Chlorine Dioxide Tablets:** More stable and broad-spectrum than iodine. Kills viruses and bacteria without excessive chemical taste.
    2. **Straw Filter (Activated Carbon):** For drinking directly from questionable sources by filtering out metals and particulates.

PART 2: THE PHARMACOLOGICAL & NOOTROPIC AIRBAG

Warning: Powerful molecules should *only* be used in cases of critical system failure and under medical supervision.

2.1 Adrenaline Blocker (Propranolol)

If you have to perform a task requiring surgical precision under stress, adrenaline causes tremors.

- **The Hack:** Beta blockers (micro-dose) block the physical receptors of adrenaline. Calm heart, steady hand, clear mind.

2.2 The "Panic Kill Switch"

- **Respiratory Action:** Box Breathing (4-4-4-4).
- **Chemical Action (Extreme Measure):** Micro-dose of sublingual benzodiazepine. Use only if collapse is imminent.

2.3 Sustained Ops ("No-Sleep" Protocol)

In a prolonged crisis (evacuation, forced night driving), sleep is not an option.

- **Modafinil (Provigil):** Military eugeroic. Maintains operational wakefulness for 12+ hours without the "jitter" of caffeine.
- **Tactical Nicotine (Gum/Spray):** 1-2mg for immediate cognitive boost. Enhances acetylcholine. ***Safety:*** Highly addictive, use only in crisis.

PART 3: TRAUMA MODULE (MARCH PROTOCOL)

A band-aid is not a medical kit. A biohacker uses the military **MARCH** protocol (Massive hemorrhage, Airway, Respiration, Circulation, Hypothermia).

3.1 Massive Hemorrhage (Stop The Bleed)

- **Tourniquet (CAT Gen 7):** Learn how to apply it in <30 seconds. Blocks arterial flow to limbs.
- **Hemostatic Gauze (QuikClot/Celox):** Coagulates blood on contact.

3.2 Airway & Respiration (Do not suffocate)

- **NPA (Nasopharyngeal Cannula):** Soft nasal tube to keep the airway open in unconscious patients.
- **Chest Seals (HyFin Vent):** Valved adhesive patches for chest wounds. Prevents tension pneumothorax.

3.3 Shock Management (Volume & Temp)

The silent killer in trauma is temperature collapse (Triad of Death: Acidosis, Coagulopathy, Hypothermia).

- **Bio-Safety: Coagulopathy Index (LaTeX):** The blood's ability to clot declines if temperature and pH drop.
- **Safety Insight:** If you do not thermally isolate the injured person, your work with hemostatic gauze will be useless. Cold disables coagulation enzymes. Warming is healing.

- **Apex Action (Space Blanket):** A high-quality isothermal blanket. Insulate the hardware immediately.

PART 4: CBRN & ENVIRONMENTAL DEFENSE

Chemical, Biological, Radiological, and Nuclear Protection.

4.1 Fire & Smoke (The Silent Killer)

In a fire, smoke and CO kill before flames.

- **Smoke Hood (iEvac):** Hood mask with catalytic filters. Gives you 15-20 minutes of breathable air.

4.2 Burn and Thermal Injury Management

Burns are the second fastest killer, causing shock due to fluid loss.

- **Apex Action (Hydrogel Module):** Insert **hydrogel** dressings (e.g., BurnFree/BurnShield) into the Trauma Module. They cool instantly without water (which could be contaminated) and stop the progression of heat into deep tissues.

4.3 Viral Defense

- **Iodine/Xylitol Nasal Spray:** Disinfects the viral entry point.
- **Shock D3:** 50,000 IU of Vitamin D3 at the first symptom.

4.4 The "Radiation & Tox" Module (CBRN Specialist)

- **Potassium Iodide (KI):** Saturates the thyroid, preventing the absorption of environmental radioactive iodine.
- **Methylene Blue (USP Grade):** The "Swiss Army knife." Antidote for metabolic poisons and mitochondrial booster in hypoxia.

PART 5: NEURO-RESILIENCE & TECH

5.1: "Ghost Protocol" & Biometric Triage

- **Panic Button:** 5 clicks on the side button for SOS.
- **Immediate Biometric Triage:** In a crisis, don't "feel" your pulse by hand. Use wearable sensors to instantly monitor **Saturation (SpO2)**. In case of smoke inhalation or shock, it is your early indicator of cerebral hypoxia before mental confusion sets in.
- **Faraday Bag:** Total digital invisibility.

5.2 Vision and Light: The Domain of Darkness

In any crisis, light is either a weapon or a target. White light destroys night vision (rhodopsin).

- **Apex Action (Tactical Red Light):** Insert an elite headlamp with **dedicated red LED**. Red light does not degrade rhodopsin and is not visible at long distances, allowing you to operate on medical kits without becoming a beacon for external threats.

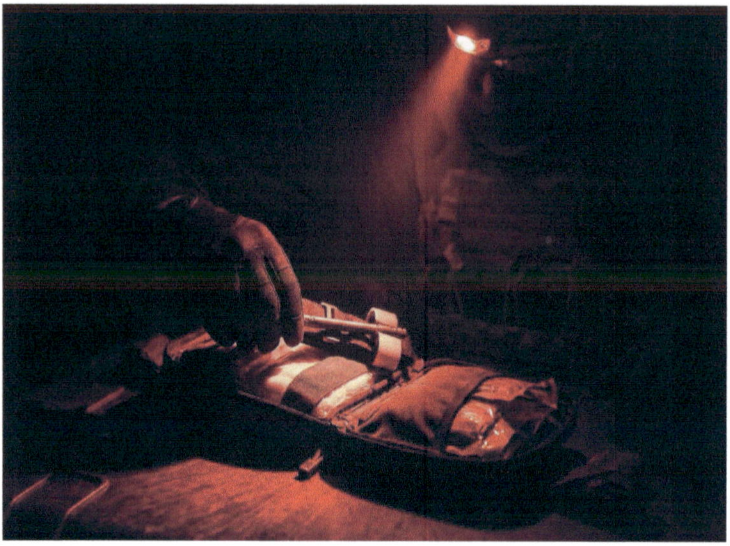

5.3 Mesh Networking & Signaling (Offline Comms)

- **Apex Action (Mesh Apps):** Download **Briar** or **Meshtastic**. They use your smartphone's Bluetooth/Wi-Fi to create a private local network without the internet.
- **Signal Audit (Low Tech):** Keep a **high-frequency whistle** in your kit.

PART 6: POST-CRISIS DECOMPRESSION (SYSTEM REBOOT)

After the adrenaline rush subsides, the crash comes.

6.1 Shake It Off (Neurogenic Tremor)

Shake your body violently for 2 minutes after the event to release the sympathetic nervous system.

6.2 Magnesium & Glycine

On the evening after the crisis, triple your magnesium dose. Recharge your neural batteries.

SAFETY OFFICER'S WORD

"The Safety Biohacker is not paranoid; he is a contingency professional.

Having a tourniquet or a smoke mask does not mean you want disaster. It means that if the Black Swan arrives, you are an asset to yourself and your family, not a victim waiting for rescue.

Hope is not a strategy. The kit is."

✅ SAFETY CHECKLIST: CHAPTER 20

Tactical Validation. Will your backpack save you, or is it just dead weight? If you have fewer than 5 green check marks, you need to upgrade your backpack.

- [ ] **TRAUMA (MARCH):** Do you have a tourniquet, chest seals, and hydrogel for burns?
- [ ] **SHOCK:** Do you have a space blanket?
- [ ] **HYDRATION:** Do you have chlorine dioxide and a filter straw?
- [ ] **FUEL:** Do you have exogenous ketones for your brain in glycemic blackout?
- [ ] **VISION:** Do you have a red light flashlight to protect your rhodopsin?
- [ ] **TRIAGE:** Do you know how to use wearable devices to monitor SpO2 in an emergency?

Safety Status:

🔴 **RED:** No kit, panic, cloud-dependent phone, dehydration, shock hypothermia.

🟢 **GREEN:** MARCH+CBRN kit, safe water, ketones, biometric triage, active night vision, operational mindset.

PART 6: STRATEGIC INTEGRATION (EXECUTION)

From Analysis Paralysis to Operational Protocol.

THE "BOTTLE NECK" OF EXECUTION

Knowing that there are products to take (previous chapters) is useless if you don't know *what* to actually take, *when* to take it, *how much* to take, and *how* to cycle it.

The human body is not a bucket to be filled; it is a rhythmic symphony.

- A powerful supplement taken at the wrong time becomes a sleep destroyer.
- A miracle peptide taken without the right co-factors is a waste of money.
- A protocol costing $500 or more per month is unsustainable if you don't have a clear ROI (Return on Investment).

THE ARCHITECTURE OF THE SYSTEM

In this final part, we stop adding information and start **removing the superfluous**. We will move from theory to pure logistics. We will build your "War Routine."

Here's how we'll turn knowledge into action:

1. **Selection (Chapter 21):** We will analyze the definitive "Gold Standard." We will remove the marketing and keep only the molecules that have passed clinical and safety screening. Which are the "Must Haves" and which are the "Nice to Haves"?

2. **Timing (Chapter 22):** Applied chronobiology. We will build the **Master Schedule Plan**. From waking up to deep sleep, we will position each intervention at the exact moment when your biology is ready to receive it.

3. **Budget (Chapter 23):** Biohacking should not be a luxury for the few. We will define the **MVP (Minimum Viable Protocol)**: how to achieve 80% of the results with 20% of the expense. We will talk about health ROI.

4. **Periodization (Chapter 24):** You can't do everything, all year round. We will create the **Annual Roadmap**, alternating between boost phases, detox phases, and washout phases.

5. **Biohacking for the Masses (Chapter 25)**: Health ROI even for those with zero budget

OPERATIONAL WARNING

Forget the idea of "taking a magic pill." We are about to build a **system**. A system requires discipline, monitoring, and constant adjustments. You are no longer a passenger in your own body. You are the pilot. And this is your takeoff checklist. Supplements and peptides are not candy. It is a good idea to make your primary care physician your ally so that you have constant medical supervision.

Welcome to the control room.

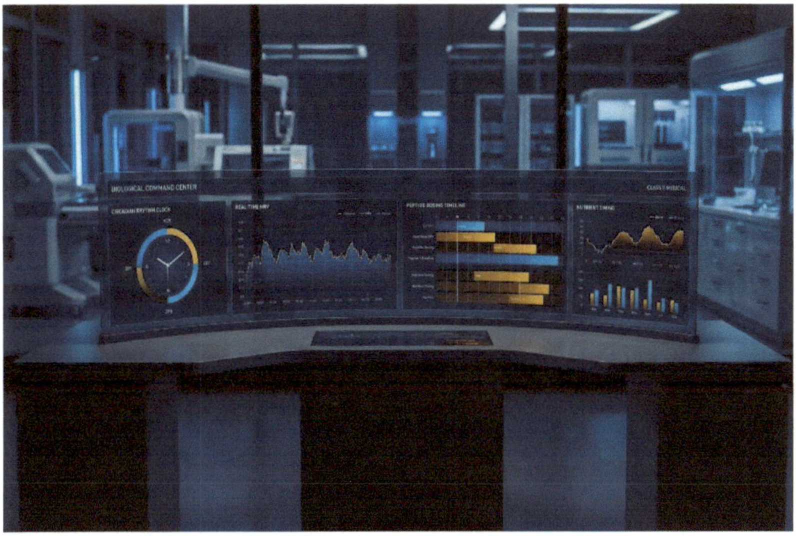

CHAPTER 21

ELITE SUPPLEMENTS AND PEPTIDES: (THE ONES YOU REALLY NEED)

"If you haven't cleaned up the air you breathe, the water you drink, and the sleep you get, close this chapter. You can't buy health in pills if your lifestyle is selling it short. Supplementing a toxic body only produces one thing: expensive urine and a stressed liver."

Before reading a single line of this list, you must pass the **Safety Checkpoint**. This chapter is reserved for Operators who have already implemented the protocols in Parts 1, 2, and 3.

THE "RED FLAG" AUDIT: If you skipped the previous steps, here's what happens if you take supplements now:

1. **Dirty Filters (Chapters 1-2):** If you are full of heavy metals or breathe mold, the antioxidants you take will bind to toxins instead of repairing cells, instantly depleting themselves.
2. **Leaky** Gut **(Chapter 4):** If you have leaky gut, expensive molecules are not absorbed or, worse, pass whole into the bloodstream, triggering autoimmune reactions.
3. **Broken Rhythm (Chapter 5):** If your cortisol is inverted (high in the evening), nootropic stimulants will send you into adrenal burnout.

4. **Depleted Cells (Chapter 9):** If your membrane voltage is low, nutrients will not enter the cell via electrical gradient. They will float around until your kidneys expel them.

If, on the other hand, you have done your homework and passed all the Safety Checklists in parts 1-2-3, then your body is fertile ground. Now, and only now, can we talk about high-yield fertilizers.

In this list, you will find no advertising promises, only the science of facts. I have selected the elite peptides and supplements that form the backbone of a superior biohacking plan, discarding the background noise of commercial 'all-in-one' formulas and useless or ineffective supplements. These molecules are the only ones that are truly reliable, backed by clinical studies and tested to ensure measurable biological transformation.

PART 1: THE "SOURCE CODE" (FUNDAMENTAL MOLECULES)

These molecules are not over-the-counter multivitamins; they are signaling molecules that act on the primary pathways of energy, inflammation, and genomic repair.

1. MOLECULAR HYDROGEN (H2)

- **Role:** The "Sniper" of Free Radicals.
- **The Mechanism:** Unlike classic antioxidants (such as Vitamin C) that neutralize everything indiscriminately (risking shutting down useful signals), H2 is a **selective antioxidant**. It only targets hydroxyl (OH) and

peroxynitrite (ONOO-) radicals, which are the most cytotoxic and harmful to DNA, leaving radicals useful for cell signaling intact. It also activates the **Nrf2** pathway, triggering endogenous glutathione production.

- **Elite Note:** Do not rely on electrolyte bottles of dubious origin. Certified ones are helpful, but the best method is to use effervescent tablets of elemental magnesium that release certified ppm (parts per million) into water.

2. AKKERMANSIA MUCINIPHILA (UNPASTEURIZED)

- **Role:** The "Guardian of the Barrier."
- **Mechanism:** This bacterium is not a simple probiotic; it is a symbiont that lives in the mucus layer of the intestine. Its function is to thicken the mucosal barrier, drastically reducing "Leaky Gut" (intestinal permeability) and metabolic endotoxemia. It also stimulates the secretion of **GLP-1** (the same hormone found in weight loss drugs), improving insulin sensitivity.
- **Elite Note:** The unpasteurized form is often more effective than the pasteurized form, although it slightly increases the risk of uncontrolled proliferation of (only in individuals with compromised immune systems).

3. NAD+ (PRECURSORS: NR or NMN) & SPERMIDINE

- **Role:** The "Longevity Stack" (Energy + Cleansing).
- **The Mechanism:**

- NAD+ (Nicotinamide Adenine Dinucleotide): It is the fuel of mitochondria and the substrate needed by Sirtuins (longevity genes) to repair DNA. Without NAD+, the cell goes into senescence.
- **Spermidine:** It is a polyamide that induces **autophagy** (the recycling of cellular waste). It mimics the effects of fasting, cleaning cells of misfolded proteins.

- **Elite Note:** Taking them together creates a powerful synergy: NAD+ provides energy for repair, while spermidine removes debris that hinders the process.

4. VITAMIN B COMPLEX (METHYLATED)

- **Role:** The "Methylation Engine."
- **The Mechanism:** It is not used to "provide energy," but to drive the methylation cycle. This process controls over 200 functions, from hormone detoxification to neurotransmitter synthesis. It is crucial for lowering homocysteine (a cardiovascular risk factor).
- **Elite Note:** If you have the MTHFR genetic mutation (very common), synthetic folic acid is toxic to you. You must strictly use **methylfolate (5-MTHF)** and **methylcobalamin** (active B12). Read the label: if it says "Folic Acid," throw it away.

5. TMG (TRIMETHYLGLYCINE OR ANHYDROUS BETAINE)

- **Role:** The "Reserve Donor."
- **Mechanism:** Works in tandem with B Complex. TMG donates methyl groups to convert toxic homocysteine into useful methionine. It is also a powerful osmolite: it protects cells from dehydration and heat stress.
- **Elite Notes:** Essential if you take NAD+ precursors, as NAD+ production consumes methyl groups. TMG replenishes supplies, preventing liver fatigue.

6. METHYLENE BLUE (USP PHARMACEUTICAL GRADE)

- **The Role:** The "Electron Accelerator."
- **The Mechanism:** A unique synthetic molecule that acts directly in the electron transport chain (Mitochondrial Complex IV). Increases ATP production and brain oxygen consumption, improving memory and focus. It is also a powerful antimicrobial.
- **Elite Note: Safety Warning.** Use ONLY USP (ultra-pure) grade. The "chemical" or "laboratory" grade contains heavy metals (arsenic, lead). It should be dosed in drops and never taken if you are taking SSRI antidepressants (risk of serotonin syndrome). **The scientifically proven therapeutic dose is 0.8mg/kg.**
- **Safety Warning:** Do not start at the maximum dosage, start with 20 drops and double weekly. If you experience adverse symptoms, discontinue use. Given the potency

of the molecule, it is advisable to consult with your doctor to verify that it does not interact with any medications you are taking or with your physical condition.

7. OMEGA-3 (HIGH POTENCY EPA/DHA)

- **Role:** The "Architect of Membranes."
- **The Mechanism:** It is not just an anti-inflammatory. EPA and DHA are incorporated into cell membranes, making them fluid. A fluid membrane allows receptors (insulin, neurotransmitters) to function properly. Without Omega-3, the membrane is rigid and the cell is "deaf" to signals.
- **Elite Note:** Ignore the "total" dosage of fish oil. Look at the sum of EPA+DHA. The Elite target is **2-3 grams of active ingredients** per day. It must be IFOS 5-Star certified to ensure the absence of mercury and oxidation.

8. TRANS-RESVERATROL (MICRONIZED)

- **Role:** "Stress Mimic."
- **The Mechanism:** A polyphenol that tricks the body into thinking it is under stress (calorie restriction mimetic), activating **Sirtuins (SIRT1)**. This improves mitochondrial biogenesis and antioxidant defense.
- **Elite Note:** Standard resveratrol is useless (bioavailability <1%). You must use the **micronized** or

lipid-matrix-delivered form **of trans-resveratrol**, and always take it with a source of fat (olive oil or Greek yogurt).

9. HYDROLYZED COLLAGEN PEPTIDES

- **Role:** The "structural scaffold."
- **The Mechanism:** After age 25, you lose 1% of collagen per year. Supplementation provides specific amino acids (glycine, proline, hydroxyproline) that act as a signal to fibroblasts: "Rebuild now." Essential for skin, tendons, and intestinal permeability.
- **Elite Note:** Look for low molecular weight peptides (<3000 Daltons) for absorption. Types I and III are for skin/organs, type II for cartilage.

10. HMB (HYDROXYMethylBUTYRATE)

- **Role:** The "Muscle Shield."
- **The Mechanism:** Active metabolite of Leucine. It is the most powerful natural anti-catabolic. It signals the body **not** to **burn muscle** for energy, even under conditions of stress, fasting, or intense training.
- **Elite Note:** Essential on days of intermittent fasting or if you are over 40, to counteract sarcopenia (age-related muscle loss) without having to eat protein every 2 hours.

11. CREATINE MONOHYDRATE & ACETYL-L-CARNITINE (ALCAR)

- **Role:** The Neuromuscular "Power Bank."
- **The Mechanism:**
    - **Creatine:** Not just for muscles. It provides phosphate groups to regenerate ATP in the brain. It is the most underrated nootropic for mental fatigue and sleep deprivation.
    - **ALCAR:** Transports fatty acids into the mitochondria (fat burning) and provides acetyl groups to synthesize acetylcholine (neurotransmitter for memory and speed of thought).
- **Elite Note:** Use only **Creapure®** Creatine (German purity). ALCAR should be taken in the morning (it is a stimulant), Creatine whenever you want (the important thing is chronic saturation).

12. BERBERINE (PHYTOSOME OR HCL)

- **Role:** "Natural Metformin" (carbohydrate control).
- **Mechanism:** Activates **AMPK**, the cell's "energy reserve" sensor. This dramatically improves insulin sensitivity, lowers postprandial blood sugar, and improves the lipid profile. It also has powerful antimicrobial effects on the gut.

- **Elite Notes:** To be used strategically before carbohydrate-rich meals ("Carb Blocker"). The Phytosome form (bound to phospholipids) solves the problem of low absorption and gastrointestinal disorders typical of the basic version.

13. ALPHA-KETOGLUTARATE CALCIUM (Ca-AKG)

- **Role:** The Biological Age Reverser.
- **The Mechanism:** AKG is a key metabolite in the Krebs cycle (energy), but its levels drop with age. Reintroducing it acts as **a demethylase**, removing the incorrect chemical "tags" from DNA that accumulate with aging.
- **Elite Note:** It is the key molecule in the *Rejuvant* study, which has been shown to reduce biological age (Horvath test) by approximately 8 years in 7 months. It is not a simple calcium supplement; it is an epigenetic modulator.

14. GLUCOSAMINE/CHONDROITIN (SULFATE)

- **Role:** The "Low-Carb Diet Mimic" (and joint protector).
- **The Mechanism:** In addition to lubricating the joints by providing cartilage precursors, Glucosamine interferes with glycolysis (the use of sugar), forcing the mitochondria to burn fat and activating **Mitofagia** (mitochondrial cleaning).

- **Elite Notes:** Massive epidemiological studies show a reduction in all-cause mortality comparable to regular exercise. Use strictly the **sulfate** form.

15. LIPOSOMAL GLUTATHIONE

- **Role:** The "Master of Detox."
- **The Mechanism:** It is the body's main antioxidant, vital for neutralizing heavy metals and free radicals. Standard ("reduced") glutathione is destroyed by gastric juices in seconds.
- **Elite Note:** The "Liposomal" specification is non-negotiable. The molecule is encapsulated in a sphere of fat (phospholipids) that bypasses the stomach and fuses directly with cell membranes, ensuring 90% absorption compared to <10% for normal powder.

16. VITAMIN D3

- **Role:** The "Genomic Hormone."
- **The Mechanism:** It is not a vitamin, it is a steroid hormone that regulates the expression of over 1000 genes, including those of the immune system and mood. Without D3, the immune "software" does not update.
- **Elite Note:** Never take it alone. It requires "Super K" (see below) to direct calcium, otherwise you risk calcification

of the arteries instead of the bones. Blood Target Safety: 60-80 ng/ml.

17. SUPER K (K1 + K2 COMPLEX)

- **Role:** The "Calcium Traffic Cop."
- **Mechanism:** While D3 absorbs calcium, Vitamin K activates proteins (Osteocalcin and MGP) that take that calcium and "glue" it into the bones, removing it from soft tissues (arteries, kidneys).
- **Elite Note:** "Super K" refers to an advanced formula that combines **K1** (for coagulation), **K2 MK-4** (short half-life, tissue-specific), and **K2 MK-7** (long half-life, systemic). It is life insurance for your arteries.

18. UBIQUINOL (WITH MITOCHONDRIAL SUPPORT)

- **Role:** The cell's "spark plug."
- **The Mechanism:** Essential in the electron transport chain to produce ATP. Without CoQ10, the heart and brain (high-energy organs) stall.
- **Elite Notes:** I have specified **Ubiquinol** (the reduced/active form), which is up to 8 times more absorbable than standard (oxidized) Ubiquinone, especially after age 40. "Mitochondrial support" usually refers to the addition of **Shilajit (Fulvic Acid)**, which stabilizes the molecule and increases its effectiveness.

19. PQQ (PYRROLOQUINOLINE QUINONE)

- **Role:** The "Engine Generator" (Mitochondrial Biogenesis).
- **The Mechanism:** While CoQ10 makes existing mitochondria work better, PQQ activates the **PGC-1alpha** gene, instructing the cell to build *new* mitochondria from scratch.
- **Elite Note:** It is the only known nutritional molecule capable of generating new mitochondria in vivo. It works in perfect synergy with Ubiquinol: one builds the engine, the other puts in the fuel.

20. TAURINE

- **Role:** The "Osmolite of Longevity."
- **The Mechanism:** Regulates cellular hydration, balances electrolytes, and calms the nervous system (GABA agonist). Studies published in *Science* in 2023 showed that taurine supplementation dramatically extends the average lifespan in animals by correcting a deficiency that worsens with age.
- **Elite Notes:** Essential for athletes (cardiac function) and those who work hard (mitochondrial protection from stress). Inexpensive but irreplaceable.

21. OPTIMIZED BROCCOLI (SULFORAPHANE)

- **Role:** The "Detox Switch" (Nrf2 Activator).

- **The Mechanism:** The active ingredient is not in broccoli, but is formed by chewing it: glucoraphanin meets the enzyme myrosinase and creates **sulforaphane**. This activates the **Nrf2** pathway, which triggers the internal production of massive antioxidants.
- **Elite Note:** "Optimized" means that the supplement contains the added enzyme **myrosinase**. Without the enzyme (destroyed by cooking or absent in cheap pills), broccoli extract is inert.

22. BENFOTIAMINE

- **Role:** The "Anti-Sugar Shield" (Anti-Glycation).
- **The Mechanism:** It is a synthetic fat-soluble form of Vitamin B1 (Thiamine). Unlike normal B1, it penetrates the fatty membranes of nerves and blocks the formation of **AGEs** (advanced glycation end products) - the "rust" caused by sugar that destroys nerves and blood vessels.
- **Elite Note:** Essential for protecting the brain (often called "Type 3 Diabetes") and for those who want to prevent metabolic damage even with normal blood sugar levels.

23. HYALURONIC ACID (HIGH MOLECULAR WEIGHT)

- **Role:** The "Systemic Moisturizer" (Extracellular Matrix).
- **The Mechanism:** Not just for wrinkles. It is the lubricant of the joints and the main component of the "glue" that

holds cells together. One molecule retains 1000 times its weight in water. Ingesting it hydrates deep tissues where water alone cannot reach.

- **Elite Note:** Look for the specific **High Molecular Weight** (>1 Million Daltons). It is absorbed by the intestinal lymphatic system and signals fibroblasts to produce more endogenously, reversing skin and joint atrophy.

24. DECAFFEINATED GREEN TEA EXTRACT (EGCG - MEGA GREEN TEA)

- **Role:** The "Metabolic Chemopreventive."
- **The Mechanism:** The active ingredient is **EGCG (Epigallocatechin-3-gallate)**. It acts on three fronts:
    1. It induces apoptosis (death) in nascent cancer cells.
    2. It increases fat oxidation at rest (thermogenesis).
    3. It inhibits the COMT enzyme, prolonging the action of dopamine and adrenaline (mental focus).
- **Elite Note:** "Mega" indicates a high titration (e.g., 98% polyphenols, 45% EGCG). Choose the **decaffeinated** version so you can take it in the afternoon without disturbing your deep sleep.

25. NATURAL ASTAXANTHIN

- **Role:** "Internal Sunscreen."
- **Mechanism:** It is the red carotenoid that protects algae (and salmon) from UV rays. Unlike other antioxidants, it is located *throughout* the entire cell membrane (inside and outside), protecting the mitochondria from damage caused by sunlight and oxidative stress.
- **Elite Note:** Essential in summer (prevents sunburn from within) and for eye health (crosses the retinal barrier). **Elite Dosage:** 8-12mg per day.

26. SILIMARIN PHYTOSOME (ADVANCED MILK THISTLE)

- **Role:** The "Armor of the Liver."
- **Mechanism:** Extracted from milk thistle, it contains silibin and isosilibin. It stimulates protein synthesis in hepatocytes (liver cells), accelerates the regeneration of damaged liver tissue, and prevents toxins from binding to cell receptors.
- **Elite Note:** The words "Advanced" or "Phytosome" are crucial. Standard silymarin is poorly absorbed. The phospholipid-bound form (Phytosome) has up to 10 times higher bioavailability, reaching therapeutic concentrations in the liver.

27. UROLITHIN A (LIPO UROLITHIN A)

- **The Role:** The "Mitochondrial Incinerator."

- **The Mechanism:** Derived from pomegranates (but only if you have the right bacteria to convert it, which is rare), Urolithin A activates **Mitophagy**: the process by which the cell identifies old and defective mitochondria and recycles them. It is essential for maintaining muscle strength and endurance as we age.
- **Elite Note:** Since few people have the right microbiome to produce it from food, direct supplementation (preferably in liposomal/lipo form for absorption) is the only sure way to obtain it.

28. ELITE CURCUMIN (PHYTOSOME/GALACTOMANNANS)

- **Role:** Systemic Fire Extinguisher (Anti-Inflammation).
- **The Mechanism:** The most powerful natural molecule for inhibiting the **NF-kB** pathway, the master switch of chronic inflammation. Protects the brain, joints, and blood vessels.
- **Elite Notes:** Turmeric powder used in cooking is not absorbed (bioavailability 1%). "Advanced/Elite" refers to patented technologies (such as Meriva or CurQfen) that bind curcumin to lecithin or fenugreek fiber, increasing absorption by 45-270 times.

29. ZINC (PICOLINATE OR BISGLYCINATE)

- **Role:** The "Immune & Hormonal Architect."

- **The Mechanism:** Cofactor for 300 enzymes. Without zinc, you cannot produce testosterone, repair DNA, and your immune system (T cells) will not function.
- **Elite Notes:** Avoid zinc oxide or sulfate (low absorption, nausea). Use chelated forms (picolinate, bisglycinate, monomethionine) for maximum bioavailability. **Always balance with copper if taken long-term (zinc/copper ratio 15:1).**

30. BORON

- **Role:** The "Testosterone Liberator."
- **The Mechanism:** An often overlooked trace mineral. It reduces levels of **SHBG** (Sex Hormone Binding Globulin), the protein that "traps" testosterone. Less SHBG means more free (active) testosterone in circulation.
- **Elite Notes:** Also essential for bone density and magnesium absorption. Just 3-6mg per day is enough to make a difference.

31. SELENIUM (SE-METHYLSELENOCYSTEINE OR YEAST)

- **Role:** The "thyroid converter."
- **The Mechanism:** The thyroid produces T4 (inactive). To become T3 (active, which gives energy and burns fat), a selenium-dependent enzyme is needed. It is also the

engine of glutathione peroxidase, the enzyme that detoxifies hydrogen peroxide in cells.

- **Elite Notes:** Be careful with the dosage. Selenium has a narrow therapeutic window (too much becomes toxic). **200 mcg/day is the gold standard.** Brazil nuts are unreliable (too much or too little), so a titrated supplement is better.

32. CHROMIUM (PICOLINATE OR GTF)

- **Role:** Insulin sensitizer.
- **Mechanism:** Enhances the action of insulin on the cell membrane, helping glucose enter the muscles instead of remaining in the blood (and becoming fat). Reduces sugar cravings.
- **Elite Note:** "Optimized" often includes **Crominex 3+** (a stable form with Amla and Shilajit) which is clinically tested for endothelial as well as glycemic health.

33. COPPER (BISGLYCINATE OR CHELATE)

- **Role**: The "Architect of the Matrix" and Mineral Balancer.
- **Mechanism**: Acts as an essential cofactor for the enzyme *lysyl oxidase*, which acts as a "molecular welder" to create cross-links in collagen and elastin fibers. This ensures the structural integrity of tendons, blood vessels, and skin. It is also essential for the functioning of mitochondrial cytochrome C oxidase (ATP

production) and for the incorporation of iron into hemoglobin.

- **Elite Note**: In an elite protocol that includes 50mg of zinc supplementation, copper is a **mandatory PPE (Personal Protective Equipment)** to maintain the **15:1 safety ratio**. Without this balance, zinc can induce copper deficiency, sabotaging tissue repair. The bisglycinate form ensures superior absorption without interfering with other minerals.

34. SUNFIBER (PARTIALLY HYDROLYZED GUAR GUM - PHGG)

- **Role:** "Precision Fertilizer" (Prebiotic).
- **The Mechanism:** Unlike traditional fibers that swell and cause gas, PHGG is an "invisible" fiber that does not gel. Its superpower is to increase the production of **butyrate**, the short-chain fatty acid that nourishes colonocytes (intestinal cells) and seals the intestinal barrier (Leaky Gut). It also regulates the glycemic index of meals without blocking the absorption of minerals.
- **Elite Note:** It is the only certified *Low-FODMAP* fiber, therefore safe even for those suffering from irritable bowel syndrome (IBS) or SIBO, where other fibers would cause damage.

35. VITAMIN C (LIPOSOMAL OR HYDROGEL 24H)

- **Role:** The "Persistent Water-Soluble Shield."

- **The Mechanism:** Vitamin C has a ridiculously short half-life: it is eliminated in the urine after 2 hours. To get real antioxidant coverage, you need technology.
    - **Liposomal:** Wrapped in fats to enter cells.
    - **Hydrogel (Fenugreek):** A matrix that releases the vitamin slowly over 24 hours.
- **Elite Notes:** Essential for collagen synthesis and cortisol management. Without sustained-release C, your adrenals are exposed for most of the day.

36. NATTOCHINASE

- **Role:** The "Vascular Scavenger" (Fibrinolytic).
- **The Mechanism:** Enzyme extracted from fermented soybeans (Natto). It is not a simple blood thinner; it is a **fibrinolytic h** . It "eats" excess fibrin in the blood, dissolving micro-clots and reducing blood viscosity. It also has the unique ability to break down bacterial **biofilms**, making latent infections vulnerable to the immune system.
- **Elite Note:** Dosage in FU (Fibrinolytic Units). **Target: 2000-4000 FU** between meals. ***Safety:*** Avoid if taking pharmaceutical anticoagulant drugs.

37. LUTEOLIN (BIO-LUTEOLIN)

- **Role:** The "Brain Cooler."

- **Mechanism:** A flavonoid that penetrates the brain and calms the **microglia** (the brain's immune cells). When the microglia is hyperactive (neuroinflammation), you experience "brain fog" and depression. Luteolin extinguishes this fire. It also lowers uric acid, protecting the metabolism.
- **Elite Notes:** Often found in synergy with rutin. It is the daytime complement to nighttime apigenin.

38. MELATONIN (IR/XR - DUAL RELEASE)

- **Role:** The "Architect of Sleep" (and Mitochondrial Antioxidant).
- **The Mechanism:** Many people make the mistake of taking "pure" melatonin, which lasts 4 hours, causing them to wake up at 3 a.m.
    - **IR (Immediate Release):** Makes you fall asleep.
    - **XR (Extended Release):** Keeps you asleep, mimicking the body's natural curve.
- **Elite Note:** The Elite dosage is **Micro** (300mcg - 1mg) for sleep, or **Macro** (10mg+) for anti-cancer/anti-aging protocols (as at high doses it becomes a powerful antioxidant that penetrates the mitochondria). For sleep, "Less is More."

39. ORAL PROBIOTICS (FLORASSIST HYGIENE - BLIS K12/M18)

- **Role:** The "Oral Gateway Firewall."
- **The Mechanism:** From Chapter 3, we know that the mouth is the gateway to heart disease. These are not probiotics to be swallowed, but lozenges to be dissolved in the mouth containing specific strains (**S. Salivarius K12 and M18**). They colonize the oral cavity and throat, killing pathogenic bacteria that cause tooth decay, bad breath, and gum inflammation.
- **Elite Note:** Use them in the evening after brushing your teeth. They are your insurance against bacterial migration to the heart.
- **Warning:** Absolutely no mouthwashes, especially those containing alcohol

PART 2: ELITE & SENOLYTIC PEPTIDES (GENOMIC REPROGRAMMING)

In this section, we discuss molecules that act on cellular aging (senescence), telomere length, and direct tissue regeneration. We move from supplementation to remodeling.

1. BIO-FISETIN (THE "MAYO CLINIC" PROTOCOL)

- **Role:** The "Zombie Cell Killer" (Senolytic Agent).
- **The Concept:** With age, some cells stop dividing but do not die. They become "senescent" (zombie) and secrete inflammatory toxins (SASP) that age nearby healthy cells. Fisetin induces apoptosis (programmed death) *only* in these cells, cleaning up the tissue.

- **The Technology:** Free fisetin has very poor bioavailability. **Bio-Fisetin** uses galactomannan (fenugreek) fiber technology that increases its absorption by 25 times.

- **THE "HIT & RUN" PROTOCOL (MAYO CLINIC):**
  - ***The Common Mistake:*** Taking it every day. Wrong. When taken chronically, it inhibits mTOR (necessary for muscles) and can slow down stem cell regeneration.
  - ***The Strategy:*** You have to hit hard, clean up, and then run away to make room for regrowth.
  - ***Dosage (Standard Fisetin):*** The Mayo study uses ~20mg/kg of body weight (e.g., 1500mg for a 75kg man).
  - ***Dosage (Bio-Fisetin):*** Thanks to increased absorption, **2-3 capsules (100mg)** per day are sufficient.
  - ***Timing:*** Take the dose for **2 consecutive days** (e.g., Sat-Sun). Then **STOP COMPLETELY** for 28-30 days. Repeat the cycle every month. Always take with fats (olive oil/yogurt) in the morning.

2. EPITHALON (THE "TIME DILATOR")

- **Role:** Telomerase activator and circadian reset.

- **The Mechanism:** Discovered by Dr. Khavinson (Russia), it is a synthetic tetra-peptide (4 amino acids) that mimics the action of the pineal gland.

  It acts on two strategic fronts:

  1. **Telomeres:** Stimulates the production of telomerase, the enzyme that "lengthens" the protective caps of DNA, theoretically extending the maximum limit of cell division (known as *the Hayflick Limit*).
  2. **Pineal** gland**:** It restores the sensitivity of the pineal gland, resetting circadian rhythms and endogenous melatonin production (which drops dramatically after age 40).

- **Operating Protocol (The Khavinson Protocol):**
  - **Method:** Strictly subcutaneous injection (Sub-Q).
  - **Elite Dosage:** 10 mg per day.
  - **Attack Cycle:** Take for 10 consecutive days (Total cycle: 100 mg).
  - **Timing:** Preferably in the evening, 1-2 hours before bedtime, to synchronize with the natural release of the pineal gland.
  - **Frequency:** Repeat the full cycle every 6 months.

- **Financial Savings Protocol:**
    - **If you are under 50:** 5 mg per day for 10 days (50 mg total) is considered the optimal "saturation point." Exceeding this dose would now provide minimal marginal benefits at double the cost. This is the smartest approach for those seeking excellent but affordable products.
    - **Aged 50 and over:** As biological age increases, pineal calcification and telomere shortening become critical. At this stage, switching to the Original Khavinson Protocol of 10 mg per day (100 mg total) is the safest choice. Russian clinical studies that showed a 30-50% reduction in mortality were conducted on elderly populations using exactly that high dosage.

- **Elite Notes & Safety Warning:**
    - **The Myth of Nasal Spray:** Unlike smaller neuroactive peptides, nasal spray is NOT a viable alternative for Epitalon. Absorption is estimated to be poor, between 10% and 30%. To replicate the clinical dose of 10mg (necessary for telomerase activation), you would need to use massive amounts of spray, making the protocol ineffective and expensive. Injection is the only way to ensure 100% bioavailability.
    - **Visible effect:** Many users report an immediate improvement in sleep depth and skin quality

(brightness) as early as the 3rd-4th day of the cycle.

3. BPC-157 (BODY PROTECTION COMPOUND)

- **Role:** The "Systemic Healer."
- **Mechanism:** A peptide of gastric origin that signals massive angiogenesis (formation of new blood vessels) and up-regulates growth hormone (GH) receptors specifically in tendon and ligament fibroblasts. It is the biological signal for "immediate reconstruction" of poorly vascularized tissues.
- **Operating Protocol (The Wolverine Protocol):**
    - **Oral (Intestinal Target):** Strictly requires the "Stable Arginate Salt" form.
        - ***Dosage:*** 500 mcg twice daily (morning and evening).
        - ***Objective:*** Repair of leaky gut, ulcers, reflux, and IBS.
    - **Sub-Q Injection (Structural Target):** Subcutaneous injection.
        - ***Elite Dosage:*** 250 mcg twice daily (total 500 mcg/day). For severe injuries, dosage may be increased to 1 mg/day for short periods (1 week).

        - ***Method:*** Inject locally near the area of pain (paracrine effect) if possible; otherwise, into abdominal fat (systemic).
        - ***Cycle:*** 4 weeks ON, 2 weeks OFF.
    - **Nasal Spray (Neural Target):** BPC crosses the blood-brain barrier.
        - ***Dosage:*** 1-2 puffs per nostril per day (approximately 200-400 mcg total, depending on the concentration of the spray).
        - ***Objective:*** Reduction of acute (e.g., post-concussion) or chronic (brain fog) neuroinflammation.
- **Elite Note & Safety Warning:**
    - **It is not a pain reliever:** Unlike NSAIDs (e.g., ibuprofen) that *block* inflammation (and often slow healing), BPC *accelerates* the repair cycle. It does not mask the damage, it resolves it.
    - **Synergy:** For severe musculoskeletal injuries, effectiveness doubles when stacked with TB-500 (2.5 mg per week).

4. THYMALIN

- **Role:** The "Immune Architect."
- **The Mechanism:** The thymus is the gland where T lymphocytes (the "soldiers" of the immune system) are

trained to recognize enemies. After the age of 40, the thymus atrophies (involutes) and is replaced by fat, causing immunosenescence. Thymalin partially reverses this process, reactivating the production and, above all, the *differentiation* of T cells, making the immune system "smarter."

- **Operating Protocol (The Russian Standard):**
  - ***Method:*** Subcutaneous (Sub-Q) or Intramuscular (IM) injection.
  - ***Attack Cycle:*** 10 mg per day for **10 consecutive days** (total 100 mg). To be taken in the morning.
  - ***Frequency:*** This is not a peptide to be taken continuously. The 10-day cycle is performed **every 6 months**. It is a "six-monthly reset" of the immune system.
  - ***Spray Alternative:*** Not effective; injectable Thymalin (purified bovine extract or synthetic tetra-peptide) remains the clinical gold standard.
  - **The Golden Synergy:** Russian protocols (St. Petersburg Institute of Bioregulation) involve the simultaneous use of **Epitalon + Thymalin**. One works on the neuroendocrine system (pineal gland), the other on the immune system (thymus gland). Together, they have been shown to massively reduce all-cause mortality in the elderly by acting on the two main biological clocks.

5. **MOTS-c (MITOCHONDRIAL OPEN READING FRAME)**
    - **Role:** "Physical Exercise in a Bottle."
    - **The Mechanism:** It is a unique peptide because it is not encoded in the DNA of the nucleus, but in the DNA of the mitochondria. It acts as a mitochondrial hormone: it dramatically increases insulin sensitivity, promotes fat oxidation, and prevents the accumulation of visceral fat even on a high-calorie diet. It moves into the cell nucleus to regulate the response to metabolic stress.

    - **Operating Protocol (Metabolic Drive):**
        - ***Method:*** Strictly **subcutaneous injection (Sub-Q)**. (The nasal spray has dubious efficacy for this molecule).
        - ***Elite Dosage:*** 5 mg per week (for maintenance) or 10 mg per week (for aggressive fat loss).
        - ***Timing:*** The dose should be taken **immediately before training** (endurance or weights) to maximize mitochondrial translocation.
        - **Example:** 5mg in a single pre-workout injection, once a week. Or 2mg every other day.
        - ***Cycle:*** 4-8 weeks on, 4 weeks off.

- **Elite Notes & Safety Warning:**
  - **Fragility:** Reconstituted MOTS-c (liquid) degrades quickly. It should be kept in the refrigerator and used within 2 weeks. Never shake the vial.
  - **The "Spicy Poke":** Unlike other painless peptides, MOTS-c injections sting slightly and may leave a redness similar to an insect bite (local histamine reaction) for 30-60 minutes. This is normal. Don't be alarmed, but be prepared.

TECHNICAL BOX: DIY BIOHACKING (NASAL SPRAY PROTOCOL)

Injection is the gold standard, but not everyone is comfortable with it. The Elite solution is **Nasal Spray**. The nasal mucosa is richly vascularized and allows direct access to the brain (bypassing the blood-brain barrier) and the systemic circulation.

CAUTION: *This procedure requires absolute sterility. You are responsible for your own safety.*

EQUIPMENT:

1. **Peptide in a lyophilized vial** (sterile vacuum-packed powder, e.g., 10mg).

2. **Bacteriostatic water** (sterile water with 0.9% benzyl alcohol to prevent bacteria). *NEVER use physiological water if you want to store it for more than 24 hours.*

3. **Insulin syringe** (for mixing).

4. **Empty nasal spray bottle** (sterile, amber glass preferred).

THE MATHEMATICS OF THE SPRAY:

Most sprays deliver **0.1 ml per spray (puff).**

- ***Goal:*** We want a total of 10mg of Epitalon.
- ***Dilution:*** If we add **5 ml** of bacteriostatic water to the spray bottle along with the powder (10 mg).
- ***Concentration:*** 10mg / 5ml = **2 mg/ml.**
- ***Dosage per Puff:*** If 1 ml = 2 mg, then 0.1 ml (one puff) = **0.2 mg (200 mcg).**

CREATION PROCEDURE:

1. Clean all surfaces and vial caps with isopropyl alcohol.
2. Draw up the Bacteriostatic Water with the syringe.
3. Inject it slowly into the peptide vial (the powder will dissolve almost instantly). Do not shake violently (peptides are fragile), rotate gently.
4. Draw up the mixed solution with the syringe and transfer it to the nasal spray bottle.

5. Close. Store in the refrigerator (**mandatory**).

COMPARATIVE ABSORPTION:

- **Oral:** < 1% (Destroyed).
- **Sublingual:** 15-20% (Variable).
- **Nasal:** 20-50% (Excellent for neuroactive peptides).
- **Subcutaneous (injection):** 100%.

Safety Rule: If using the spray, double or triple the recommended injection dose to compensate for lower absorption.

Example: If the injection dose is 300 mcg, administer 3-4 nasal puffs (total 600-800 mcg).

CHAPTER 22

THE CHRONOBIOLOGY OF SUPPLEMENTATION (THE MASTER TIME PLAN)

"The human body is not a bucket to be filled whenever it happens. It is an orchestra. If you play the drum (stimulant supplements) during the lullaby (evening phase), you ruin the symphony. The 'When' is as powerful as the 'What'."

You understand which molecules are right (Chapter 21). Now you need to learn how to place them on the timeline.

Many biohackers fail here: they take everything at breakfast "for convenience." The result? Competition for absorption, incorrect blood sugar spikes, and confused hormonal signals.

The following Master Plan is not random. It is designed to take advantage of your body's metabolic windows:

1. **Morning (7:00-9:00 a.m.):** Mitochondrial activation and membrane protection.
2. **Anabolic window (11:00 a.m.):** Structural repair during partial fasting.
3. **Lunch (1:00 p.m.):** Glycemic management and lipid loading.
4. **Evening (8:00-10:30 p.m.):** Deep detox, vascular cleansing, and sleep induction.

Here is your Operating Protocol.

PHASE 1: AWAKENING (MITOCHONDRIAL STARTUP)

Objective: Start the engines, hydrate, and signal the start of the day.

7:45 a.m. - THE START SIGNAL

- **Molecular Hydrogen (H2):** As soon as you wake up, on an empty stomach.
    - ***Why now:*** The brain is dehydrated and full of metabolic waste from the night. Hydrogen dissolves the oxidative "fog" and penetrates cells in milliseconds, signaling the mitochondria to wake up without the shock of cortisol.

08:00 - THE INTESTINAL GUARDIAN

- **Akkermansia Muciniphila:** 15 minutes after water, before eating.
    - ***Why now:*** It must reach the intestine when the stomach is still empty (or almost empty) to colonize the mucosa. It strengthens the barrier before food arrives.

PHASE 2: BREAKFAST (GENOMIC & MEMBRANE LOAD)

8:30 a.m. - WITH THE FIRST MEAL (NECESSARY FATS)

This is the heaviest stack of the day. It requires fats (eggs, avocado, oil) for absorption.

- **NAD+ & Spermidine:**
  - ***The Logic:*** Pure energy (NAD+) and cellular cleansing (Spermidine). Take them now to get your energy peak in the middle of the morning, when you are most productive.

- **B Complex (Methylated) + TMG (Betaine):**
  - ***The Logic:*** B vitamins are energy cofactors. If you take them in the evening, you risk insomnia. TMG supports the methylation cycle that NAD+ stresses.

- **Methylene Blue:**
  - ***The Logic:*** It boosts the electron transport chain. You need it for cognitive work over the next 8 hours.

- **Fish Oil (Omega-3) + Trans-Resveratrol:**
  - ***The Logic:*** They are 100% fat-soluble. Without the fats in your breakfast, you won't absorb them. Resveratrol mimics metabolic fasting while you eat.

PHASE 3: THE ANABOLIC WINDOW (STRUCTURAL REPAIR)

11:00 a.m. - AWAY FROM MEALS

Mid-morning, your stomach is empty. It's the perfect time for pure amino acids that would otherwise compete with the proteins in food.

- **Hydrolyzed Collagen:**
    - ***The Logic:*** Taken alone, it is better absorbed and sent to the tendons/skin.

- **HMB (Hydroxymethylbutyrate):**
    - ***The Logic:*** Signals to the body "Don't burn muscle" while you are between meals. Essential for preventing catabolism.

- **Creatine & Acetyl-L-Carnitine (ALCAR):**
    - ***The Logic:*** ALCAR gives a second boost of mental focus to get you to lunch sharp. Creatine replenishes muscle and brain ATP stores.

PHASE 4: BEFORE LUNCH

12:45 p.m. - THE "CARB BLOCKER" (15 min BEFORE your meal)

- **Berberine (Phytosome or HCL):**

- *The Tactical Logic:* It must be in the bloodstream before the sugar from lunch arrives. It acts like Metformin: it prepares muscle cells to "suck up" glucose, flattening the post-prandial insulin spike that causes drowsiness and fat accumulation.

PHASE 5: LUNCH

1:00-2:00 p.m. - WITH MEAL (LIPID ABSORPTION)

This block uses fats from lunch to absorb fat-soluble nutrients and support active metabolism.

- **Calcium AKG (Alpha-Ketoglutarate):**
  - *The Logic:* An epigenetic modulator that requires an active gastric environment (full stomach) to avoid acidity disorders and maximize absorption.

- **Fish Oil (Omega-3) – Second dose**
  - *The Logic:* It is 100% fat-soluble. Without the fats from breakfast, you cannot absorb it.

- **Glucosamine and Chondroitin Sulfate:**
  - *The Logic:* Joint structural support that works in synergy with meals to activate the metabolic pathway of mitophagy (simulating fasting).

- **Liposomal Glutathione:**
    - ***The Logic:*** The "Master Antioxidant" is provided during the digestive peak to protect the liver from the metabolic load of lunch.

- **Vitamin D3:**
    - ***The Logic:*** 100% fat-soluble. Taken with lunch (which contains fats) to ensure optimal absorption without interfering with sleep at night.

- **Super K (K1 + K2):**
    - ***The Logic:*** The "Calcium Guardian." Needed at the same time as D3 and calcium from meals to ensure that minerals go to the bones and not the arteries.

- **Ubiquinol (CoQ10):**
    - ***The Logic:*** Mitochondrial fuel. Taking it at lunch provides sustained energy to get through the afternoon without cognitive decline.

- **PQQ (Pyrroloquinoline Quinone):**
    - ***The logic:*** Stimulates the growth of new mitochondria. Combined with Ubiquinol, it creates perfect energy synergy.

- **Taurine:**
    - ***The Logic:*** Cellular osmolite and nervous system calming agent. Helps manage the metabolic stress of eating and hydrates cells.

- **Sulforaphane (Optimized Broccoli):**
    - ***The Logic:*** Nrf2 activator for deep detoxification. Taken with meals, it reduces the risk of gastric bloating typical of cruciferous vegetables.

- **Benfotiamine Mega (Fat-soluble B1):**
    - ***The Logic:*** Protects blood vessels and nerves from damage caused by sugars (glycation/AGEs) ingested with lunch.

- **Hyaluronic Acid:**
    - ***The Logic:*** Systemic hydration and lubrication of connective tissues.

- **Mega Green Tea (Decaffeinated EGCG):**
    - ***The Logic:*** Increases postprandial thermogenesis (fat burning) and provides powerful antioxidants without stimulating caffeine.

- **Astaxanthin:**
    - ***The Logic:*** "Internal sunscreen." Being a carotenoid, it absolutely requires fats to be absorbed.

- **Silymarin (Advanced Milk Thistle):**
    - ***The Logic:*** Direct liver support to help the liver process nutrients and food toxins.

- **Lipo Urolithin A:**
    - ***The Logic:*** Muscle mitophagy inducer. Optimal at lunchtime to support muscle function throughout the day.

- **Curcumin Elite:**
  - ***The Logic:*** Powerful systemic anti-inflammatory. Taken with food, it dramatically improves bioavailability.

- **Zinc:**
  - ***The Logic:*** Essential for the immune and hormonal systems. Taking it on a full stomach prevents the nausea typical of zinc on an empty stomach.

- **Boron:**
  - ***The Logic:*** Modulator of free testosterone and bone health.

- **Copper:**
  - ***The Logic:*** Architect of the collagen matrix and critical balancer of the 15:1 safety ratio with zinc for vessel and tissue integrity.

- **Selenium:**
  - ***The Logic:*** Supports the conversion of thyroid hormones (T4->T3) to maintain high metabolism.

- **Chromium:**
    - ***The Logic:*** Insulin sensitizer. Helps manage blood sugar after meals by pushing glucose into the muscles.

STEP 6: AFTERNOON (REDOX RESET)

5:00 p.m. - THE SECOND BREATH

- **Molecular Hydrogen (H2) - Second Dose:**
    - ***The Logic:*** At the end of the working day, oxidative stress is high and mental fatigue (adenosine) increases. Hydrogen resets the accumulated free radicals, giving you clarity for the evening without using caffeine (which would ruin your sleep).

PHASE 7: BEFORE LUNCH

7:45 p.m. - THE "CARB BLOCKER" (15 min BEFORE the meal)

- **Berberine (Phytosome or HCL):**
    - ***The Tactical Logic:*** It must be in the blood before the sugar from lunch arrives. It acts like Metformin: it prepares muscle cells to "suck" glucose, flattening the postprandial insulin spike that causes drowsiness and fat accumulation.

PHASE 8: DINNER

8:00 p.m. - FIBER LOADING (WITH DINNER)

- **Hydrolyzed Guar Gum (PHGG/Sunfiber):**
  - ***The Logic:*** It nourishes good bacteria during the night and regulates the absorption of dinner. It does not cause bloating.

PHASE 9: PRE-BED

10:30 p.m. - THE NIGHT-TIME "NUCLEAR STACK" (ON AN EMPTY STOMACH 3 HOURS AFTER DINNER)

This is the most important time for longevity and cleansing. The body enters "Maintenance" mode.

- **Magnesium L-Threonate (Neuro-Mag):**
  - ***The Logic:*** The only magnesium that enters the brain. Calms neural excitation and prepares for deep sleep.

- **Glycine (High Dose) + NAC:**
  - ***The Logic (GlyNAC):*** During the night, the liver does the dirty work. We give it the building blocks (Glycine+NAC) to produce Glutathione and detoxify the body while we sleep. Glycine also lowers body temperature, promoting sleep.

- **Nattokinase:**
    - ***The Logic:*** **Crucial.** It should be taken between meals (otherwise it digests food instead of fibrin). At night, blood is more viscous and cardiovascular risk increases. Nattokinase keeps the blood fluid and cleans the vessels while you are lying down.

- **Luteolin & Apigenin:**
    - ***The Logic:*** They turn off brain inflammation (neuroinflammation) and calm the microglia. Apigenin also inhibits CD38, raising nighttime NAD+.
- **Liposomal Vitamin C (24 hrs Hydrogel):**
    - ***The Logic:*** At night, cortisol must drop to a minimum, but the adrenals need support for regeneration. Vitamin C is the fuel for the adrenal glands and the cofactor necessary for collagen synthesis (which occurs mainly during sleep). Hydrogel/Liposomal technology is crucial here: normal vitamin C would be expelled in 2 hours; this covers the entire night, protecting cells from the oxidative stress of the cleansing metabolism.

- **Melatonin (Dual Release IR/XR):**
    - ***The Logic:*** The final shutdown signal. The dual-release version puts you to sleep immediately (IR) and keeps you asleep (XR), preventing you from waking up at 3 a.m.

- **Florassist Hygiene (Oral Probiotics):**
    - ***The Logic:*** The Final Gesture. Taken after brushing your teeth, it dissolves slowly in your mouth while you are already in bed. The BLIS K12 and M18 strains colonize the oral cavity during the night, creating a shield against pathogens that cause gum and systemic inflammation. It is the final "checkpoint" to protect the heart from oral bacteria.

VISUAL SUMMARY: THE WORKFLOW

Time	Substance
07:45	Hydrogen (H2)
08:00	Akkermansia
08:30	NAD+ & Spermidine
08:30	B-Complex
08:30	TMG (Betaine)
08:30	Methylene Blue
08:30	Super Omega-3
08:30	Resveratrol
11:00	Collagen

Time	Substance
11:00	HMB
11:00	Creatine and Acetyl L Carnitine
12:45	Berberine Advanced
1:00-2:00	Calcium AKG
1:00-2:00	Super Omega-3
1:00 p.m.	Glucosamine/Chondroitin
1:00 p.m.	Liposomal Glutathione
1:00 p.m.	Vitamin D3
1:00 p.m.	Super K
1:00 p.m.	Ubiquinol with mitochondrial support
1:00 p.m.	PQQ
1:00 p.m.	Taurine
1:00 p.m.	Sulforaphane
1:00 p.m.	Benfotiamine
1:00 p.m. to 2:00 p.m.	Hyaluronic acid
1:00 p.m.	Green Tea
1:00 p.m.	Astaxanthin
1:00 p.m.	Silymarin
1:00 p.m.	Lipo Urolithin A
1:00 p.m.	Advanced Curcumin
1:00 p.m.	Zinc
1:00 p.m.	Boron
1:00 p.m.	Copper
1:00 p.m. to 2:00 p.m.	Selenium
1:00 p.m. to 2:00 p.m.	Chromium
5:00	Hydrogen (H2)

Time	Substance
7:45	Berberine Advanced
8:00	Sunfiber
10:30	Magnesium L-Threonate
10:30	Glycine
10:30	Liposomal Vitamin C 24 hrs hydrogel
10:30	NAC
10:30	Nattokinase
10:30	Bio-Luteolin
10:30	Melatonin (IR/XR)
10:30	Liposomal Apigenin
10:30	Florassist Hygiene

CHAPTER 23

THE BEST SUPPLEMENTS AND DOSAGES: TECHNICAL DATA SHEETS & WEIGHT SCALING

"Standard medicine is wrong because it treats a 110kg man as if he were a 30g mouse. At Biohacking Elite, we use Scientific Dosimetry. Here you won't find 'take 1 pill'. You'll find the active ingredient per kg of mass, translated into practical action."

1. MOLECULAR HYDROGEN (H2)

- **Selected Product: H2 Elite**
- **Brand: Quicksilver Scientific**
- **The Audit (Why Best):** Hydrogen is only effective if it reaches an immediate peak concentration. Cheap tablets generate <1 ppm (parts per million). H2 Elite uses a patented elemental hydrogen matrix that generates **8-10 ppm** in 500ml of water and is also in liposomal form to ensure maximum absorption. This is the therapeutic range used in studies for Nrf2 activation.
- **Therapeutic Range:** Effectiveness does not depend strictly on weight, but on distribution volume and oxidative stress. The clinical standard is **80 mg of reactive hydrogen** to generate saturation.

Weight Range	55-60 kg	70-75 kg	80-85 kg	90-95 kg	105 kg
Dosage (Capsules)	1	1	1	1	1-2

Notes: *Above 105 kg or in cases of acute inflammation/air travel, doubling the dose (2 capsules together) is safe and recommended to manage the increased oxidative load. Hydrogen is present twice in the plan, so the same dose can be maintained for each administration.*

2. AKKERMANSIA MUCINIPHILA

- **Selected Product: Akkermansia**
- **Brand: Pendulum**
- **The Audit (Why Best):** Pendulum is the only company in the world with a patent for the cultivation of the live *WB-STR-0001* strain. It is a strict anaerobe (it dies with oxygen). Other products are "pasteurized" (dead) or simple prebiotics. For real colonization, live bacteria are needed.
- **Therapeutic Range: 100 Million - 500 Million AFU** (Active Fluorescent Units). The bacterial dosage does not follow body weight, but the surface area of the intestinal mucosa (which varies little between a 60kg adult and a 100kg adult).

Weight Range	55-60 kg	70-75 kg	80-85 kg	90-95 kg	105 kg+
Dosage (Capsules)	1	1	1	1	1

3. NAD+ & SPERMIDINE (LIPOSOMAL)

- **Selected Product: Liposomal Spermidine NAD+ Eternal**
- **Brand: Codeage**
- **The Audit (Why Best):** This is not just a supplement, it is a **Molecular Chimera**. It combines two of the most powerful longevity activators in a single capsule , with liposomal technology (which protects NAD+ from gastric destruction).
    - **NAD+** fuels the engines (mitochondria).
    - **Spermidine** cleans the engines (autophagy).
    - **Technology:** The phospholipid matrix (non-GMO sunflower) ensures that these fragile molecules arrive intact in the bloodstream.
- **Therapeutic Range (Scientific):**
    - ***Spermidine:*** Studies on human autophagy suggest a target of **1-2 mg** per day for maintenance, up to **6 mg** for strong induction.

- *NAD+ Precursors:* The effective range starts at **200-300 mg**.
- *Product note:* Codeage uses a "Proprietary Blend." To achieve "Nuclear Grade" therapeutic levels in a large body, a single capsule is a *maintenance* dosage. For metabolic activation, you need to increase the dosage.

Weight Range	55-60 kg	70-75 kg	80-85 kg	90-95 kg	105 kg
Dosage (Capsules)	1	1	2	2	2

4. B COMPLEX (METHYLATED)

- **Selected Product: Complete B-Complex**
- **Brand: Life Extension**
- **The Audit (Why Best):** Orthomolecular (high) dosages, not minimum recommended (RDA). Uses **5-MTHF** (methylfolate) instead of folic acid (toxic to MTHFR mutants) and **methylcobalamin** (B12). It is the fuel for methylation.
- **Therapeutic Range:** Based on renal clearance capacity and energy requirements. Individuals with more muscle/fat mass have greater blood volume and require higher doses to maintain plasma concentration.

Weight Range	55-60 kg	70-75 kg	80-85 kg	90-95 kg	105 kg
Dosage (Capsules)	1	2	2	2	2

Notes: Life Extension recommends 2 capsules. For light weights (<60kg), 1 is sufficient and reduces unnecessary renal load (neon yellow urine). For everyone else, 2 is the standard.

5. **TMG (TRIMETHYLGLYCINE / ANHYDROUS BETAINE)**

- **Selected Product: TMG 500 mg** (Liquid Vegetarian Capsules)
- **Brand: Life Extension**
- **The Audit (Why Best):** TMG is inexpensive, but low-quality TMG is often contaminated or oxidized. Life Extension guarantees pure **Betaine Anhydrous**.
- **The Strategy (Methyl Donor):** When you take NAD+ precursors (such as Codeage's), your body consumes methyl groups to metabolize excess nicotinamide. Without TMG, you feel tired instead of energetic, and your homocysteine rises.
- **Therapeutic Range:** The functional dosage is **500mg - 1000mg** for the general population. For athletes or heavyweights (high protein turnover), it rises to **1500-2000mg**.

Weight Range	55-60 kg	70-75 kg	80-85 kg	90-95 kg	105 kg
Dosage (Capsules)	1	1	2	2	2-3

Notes: If blood tests show homocysteine > 10 μmol/L, go directly to 3 capsules (1500 mg) regardless of weight, until normalization.

6. METHYLENE BLUE (PHARMACEUTICAL GRADE)

- **Selected Product: Methylene Blue 1%**
- **Brand: MoleQlar**
- **The Audit (Why Best):** Purity. Industrial MB contains heavy metals (arsenic, cadmium). MoleQlar is **USP (Pharmaceutical Grade)** certified , tested for heavy metals. Essential for internal use.
- **Therapeutic Range (Scientific):** Studies by *Francisco Gonzalez-Lima* indicate the ideal hormetic window between **0.5 mg/kg** and **1 mg/kg**. Above 2 mg/kg, it risks inhibiting MAO-A (drug interaction) and becoming pro-oxidant. We will stay in the low range (0.5-0.8 mg/kg) for chronic safety.
- **Calculation:** 1% solution = 10 mg per 1 ml (approximately 20 drops). Therefore, **1 drop ≈ 0.5 mg**.

Weight range	55-60 kg	70-75 kg	80-85 kg	90-95 kg	105 kg
Target mg (0.5-0.8)	30	40	50	60	80-100 mg
Drops (1%)	**60**	**80**	**100**	**120**	**160**

Start-Up Protocol: **EVERYONE** starts with **10 or a maximum of 20 drops** in the first week. Increase by 10 or 20 drops per week until you reach your target range.

7. SUPER OMEGA-3 (EPA/DHA)

- **Selected Product: Super Omega-3 Plus** (with Lignans and Olive)
- **Brand: Life Extension**
- **The Audit (Why Best): IFOS 5-Star** Certification (absolute purity). Includes **Olive Polyphenols** (which protect Omega-3 from oxidation in the body) and **Sesame Lignans** (which enhance its anti-inflammatory effect). Unprotected fish oil goes rancid and causes inflammation; this one heals.
- **Therapeutic Range (Anti-Inflammatory):** To reduce systemic inflammation (hs-CRP) and optimize the Omega-3 index (>8%), the clinical dose is **30-40 mg of EPA+DHA per kg.** Inflammation is proportional to the volume of adipose tissue.

Weight Range	55-60 kg	70-75 kg	80-85 kg	90-95 kg	105 kg+
Softgel (Morning)	2	2	3	3	3
Softgel (Lunch)	0	1	0	1	3
TOTAL DAY	**2**	**3**	**3**	**4**	**6**

8. RESVERATROL ELITE

- **Selected Product: Optimized Resveratrol Elite**
- **Brand: Life Extension**
- **The Audit (Why Best):** Standard resveratrol has <1% bioavailability (useless). This formula uses **galactomannan** technology (fenugreek fiber) that increases absorption **10-fold**. It also includes quercetin phytosome.
- **Therapeutic Range:** Studies on SIRT1 activation indicate dosages equivalent to 250-500mg of trans-resveratrol with high bioavailability for an average adult.

Weight Range	55-60 kg	70-75 kg	80-85 kg	90-95 kg	105 kg
Dosage (Capsules)	1	1	1	1	2

Notes: The 2-capsule dose is reserved for heavyweights (105 kg+) or those with high blood sugar, as a greater boost is needed to activate metabolic pathways in a body with high insulin resistance.

9. HYDROLYZED COLLAGEN (PEPTIDES)

- **Selected Product: Collagen Peptides for Skin & Joints**
- **Brand: Life Extension**
- **The Audit (Why Best):**
  - **Absolute Purity:** This product is pure hydrolyzed bovine peptide powder. No flavorings, no sugars.
  - **The Technology:** It uses an enzymatic hydrolysis process that reduces the molecular weight of collagen. This is crucial: normal collagen (e.g., broth) is too large to be absorbed well. These peptides are small enough to cross the intestinal barrier and act as signaling molecules, stimulating fibroblasts to produce new matrix (skin and cartilage).
  - **Types:** Contains mainly Type I (skin/bones) and Type III (vessels/elastic tissues) collagen.
- **Therapeutic Range:**
  - **2.5 g:** Minimum cosmetic dose (skin).
  - **10-15 g:** Structural clinical dose (joints, tendons, and prevention of loose skin during weight loss).

- **Operational Calculation:** The measuring spoon included in the jar is **11 grams** (which corresponds exactly to the standard clinical dose).

Weight Range	55-60 kg	70-75 kg	80-85 kg	90-95 kg	105 kg
Measuring spoons (Scoop)	0.5 (Half)	1 (Level)	1 (Level)	1.5	1.5 - 2
Total Grams	~5.5 g	~11 g	~11 g	~16 g	~16-22 g

10. HMB (HYDROXYMethylBUTYRATE)

- **Selected Product: Wellness Code Muscle Strength & Restore Formula (Powder)**
- **Brand: Life Extension**
- **The Audit (Why Best):**
    - **The Formula:** It's not just HMB. It's a synergistic matrix that combines **3 grams of Ca-HMB** (the exact clinical dose) with **1000 IU of Vitamin D3**.
    - **The Logic:** HMB stops catabolism (muscle breakdown), but to work best, it requires optimal Vitamin D levels. Life Extension has combined them in powder form to maximize immediate absorption after ingestion.
    - **Format:** The unflavored powder (or lightly flavored with vanilla, depending on the batch)

dissolves easily and avoids having to swallow 6 huge capsules.

- **Therapeutic Range:** The "magic number" validated by dozens of studies is **3 grams** per day. Below this threshold, the anti-catabolic effect is weak.
- **Operational Calculation:** One level scoop (included in the jar) provides exactly the clinical dose (3g of HMB + 1000 IU D3).

Weight Range	55-60 kg	70-75 kg	80-85 kg	90-95 kg	105 kg
Serving size (Measuring cups)	0.5 (Half)	1 (Level)	1 (Level)	1 (Level)	1 (Level)
Net HMB	1.5 g	3 g	3 g	3 g	3 g

11. CREATINE & ACETYL-L-CARNITINE (ENERGY STACK)

- **Selected product: Creatine Acetyl-L-Carnitine Energy Plus** (Powder)
- **Brand: Life Extension**
- **The Audit (Why Best):**
    - **The Synergy:** This is not a "gym" supplement. It is pure mitochondrial fuel. It combines **5 grams of Creatine** (for rapid ATP) with **450 mg of Acetyl-L-Carnitine Arginate** (to transport fats into the mitochondria and increase mental focus) and

PepZinGI® (Zinc-Carnosine) to protect the stomach.

- **The Advantage:** Having everything in one scoop simplifies intake on an empty stomach and ensures the correct ratio of molecules. The powder is absorbed immediately.

- **Therapeutic Range:**
  - **Creatine:** 5 g (standard clinical dose for muscle and cognitive saturation).
  - **ALCAR:** 500-1000 mg (Focus). Here we are at 450-900 mg depending on the scoops.
- **Operational Calculation:** One level scoop (approximately 7 grams of powder) provides exactly 5g of pure creatine.

Weight Range	55-60 kg	70-75 kg	80-85 kg	90-95 kg	105 kg
Serving size (Measuring cups)	0.5 - 1	1	1	1	1 - 1.5
Net creatine	2.5 - 5 g	5 g	5 g	5	5 - 7.5 g

12. BERBERINE (GLUCOSE DISPOSAL AGENT)

- **Selected Product: Berberine Advanced (500 mg)**
- **Brand: California Gold Nutrition**

- **The Audit (Why Best):**
    - **The Strategy:** Berberine has notoriously low oral bioavailability. California Gold uses a standardized extract of *Berberis aristata* (the purest source) in an "Advanced" formula that ensures its potency.
    - **The Mechanism:** It works by activating AMPK (the master metabolic switch). If you take it 15-20 minutes before eating, it prepares your muscle receptors to "suck up" the glucose that is about to arrive from your food, preventing the insulin spike that makes you gain weight.
- **Therapeutic Range:**
    - **Standard:** 500 mg before main meals (total 1000-1500 mg/day).
    - **High Load:** 1000 mg in one go if the meal is a "Cheat Meal" or very rich in carbohydrates.
- **Safety Warning:** Do not take on an empty stomach unless you eat immediately afterwards, as you risk hypoglycemia (dizziness).

Weight Range	**55-60 kg**	**70-75 kg**	**80-85 kg**	**90-95 kg**	**105 kg+**
Lunch dose (capsules)	1	1	1	1	1 - 2

Weight Range	55-60 kg	70-75 kg	80-85 kg	90-95 kg	105 kg+
Dinner dose (capsules)	1	1	1	1	1 - 2

13. CALCIUM ALPHA-KETOGLUTARATE (Ca-AKG)

- **Selected Product: Liposomal Calcium AKG**
- **Brand: Codeage**
- **The Audit (Why Best):**
    - **The Problem:** Alpha-ketoglutarate is an acidic and fragile molecule. Most AKG supplements are destroyed by stomach acids before reaching the cells.
    - **The Solution:** Codeage uses a **liposomal matrix** that envelops the AKG. This not only protects it from the stomach, but allows it to enter directly into the cells where it acts as a demethylase (removing aging tags from DNA).
- **Therapeutic Range:** The *Rejuvant* clinical study (which showed an 8-year reduction in biological age) used approximately **1000 mg** of Ca-AKG per day.
- **Operational Calculation:** This Codeage product provides 1000 mg of Ca-AKG per **2 capsules**.

Weight Range	55-60 kg	70-75 kg	80-85 kg	90-95 kg	105 kg
Dosage (Capsules)	1	2	2	2	2
AKG Net	500 mg	1000 mg	1000 mg	1000 mg	1000 mg

14. GLUCOSAMINE & CHONDROITIN (SULFATE)

- **Selected Product: Glucosamine/Chondroitin Capsules**
- **Brand: Life Extension**
- **The Audit (Why Best):**
    - **Chemical Form:** It must be strictly **SULFATE**. Many products use Glucosamine *Hydrochloride (HCL)* because it costs less, but it does not work as well. The "Sulfate" group is essential for the synthesis of GAGs (the structure of cartilage).
    - **Longevity:** In addition to joints, this stack (at clinical dosage) mimics a low-carb diet, activating mitophagy and reducing all-cause mortality (large-scale epidemiological studies).
- **Therapeutic Range:** The fixed dose validated by studies (e.g., GAIT trial) is **1500 mg glucosamine** + **1200 mg chondroitin**.

- **Operational Calculation:** Life Extension has formulated the capsules to achieve this exact target with **4 capsules**.

Weight Range	55-60 kg	70-75 kg	80-85 kg	90-95 kg	105 kg
Dosage (Capsules)	2	4	4	4	4

Notes: *Do not exceed 4 capsules even at 130 kg. Intestinal transporters become saturated at this dosage.*

15. LIPOSOMAL GLUTATHIONE

- **Selected product: Liposomal Glutathione**
- **Brand: Codeage**
- **The Audit (Why Best):**
    - **Technology:** "Reduced" (standard) glutathione powder is useless; it is destroyed by the stomach in seconds. The only oral route that works is **liposomal** (or S-Acetyl). Codeage offers high-quality liposomes (non-GMO sunflower phospholipids).
    - **The Load:** One capsule contains **500 mg** of glutathione (Setria®), which is a very high dose.
- **Therapeutic Range:**

- **250-500 mg:** Maintenance and skin health.
- **500-1000 mg:** Active detoxification, fatty liver disease, obesity (where oxidative stress is systemic).

Weight Range	**55-60 kg**	**70-75 kg**	**80-85 kg**	**90-95 kg**	**105 kg**
Dosage (Capsules)	1	1	1	1 - 2	2
Net Glutathione	500 mg	500 mg	500 mg	500-1g	1000 mg

Notes: *Adipose tissue generates inflammatory cytokines 24 hours a day. If you are obese or overweight, your "engine" produces a lot of smoke (free radicals). Two capsules (1000 mg) are the correct tactical dose until you lose weight.*

16. VITAMIN D3 (SUN HORMONE)

- **Selected product: Vitamin D3 5000 IU** (or 1000/7000 depending on weight)
- **Brand: Life Extension**
- **The Audit (Why Best):**
  - **Purity:** Life Extension dissolves D3 (cholecalciferol) in high-quality extra virgin olive oil, not in inflammatory seed oils (such as

soybean or corn) used by cheaper brands. Being fat-soluble, the vehicle is crucial.

  - **The Logic:** D3 is not a vitamin, it is a steroid hormone that regulates 3000 genes.

- **Therapeutic Range:** The functional dose to achieve the optimal blood target (60-80 ng/ml) is **40-60 IU per kg** of body weight.
  - ***Caution:*** Adipose tissue "sequesters" vitamin D. The more fat you have, the less D3 circulates in your blood; therefore, you need to take much more to have the same effect as a lean person.

Weight Range	**55-60 kg**	**70-75 kg**	**80-85 kg**	**90-95 kg**	**105 kg**
Target UI	2000 - 3000 IU	4000 IU	5000 IU	5000 - 6000 IU	7000 - 8000 IU
Capsules (Ref. 5000)	1 every other day	1 (excluding weekends)	1	1	1.5

Practical Strategy: Buy the **5000 IU** jar.

- **Lightweights:** Take it Mon-Wed-Fri (or every other day).
- **Medium Weight (176 lbs):** Every day.
- **Heavyweights (105kg+):** Every day. If tests show <50 ng/ml, increase the dosage.

17. SUPER K (THE CALCIUM GUARDIAN)

- **Product of Choice: Super K**
- **Brand: Life Extension**
- **The Audit (Why Best):**
    - **The Formula:** Don't just buy "K2." You need all three bioactive forms, and Super K has them all in one softgel:
        1. **K1 (1500 mcg):** For coagulation.
        2. **K2 MK-4 (1000 mcg):** Short half-life, penetrates tissues and bones quickly.
        3. **K2 MK-7 (100 mcg):** Long half-life (24h+), protects arteries from calcification all day long.
    - **Safety:** Without K2, Vitamin D3 is dangerous because it increases calcium in the blood but does not tell it *where* to go (risk of stones/plaques). K2 activates Osteocalcin, which "cements" calcium into the bone.
- **Therapeutic Range:** 1 capsule of Super K provides a "high-end" clinical dose that covers any requirement.

Weight Range	55-60 kg	70-75 kg	80-85 kg	90-95 kg	105 kg+
Dosage (Softgel)	1	1	1	1	1

Notes: The dose is standard for everyone. There is no known toxicity for K2.

18. UBIQUINOL (ACTIVE CoQ10)

- **Product of Choice: Super Ubiquinol CoQ10 with Enhanced Mitochondrial Support™ (100 mg)**
- **Brand: Life Extension**
- **The Audit (Why Best):**
    - **The Form:** After age 40, the body struggles to convert normal CoQ10 (Ubiquinone) into its active form. You must take **Ubiquinol** directly. Life Extension uses **Kaneka Ubiquinol™** (Japan) raw material, the only one that is stable in air.
    - **Support:** It also contains **Shilajit PrimaVie®** (fulvic acid), which stabilizes Ubiquinol in the stomach and doubles its mitochondrial effectiveness.
- **Therapeutic Range:**
    - **100 mg:** Maintenance dose for healthy adults.
    - **200 mg:** Dosage for athletes, people weighing over 90 kg, or those taking statins (which destroy CoQ10) or who have heart problems.

Weight range	55-60 kg	70-75 kg	80-85 kg	90-95 kg	105 kg
Dosage (Capsules)	1	1	1	2	2
Net Mg	100 mg	100 mg	100 mg	200 mg	200

Notes: *If you are obese, your heart pumps for two. 200 mg is essential to support cardiac output and cellular energy.*

19. PQQ (MITOCONDRIAL BIOGENESIS)

- **Selected Product: PQQ Caps (10 mg)**
- **Brand: Life Extension**
- **The Audit (Why Best):**
  - **Function:** While CoQ10 makes your existing mitochondria work better, PQQ (pyrroloquinoline quinone) activates genes to **grow new ones** (biogenesis).
  - **Quality:** Uses purified **BioPQQ®**, tested for efficacy and renal safety.
- **Therapeutic Range: 10-20 mg** per day is the range used in clinical studies for cognitive and mitochondrial function.

Weight Range	55-60 kg	70-75 kg	80-85	90-95 kg	105 kg
Dosage (20 mg capsules)	1	1	2	2	2

20. TAURINE (THE OSMOLITE OF LONGEVITY)

- **Selected Product: Taurine 1000 mg**
- **Brand: Life Extension**
- **The Audit (Why Best):**
    - **The Scientific Case:** Until recently, taurine was considered just an ingredient in energy drinks . A landmark study in *Science (2023)* revealed that taurine deficiency is one of the primary drivers of aging. Replenishing it significantly extended healthy life in animals.
    - **Function:** It is an osmolite (keeps cells hydrated and full), calms the nervous system (GABA agonist), and protects mitochondria from stress. Life Extension offers **1000 mg** (1 g) pure capsules with no unnecessary additives.
- **Therapeutic Range: 1000 mg - 3000 mg** per day. Higher doses (up to 6g) are used by athletes for cardiac performance, but 1-3g is the longevity range.

Weight Range	55-60 kg	70-75 kg	80-85 kg	90-95 kg	105 kg
Dosage (Capsules)	1	1	2	2	3
Net Grams	1 g	1 g	2 g	2 g	3 g

21. OPTIMIZED BROCCOLI (ACTIVE SULFORAPHANE)

- **Selected Product: Optimized Broccoli and Cruciferous Blend**
- **Brand: Life Extension**
- **The Audit (Why Best):**
    - **The Chemical Secret:** Sulforaphane does not exist in whole broccoli. It is only formed when *glucoraphanin* encounters the enzyme *myrosinase* (during chewing). But cooking destroys myrosinase, rendering cooked broccoli useless for this purpose.
    - **The Solution:** Life Extension separates glucoraphanin and myrosinase into two different layers of the tablet. They only mix in your stomach, ensuring explosive production of real sulforaphane. It is the most powerful Nrf2 activator in nature (deep detox).

- **Therapeutic Range: 1 tablet** per day is sufficient to activate detoxification genes (glutathione-S-transferase).

Weight Range	55-60 kg	70-75 kg	80-85 kg	90-95 kg	105 kg
Dose (Tablets)	1	1	1	1	1

Notes: *The dose does not scale with weight. 1 tablet activates the genetic cascade pathway.*

22. MEGA BENFOTIAMINE (ANTI-SUGAR SHIELD)

- **Selected Product: Mega Benfotiamine 250 mg**
- **Brand: Life Extension**
- **The Audit (Why Best):**
    - **The Problem:** Normal vitamin B1 (thiamine) is water-soluble. It provides little protection for peripheral nerves and the retina, which are rich in fat.
    - **The Solution:** Benfotiamine is a synthetic **fat-soluble** form of B1. It penetrates fatty membranes and neutralizes the end products of glycation (AGEs) right where they do the most damage (nerves, eyes, kidneys). It is essential for those who have (or have had) a diet rich in carbohydrates or insulin resistance.

- **Therapeutic Range:**
    - **250 mg:** Standard prevention.
    - **500-1000 mg:** For those with high fasting blood sugar, neuropathy, or retinopathy.

Weight Range	55-60 kg	70-75 kg	80-85 kg	90-95 kg	105 kg+
Dosage (Capsules)	1	1	1	1	2
Net Mg	250 mg	250 mg	250 mg	250 mg	500 mg

23. HYALURONIC ACID (STRUCTURAL HYDRATION)

- **Selected Product: Hyaluronic Acid Capsules**
- **Brand: Life Extension**
- **The Audit (Why Best):**
    - **The Problem:** Hyaluronic acid is a huge molecule. If you take a generic one, it won't pass through your intestines.
    - **The Solution:** Life Extension uses a specific low molecular weight fermented form (not from rooster combs), enriched and formulated to maximize oral absorption.
    - **The Function:** It's not just for wrinkles. It's the lubricant for your joints (synovial fluid) and,

crucially for your weight loss phase, it keeps the extracellular matrix hydrated to support skin elasticity as your body volume decreases.

- **Therapeutic Range: 100–200 mg** per day.

Weight Range	55-60 kg	70-75 kg	80-85 kg	90-95 kg	105 kg
Dosage (Capsules)	1	1	1	1	1-2

Elite Note (105+kg): *1 capsule is sufficient. If your joints feel "dry" or creaky, increase to 2 capsules for one month.*

24. MEGA GREEN TEA (DECAFFEINATED FAT BURNER)

- **Selected Product: Mega Green Tea Extract (Decaffeinated)**
- **Brand: Life Extension**
- **The Audit (Why Best):**
    - **Potency:** A single capsule contains **725 mg** of pure extract, standardized to **98% polyphenols** and **45% EGCG** (epigallocatechin-3-gallate).
    - **The Comparison:** To get this dose of EGCG (326 mg), you would need to drink about 3-4 cups of high-quality matcha green tea.

- **The Advantage:** It is **decaffeinated.** This is crucial because you have already activated your nervous system at lunch; adding caffeine now would only increase cortisol. Here we only want the metabolic (thermogenesis) and antioxidant effects, without the agitation.

- **Therapeutic Range: 300-600 mg of EGCG** to activate fat oxidation.

Weight Range	55-60 kg	70-75 kg	80-85 kg	90-95 kg	105 kg
Dosage (Capsules)	1	1	1	1	1

Notes: *The dose is standard for all weights. Do not exceed 1 capsule on an empty stomach (may cause slight nausea), always take with food.*

25. ASTAXANTHIN (THE INTERNAL SUNSCREEN)

- **Selected Product: Astaxanthin with Phospholipids (4 mg)**
- **Brand: Life Extension**
- **The Audit (Why Best):**
    - **The Molecule:** It is the red carotenoid that gives salmon the strength to swim upstream. It is 6000

times more powerful than Vitamin C as a singlet antioxidant.

- **The Technology:** Astaxanthin is fat-soluble but difficult to absorb. Life Extension blends it with **phospholipids** (lecithin). This "tricks" the intestine and dramatically increases its entry into the bloodstream.
- **Function:** It protects the mitochondria (your powerhouses) from "overheating" and acts as systemic sunscreen for the skin and eyes.

- **Therapeutic Range:**
    - **4 mg:** Basic dose for vision and maintenance.
    - **12 mg:** "Athlete" dose or for those with a lot of visceral fat (which is inflammatory).

Weight Range	**55-60 kg**	**70-75 kg**	**80-85 kg**	**90-95 kg**	**105 kg**
Dosage (Capsules)	1	1	1	2	2-3
Net Mg	4 mg	4 mg	4 mg	8 mg	8-12 mg

Elite Note (105 kg+): *At this weight, systemic oxidative stress is high. 2 capsules (8 mg) are the minimum requirement. If you spend a lot of time in the sun or at the computer, 3 capsules (12 mg) are ideal.*

26. SILIMARIN (LIVER SHIELD)

- **Selected Product: Advanced Milk Thistle**
- **Brand: Life Extension**
- **The Audit (Why Best):**
    - **The Problem:** Standard silymarin extracted from milk thistle has terrible bioavailability. You absorb maybe 5% of it.
    - **The Solution:** Life Extension uses **Siliphos®** (Phytosome) technology. Silybin (the active ingredient) is molecularly encapsulated in phosphatidylcholine ( ). This not only makes it 10 times more absorbable, but the phosphatidylcholine itself repairs liver cell membranes damaged by fat (steatosis).
- **Therapeutic Range: 760 mg** (of phytosome complex) is the dose used in studies for liver regeneration.

Weight Range	55-60 kg	70-75 kg	80-85	90-95 kg	105 kg+
Dosage (Softgel)	1	1	2	2	2

27. LIPO UROLITHIN A (MUSCLE MITOPHAGY)

- **Selected Product: Liposomal Urolithin A**
- **Brand: Codeage**

- **The Audit (Why Best):**
    - **The Revolution:** Until a few years ago, Urolithin A could only be obtained by eating pomegranates, but only if you had specific gut bacteria (which 60% of people do not have).
    - **The Effect:** It is the only known compound capable of activating selective **mitophagy**: it instructs the cell to "eat" old and defective mitochondria in order to grow new and efficient ones.
    - **The Form:** Codeage encapsulates it in liposomes to ensure it reaches the muscles.
- **Therapeutic Range: 500 mg** per day to see effects on muscle endurance in 4 weeks.

Weight Range	**55-60 kg**	**70-75 kg**	**80-85 kg**	**90-95 kg**	**105 kg**
Dosage (Capsules)	1	1	1	2	2

Notes: *The initial dose for body recomposition is 1000 mg (2 capsules).*

28. CURCUMIN ELITE (ANTI-INFLAMMATORY)

- **Selected Product: Curcumin Elite Turmeric Extract**

- **Brand: Life Extension**
- **The Audit (Why Best):**
    - **The Trap:** Free curcumin (the kind found in spices) does not enter the bloodstream. It is expelled immediately.
    - **Innovation:** This formula uses a **galactomannan** matrix (fenugreek fiber) that protects curcuminoids from degradation. Result: **45 times more bioavailable** than standard curcumin and much higher tissue levels.
- **Therapeutic Range: 500 mg - 1000 mg** to suppress inflammatory cytokines (TNF-alpha, IL-6) produced by visceral fat.

Weight Range	55-60 kg	70-75 kg	80-85 kg	90-95 kg	105 kg
Dosage (Capsules)	1	1	1	1	1 - 2

Notes (105kg+): *Obesity is technically a "low-grade chronic inflammation." 2 capsules help extinguish the systemic fire.*

29. THE MINERAL STACK (ZINC, BORON, SELENIUM, CHROMIUM)

These 5 minerals work together for hormonal metabolism, code repair, and insulin stability. We analyze them as a single block.

- **Selected Products (Life Extension):**
    1. **Zinc:** *High Potency Zinc (50 mg)* - Gluconate/Citrate.
    2. **Boron:** *Boron (3 mg)* - Glycinate/Citrate/Aspartate Complex.
    3. **Selenium:** *Super Selenium Complex (200 mcg)*
    4. **Chromium:** *Optimized Chromium with Crominex® (500 mcg).*
    5. **Copper:** Copper Caps (2 mg) - Copper Bisglycinate Chelate.
- **Audit & Strategy:**
    - **Zinc:** 50mg is a high dose (immune/testosterone booster). For light weights, it should be cycled.
    - **Boron:** Frees testosterone from SHBG. Essential while losing weight to maintain metabolic virility.
    - **Selenium:** Activates the thyroid (T4 -> T3). Without selenium, metabolism slows down.
    - **Chromium:** Sensitizes cells to insulin.
    - Cop**per:** Architect of the collagen matrix and critical balancer of the 15:1 safety ratio with zinc for vessel and tissue integrity.

Weight Range	55-60 kg	70-75 kg	80-85 kg	90-95 kg	105 kg+
Zinc (50mg)	1 every 3 days	1 every 2 days	1 per day	1 per day	1 per day
Boron (3mg)	1 capsule	1 capsule	2 caps	2 caps	2-3 caps
Selenium (200 mcg)	1 capsule	1 capsule	1 capsule	1 capsule	1 capsule
Chromium (500 mcg)	1 capsule	1 capsule	1 capsule	1 capsule	1 capsule
Copper (2mg)	1 every 3 days	1 every 2 days	1 per day	1 per day	1 per day

Safety Note: Never exceed 1 capsule of selenium per day (risk of toxicity above 400 mcg total).

30. SUNFIBER (SMART FIBER)

- **Selected Product: Doctor's Best with Sunfiber®**
- **Brand: Doctor's Best**
- **The Audit (Why Best):**
    - **The Molecule:** Not all fibers are the same. Many (psyllium, inulin) cause bloating and gas. Sunfiber® is **Partially Hydrolyzed Guar Gum**

(PHGG). It is *Low-FODMAP* certified, so it does not ferment explosively.

  - **Function:** Taken before or during dinner, it slows down sugar absorption (stable nighttime blood sugar) and feeds the bacteria that produce **butyrate**, which is essential for repairing the intestinal barrier while you sleep.

- **Therapeutic Range: 5-7 grams** (usually 1 scoop).
- **Operational Calculation:** 1 level scoop.

Weight Range	55-60 kg	70-75 kg	80-85 kg	90-95 kg	105 kg
Serving size (Measuring cup)	1	1	1	1	1 - 1.5

Notes: *The dose is standard. At 130kg, a generous scoop helps to better manage the glycemic load of dinner.*

Everything below should be taken together, approximately 30-45 minutes before bedtime, strictly away from food to maximize absorption and signal effect.

31. NEURO-MAG (CEREBRAL MAGNESIUM)

- **Product Selected: Neuro-Mag Magnesium L-Threonate Powder (Tropical Punch)**

- **Brand: Life Extension**
- **The Audit (Why Best):**
    - **The Problem:** Normal magnesium (citrate, oxide) ends up in the intestines (laxative effect) but does not reach the brain.
    - **The Solution: L-Threonate** is the only chemical form capable of crossing the blood-brain barrier in large quantities. It increases synapse density and calms neuronal excitation and NMDA receptors ( ), facilitating entry into deep sleep.
    - **Format:** The powder allows you to adjust the dose and drink a glass of water before bed (nighttime hydration).
- **Therapeutic Range: 2000 mg of Magtein™** (providing 144 mg of elemental magnesium for the brain).

Weight Range	55-60 kg	70-75 kg	80-85 kg	90-95 kg	105 kg
Serving size (Measuring cup)	1 (Level)	1 (Level)	1 (Level)	1 (Level)	1.5

32. GLYCINE (LIVER DETOX & THERMOREGULATION)

- **Selected Product: Glycine 1000 mg (Vegetarian Capsules)**
- **Brand: Life Extension**

- **The Audit (Why Best):**
  - **Function:** Glycine does two key things at night:
    1. It lowers body temperature (a biochemical signal for sleep).
    2. It is the limiting factor for glutathione production in the liver. Without glycine, the liver cannot detoxify itself.
  - **Quality:** Pure amino acid in free form.
- **Therapeutic Range: 3 grams** (Sleep) - **5 grams** (Metabolic Reset).

Weight Range	55-60 kg	70-75 kg	80-85 kg	90-95 kg	105 kg+
Dosage (Capsules)	3	3	3	4	5

33. LIPOSOMAL VITAMIN C (24 HOURS)

- **Selected Product: Vitamin C 24-Hour Liposomal Hydrogel**
- **Brand: Life Extension**
- **The Audit (Why Best):**
  - **The Limit:** Normal vitamin C is excreted in the urine after 2 hours (very short half-life). At night, you are left "unprotected."
  - **The Innovation:** This formula uses a **fenugreek hydrogel** + liposomes. It protects vitamin C and

releases it slowly. One capsule covers 24 hours, maintaining high plasma levels even at 4 a.m., when nighttime oxidative stress (repair) is at its peak.

- **Therapeutic Range: 350 mg - 700 mg** extended release.

Weight Range	55-60 kg	70-75 kg	80-85 kg	90-95 kg	105 kg+
Dosage (Capsules)	1	1	1	1	2

34. NAC (THE PRECURSOR OF GLUTATHIONE)

- **Selected Product: N-Acetyl-L-Cysteine 600 mg**
- **Brand: Life Extension**
- **The Audit (Why Best):**
    - **The Chemistry:** NAC provides cysteine, the other building block (along with glycine) for making glutathione.
    - **Synergy:** This is the famous **"GlyNAC Stack."** Clinical studies show that high doses of GlyNAC reverse many markers of aging. Taken at night, it supports liver function.
- **Therapeutic Range: 600 mg** (Maintenance) - **1800 mg** (High Load).

Weight Range	55-60 kg	70-75 kg	80-85 kg	90-95 kg	105 kg+
Dosage (Capsules)	1	1	2	2	3

Elite Note (105kg+): *3 capsules (1800mg) is the therapeutic dose for combating massive oxidative stress.*

35. NATTOKINASE (THE VASCULAR CLEANER)

- **Selected Product: Nattokinase 2000 FU**
- **Brand: Doctor's Best**
- **The Audit (Why Best):**
  - **The Mechanism:** Nattokinase is a fibrinolytic enzyme: it literally "eats" fibrin, the protein that forms clots and thickens the blood.
  - **Quality:** Doctor's Best removes Vitamin K2 from natto (which would coagulate the blood), leaving only the pure enzyme. Its activity is certified in **FU (Fibrinolytic Units)**, the only unit of measurement that matters.
  - **Timing:** Strictly on an empty stomach before bed. If you take it with food, it digests the proteins in your dinner and you waste your money. On an empty stomach, it enters the bloodstream and cleans your arteries while you sleep.

- **Therapeutic Range:**
    - **2000 FU:** Standard prevention.
    - **4000 FU:** Active protection for those at cardiovascular risk, with plaque or high blood viscosity (typical of obesity).

Weight Range	55-60 kg	70-75 kg	80-85 kg	90-95 kg	105 kg
Dosage (Capsules)	1	1	1	1	2
Total FU	2000	2000	2000	2000	4000

Elite Note (105kg+): *The blood of an obese person is hypercoagulable (thicker), 2 capsules (4000 FU) are nighttime insurance against blood clots.*

36. BIO-LUTEOLIN (NEURO-ANTI-INFLAMMATORY)

- **Selected Product: Bio-Luteolin**
- **Brand: Life Extension**
- **The Audit (Why Best):**
    - **The Target:** Luteolin is one of the few flavonoids that calms **microglia** (the brain's immune cells). When you are inflamed or stressed, microglia "eat" neural connections. Luteolin shuts this down.

- **The Technology:** Luteolin is difficult to absorb. Life Extension micronizes it to ensure it reaches the brain.

- **Therapeutic Range: 100 mg** is the clinical dose for neuroprotection.

Weight Range	55-60 kg	70-75 kg	80-85	90-95 kg	105 kg+
Dosage (Capsules)	1	1	1	1	2

Elite Note (105kg+): *Adipose tissue sends inflammatory signals to the brain (Brain Fog), 2 capsules help maintain clarity and protect neurons until systemic inflammation subsides.*

37. LIPOSOMAL APIGENIN (THE GUARDIAN OF NAD+)

- **Selected Product: Liposomal Apigenin**
- **Brand: Codeage**
- **The Audit (Why Best):**
  - **Dual Action:**
    1. **Sleep:** Acts on GABA receptors (like chamomile tea 100x stronger), inducing relaxation.
    2. **Longevity:** Inhibits **CD38**, a "parasitic" enzyme that destroys your NAD+. Less

CD38 = More NAD+ available in the morning.

- **Form:** Liposomal (Codeage) to overcome the gastric barrier.

- **Therapeutic Range: 50 - 100 mg.**

Weight Range	55-60 kg	70-75 kg	80-85 kg	90-95 kg	105 kg
Dosage (Capsules)	1	1	1	1	2

Elite Note (105kg+): *2 capsules maximize the natural sedative effect and NAD+ protection.*

38. MELATONIN (SLEEP ARCHITECTURE)

- **Selected Product: Melatonin IR/XR (Immediate & Extended Release)**
- **Brand: Life Extension**
- **The Audit (Why Best):**
    - **The Problem:** Regular melatonin makes you fall asleep, but after 4 hours it wears off and you wake up.
    - **The Solution: MicroActive®** technology releases 1.5mg immediately (to fall asleep) and another 1.5mg slowly over 7 hours (to stay asleep).

- **Therapeutic Range: 1.5 mg** is the physiological dose. **3 mg** (or more) is the "anti-aging" and mitochondrial dose, but it can cause vivid dreams.

Weight Range	55-60 kg	70-75 kg	80-85	90-95 kg	105 kg
Dosage (Capsules)	1	1	1	1	1

Elite Note (105kg+): *2 capsules. At this weight, melatonin also acts as a powerful mitochondrial antioxidant. If you tolerate intense dreams well, stick with 2. Otherwise, reduce to 1.*

39. FLORASSIST HYGIENE (THE ENTRANCE DOOR)

- **Selected Product: Florassist Oral Hygiene**
- **Brand: Life Extension**
- **The Audit (Why Best):**
    - **Common Mistake:** We take care of our intestines but ignore our mouths, which are the main entry point for heart pathogens.
    - **The Solution:** Contains **BLIS K12 and M18** (S. salivarius) strains. These bacteria colonize the mouth and kill bad bacteria that cause gum inflammation (which is directly linked to heart disease).

- **Use:** It is a lozenge to be dissolved slowly in the mouth *after* brushing your teeth, directly in bed.

- **Dosage: 1 tablet** for everyone. The bacteria multiply on their own.

Weight range	55-60 kg	70-75 kg	80-85 kg	90-95 kg	105 kg
Dose (tablet)	1	1	1	1	1

40. BIO-FISETIN (THE MAYO/SENOLYTIC PROTOCOL)

- **Selected Product:** Bio-Fisetin
- **Brand:** Life Extension
- **The Audit (Why Best):**
    - **The "Hit & Run" Strategy:** This is not a supplement to be taken every day. We follow the **Mayo Protocol**: a shock dosage for **2 consecutive days**, followed by **a 28-29 day break**.
    - **The Goal:** To create an acute blood spike that signals the body to activate apoptosis (programmed death) of senescent cells accumulated in the tissues, without interfering with healthy cell growth for the rest of the month.
    - **The Technology:** Since this formula is 25 times more bioavailable, you **don't** need the 20-30 capsules you would need with generic fisetin powder.

Therapeutic Range (Mayo Protocol): Daily dose to be taken for **2 consecutive days** per month.

Weight Range	55-60 kg	70-75 kg	80-85 kg	90-95 kg	105 kg
Dosage (Capsules)	3	4	5	5	6

ELITE NOTES: EXECUTION PROCEDURE

- **Timing**: The capsules should be taken in a single dose in the morning.
- **Lipid Co-factor**: To maximize absorption, always take with a source of healthy fats (e.g., olive oil or Greek yogurt).
- **Washout**: Do not take the product during the 28-day break.
- **Synchronization**: During the two days of the Mayo protocol, it is recommended to suspend supplements that excessively stimulate cell growth (mTOR) to maximize the cell "cleansing" effect.

Here are the supplements on the list that stimulate mTOR or promote growth and that **you should suspend for the 2 days** of Bio-Fisetin intake:

A. Muscle and Structural "Builders"

These molecules tell cells to grow and accumulate energy, the exact opposite of what we want during senolysis:

- **HMB:** One of the most powerful direct activators of mTOR.
- **Creatine:** Increases cellular ATP and muscle growth factors.
- **Collagen:** Provides amino acids that signal tissue reconstruction.
- **Glucosamine/Chondroitin:** Although they have effects on longevity, they stimulate the synthesis of the cartilage matrix.

B. Anabolic and Regenerative "Signals" (Peptides)

Almost all peptides are pro-regenerative. During the 2 "Mayo" days, their "repair/growth" signal conflicts with that of Fisetin's "disposal":

- **BPC-157:** Stimulates angiogenesis and fibroblast proliferation.
- **MOTS-c:** Boosts energy metabolism and biogenesis, prompting cells to take action.
- **Epithalon:** Acting on telomerase and the pineal gland, it regulates cell division; it is best to pause it.
- **Thymalin:** Stimulates the maturation and proliferation of T lymphocytes.

C. Hormonal and Vitamin Support for Proliferation

- **Zinc and Boron (Testosterone Boosters):** Zinc and boron serve to optimize **testosterone** levels. Testosterone is the anabolic (growth) hormone par excellence: its job is to tell cells to grow and multiply. If, during the two days you are trying to eliminate "zombie" cells (senolysis), you simultaneously send a "maximum growth" signal via testosterone, you create a conflict of signals.

  Result: fisetin works less effectively because the cell receives the order to stay alive and grow.

- **Vitamin D3 (The Genomic Regulator):** Vitamin D3 is not just a vitamin, it is a hormone that controls over **1000 genes**. Many of these genes regulate **cell proliferation** (the birth of new cells) and their survival. During senolytic cleansing, we want the system to focus only on "disposal." By pushing the transcription of genes related to life and cell division, D3 can unintentionally "protect" the senescent cells that we want to eliminate.

What you can continue to take (Team Partners)

These molecules create the ideal biochemical environment for fisetin to identify and eliminate senescent cells:

- **Berberine Advanced:** This is the key partner. It activates the **AMPK** enzyme, the master switch for energy conservation and repair, which works in perfect harmony with fisetin-induced senolysis. You can increase the dose during these 2 days of treatment.

- **Optimized Resveratrol Elite:** Contains **Quercetin Phytosome**. Quercetin is a senolytic "cousin" of fisetin; together they broaden the spectrum of "zombie" cells removed from tissues. You can maintain the standard dose.
- **Spermidine (in NAD+ & Spermidine):** While fisetin kills damaged cells, spermidine activates **autophagy**, the recycling process that "clears away" the debris left behind by senolysis. Do not change the standard dose you are taking.
- **Lipo Urolithin A:** Specifically deals with **mitophagy**, i.e., the cleaning and recycling of old mitochondria, completing the cell restoration work of fisetin. You can increase the dose during the 2-day attack phase.

Detoxification Support (Disposal)

Eliminating zombie cells generates a load of "waste" that the body must process:

- **Liposomal Glutathione:** This is the main antioxidant that protects healthy cells from oxidative stress generated during the removal of senescent cells. You can increase the dose during the 2-day attack phase.
- **Optimized Broccoli (Sulforaphane):** Activates the **Nrf2** pathway, enhancing the liver's ability to expel inflammatory toxins released by eliminated cells. Maintain the standard dose.

Hydration and Stability

- **Hydrogen (H2):** Acts as a selective antioxidant, reducing systemic inflammation during the protocol without interfering with useful repair signals. Maintain the standard dose.
- **Magnesium L-Threonate (Neuro-Mag):** Keeps the central nervous system and blood-brain barrier stable during the cleansing phase. Maintain the standard dose.

Apex Action for You:

When doing the Saturday and Sunday "Mayo," follow this **SOP (Standard Operating Procedure)**:

1. **Completely** stop: Peptides, HMB, Creatine, Collagen, and Vitamin D3.
2. **Focus mainly on**: Berberine and Spermidine.
3. **Fasting**: If possible, combine the two days with a tighter intermittent fasting window (e.g., 18:6 or 20:4) to enhance the senolytic effect.

41. EPITHALON (THE FATHER OF LONGEVITY)

- **Selected Product:** Epithalon (Synthetic Epitalon)
- **Brand:** Peptide Sciences
- **The Audit (Why Best):**

- **Telomere Reset:** It is the only peptide proven to lengthen telomeres (the "caps" of DNA) and reset cellular biological age.
- **Neuro-Endocrine:** Restores pineal gland sensitivity, normalizing natural melatonin and cortisol production (circadian rhythm).
- **Khavinson Protocol:** We follow the original Russian clinical protocol: high doses for a short period (cycle), not continuous low doses.

Therapeutic Range (Khavinson Protocol): Daily dose (single evening injection) for **10 consecutive days**.

Weight Range	55-60 kg	70-75 kg	80-85 kg	90-95 kg	105 kg
Dose (mg/day)	5	5	10 mg	10 mg	10 mg

Elite Note: Inject **1 hour before bedtime**. Repeat the 10-day cycle every 6 months. (The standard vial is often 10mg or 50mg, calculate the reconstitution accordingly).

42. BPC-157 (THE SYSTEMIC HEALER)

- **Selected Product:** BPC-157 (Arg-Salt Stable)
- **Brand:** Peptide Sciences
- **The Audit (Why Best):**

- **Rapid Repair:** Accelerates angiogenesis (new blood vessels) to repair damaged tendons, ligaments, and intestinal tissue.
- **Gut-Brain Axis:** It is essential for closing the "Leaky Gut," reducing inflammation that reaches the brain.
- **Stability:** The "Stable" version is more resistant to body pH, ensuring that it reaches the target tissues.

Therapeutic Range: Dose to be injected **twice a day** (morning and evening). The table indicates a **SINGLE** injection (to be done twice).

Weight range	**55-60 kg**	**70-75 kg**	**80-85 kg**	**90-95 kg**	**105 kg+**
Single dose (mcg)	**200 mcg**	**250 mcg**	**350 mcg**	**400 mcg**	**500 mcg**
(Daily Total)	*(400 mcg)*	*(500 mcg)*	*(700 mcg)*	*(800 mcg)*	*(1000 mcg)*

Elite Note: For specific injuries (e.g., shoulder, knee), inject subcutaneously near the area (site enhancement), even though the effect is systemic. Cycles of 4 weeks, then pause.

43. THYMALIN (THE IMMUNE ARCHITECT)

- **Selected Product:** Thymalin (or Thymogen)

- **Brand:** Peptide Sciences
- **The Audit (Why Best):**
    - **Thymus Regeneration:** Reactivates the thymus gland, which atrophies with age, increasing the production and maturation of T lymphocytes (the soldiers of the immune system).
    - **Synergy:** It is the perfect partner for Epithalon. Used together (or one after the other), they constitute the "Gold Standard" of Russian bio-regeneration.
    - **Safety:** It does not overstimulate (like generic immune boosters), but modulates.

Therapeutic Range: Daily dose (single morning injection) for **10 consecutive days**.

Weight range	55-60 kg	70-75 kg	80-85 kg	90-95 kg	105 kg
Dose (mg/day)	5	10 mg	10 mg	10 mg	10 mg

Elite Note: The standard clinical dose for adults is **10mg**. It is reduced to 5mg only for very light or hypersensitive individuals. To be taken in the morning. Cycle to be repeated every 6-12 months.

44. MOTS-c (THE MITOCHONDRIAL MOTOR)

- **Selected product:** MOTS-c

- **Brand:** Peptide Sciences
- **The Audit (Why Best):**
    - **Exercise Mimetic:** Acts directly on the mitochondrial genome, mimicking the metabolic effects of intense exercise ("Exercise in a bottle").
    - **Insulin Sensitivity:** Drastic improvement in glucose management and prevention of visceral fat accumulation, even in calorie surplus.
    - **Energy:** Increases intracellular NAD+ levels and perceived energy.

Therapeutic Range (Metabolic Drive Protocol): TOTAL WEEKLY dose.

Preferably administered in a single "Bolus" injection (or divided into two for high dosages) strictly pre-workout.

Weight Range	**55-60 kg**	**70-75 kg**	**80-85 kg**	**90-95 kg**	**105 kg+**
Weekly dose	**5 mg**	**5 mg**	**5 mg**	**10 mg**	**10 mg**
Frequency	Once a week	Once a week	Once a week	Once a week*	Once a week*

Elite Notes & Safety Warning:

- **Timing:** The injection should be administered **immediately before** the most intense workout of the week (e.g., Leg Day or Metabolic Conditioning).
- **10mg Management (*):** For the 90kg+ range, a single 10mg injection can be very painful. We recommend dividing it into **two 5mg injections** (e.g., Monday and Thursday, always pre-workout) or two simultaneous injections at different sites.
- **The "Fire":** Remember that MOTS-c burns during injection and leaves a red halo for 30-60 minutes (histamine reaction). This is normal. Never shake the vial (fragile peptide).

Final Note: This list is not sponsored. It is the result of independent audits. Formulations change: always check the updated label before purchasing. You are the final quality control before the substance enters your system.

CHAPTER 24: The Roadmap (Annual Routine)

"The amateur takes everything, all the time. The professional knows when to stop and let the body do the dirty work."

Having the best supplements in the world (like the ones we selected in previous chapters) is useless if you don't have a timing strategy. The human body is an adaptive machine: if you constantly provide it with the same external stimulus, it will stop responding (habituation) or slow down its internal mechanisms (negative homeostasis).

In **the Safety Biohacker Plan**, we apply the **Pulsing Rule**.

GROUP 1: THE PILLARS (7 DAYS A WEEK)

These are "concentrated food." They are structural. The body uses them to build bones, membranes, and neurotransmitters. They should never be suspended because the need for them is constant.

WHAT (Substance)	WHY (The Goal)
Hydrogen (H2)	Deep hydration and selective antioxidant.
Akkermansia	Intestinal colonization (must be constant).

WHAT (Substance)	WHY (The Goal)
Sunfiber	Prebiotic (food for good bacteria).
Super Omega-3	Cell membrane structure and brain.
Vitamin D3	Immunity and bones (D hormone).
Super K	Transports calcium to the bones (partner of D3).
Creatine	Muscle and cognitive energy (works by saturation).
HMB	Prevents muscle loss (anti-catabolic).
Collagen	"Glue" for skin and tendons.
Hyaluronic acid	Hydration for skin and joints.
Glucosamine/Chondroitin	Joint structure.
Calcium AKG	Bone longevity and biological age reversal.
Taurine	Electrolyte management and nervous calm.
Neuro-Mag (Magnesium)	Brain relaxation and plasticity.

WHAT (Substance)	WHY (The Goal)
Glycine	Nighttime detox and lowering of body temperature.
Melatonin (IR/XR)	Sleep signal (only if necessary).
Liposomal vitamin C.	Collagen and immunity (water-soluble, needed daily).
Florassist Hygiene	Oral hygiene/oral microbiota.

GROUP 2: ACTIVATORS (5 DAYS ON / 2 DAYS OFF)

These are "signals." They stimulate enzymes, mitochondria, and metabolism. We take a break on the weekend (Sat-Sun) to avoid habituation and let the body work on its own.

Days of intake: Monday - Friday (work routine).

Days off: Saturday - Sunday (washout).

WHAT (Substance)	WHY (The Goal)
NAD+ & Spermidine	Energy Activator and Autophagy.
TMG (Betaine)	Partner of NAD+ (methylation cycle).
B-Complex	Energy (avoid accumulation in the liver over the weekend).
Methylene Blue	Energy production

WHAT (Substance)	WHY (The Goal)
Ubiquinol (CoQ10)	Mitochondrial motor (heart/energy).
PQQ	Creates new mitochondria.
Acetyl L-Carnitine	Mental focus and fat transport.
Optimized Resveratrol	Hormetic stress (mimics fasting).
Lipo Urolithin A	Mitofagia (recycling old mitochondria).
Optimized Broccoli	Sulforaphane (cellular detox).
Mega Green Tea	Antioxidant and EGCG.
Advanced Curcumin	Systemic anti-inflammatory.
Advanced Berberine	Sugar metabolism (the biohacker's insulin).
Benfotiamine	Protection from sugar damage (glycation).
Astaxanthin	Internal sun protection and eye protection.
Zinc / Selenium / Copper	Hormonal and thyroid support.
Boron / Chromium	Free testosterone and blood sugar.

WHAT (Substance)	WHY (The Goal)
Bio-Luteolin	CD38 inhibitor (saves NAD+).
Liposomal Apigenin	Relaxant (acts on GABA). Stop to avoid addiction.
NAC	Master antioxidant. Stop to avoid blocking adaptations.
Milk Thistle	Liver detox.
Nattokinase	Blood fluidity (enzyme).

GROUP 3: SPECIAL OPS (SPECIAL PROTOCOLS)

These do not follow the weekly routine. They are tactical weapons to be used with a calendar in hand.

WHAT	THE PROTOCOL (When to take it)
Bio-Fisetin	**Mayo Protocol:** 1st weekend of the month (Sat+Sun). While using Bio-Fisetin, be sure to suspend Group 2.
MOTS-c (Peptide)	**Metabolic Drive:** 1 injection per week (e.g., Monday).
Epithalon (Peptide)	**Reset:** 10-day cycle every 6 months (e.g., January/July).

WHAT	THE PROTOCOL (When to take it)
Thymalin (Peptide)	**Immunity:** 10-day cycle every 6 months (with Epithalon).
BPC-157 (Peptide)	**Recovery:** 30-day cycle ONLY if injured or inflamed.

HOW TO READ THIS TABLE

1. **Every Day:** Take **Group 1**. It is your life base.
2. **Monday to Friday:** Add **Group 2**. You become a performance machine.
3. **Saturday and Sunday:** Take *only* **Group 1**. Your liver will thank you, and your receptors will reset.
4. **First Weekend of the Month:** Add **Bio-Fisetin** to cleanse zombie cells, make sure you have suspended Group 2 except mainly NAD+ with Spermidine and Berberine.

THE TOTAL WASHOUT WEEK

Once every 6 months (perhaps after the peptide cycle, or during a relaxing week's vacation), I recommend **Zero Week**.

- **Rule:** Zero supplements. Only real food, water, and sleep.
- **Exceptions allowed:** Magnesium and Omega-3 only.

- **Why:** This reminds your body how to function without external aids. It is the litmus test of your metabolic health. If you fall apart without supplements, there is something to review in your basic lifestyle.

Why Detox Week is crucial (Safety First):

- **The "Naked Test" (Diagnostics):** If you feel like a rag, tired, foggy, or depressed after taking away supplements for 7 days, it means that **your basic lifestyle (Sleep, Food, Light) is not working**. It means that supplements are *masking* a problem, not optimizing a healthy machine.
- *The confident biohacker must feel good "naked." Supplements should take you from 100% to 120%, not from 0% to 60%.*
- **Detox from Excipients:** Even the best supplements have capsules (cellulose), flow agents (magnesium stearate), etc. If you take 30 pills a day, you are ingesting grams of excipients. A week off allows your liver and kidneys to dispose of everything without additional load.
- **Psychological Reset:** It is essential not to become psychologically dependent on swallowing pills to feel "safe." Week zero gives you back your mental control.

CHAPTER 25

BIOHACKING FOR THE MASSES (The ROI of Health)

"Biology does not accept credit cards. It only accepts signals. If you are rich but live against your evolution, you get sick. If you have a limited budget but send the right signals, you thrive. The true Biohacker is not the one who spends the most, but the one who achieves the maximum result with the minimum energy and economic expenditure."

There is a toxic misconception in the world of wellness: the idea that it takes thousands of dollars a month to be "optimized." This is false.

In **the Safety Biohacker Plan**, we apply the financial concept of **ROI (Return On Investment)** to biology.

In this chapter, I will give you **the MVP (Minimum Viable Protocol)**: how to transform your body into a Formula 1 machine using zero-cost resources.

1. THE MVP PROTOCOL: ANCESTRAL SIGNALS (Budget €0)

In engineering, the MVP is the basic version that works perfectly. In biology, these are the signals that your DNA has been expecting for millennia.

1. **LIGHT (Morning Glory):**
    - **The Mistake:** Buying serotonin supplements but living in the dark.
    - **The Hack:** Direct exposure (no glasses, no glass) of skin and eyes to natural light for 10-20 minutes as soon as you wake up.
    - **The ROI:** Sets your circadian rhythm, produces Vitamin D (immunity), increases dopamine and serotonin for free.

2. **THE COLD (Guerrilla Thermogenesis):**
    - **The Mistake:** Thinking you need a cryochamber.
    - **The Hack:** Take your normal shower. At the end, turn the knob *to cold*. Hold for 30 seconds to 2 minutes. Or: immerse your face in a bowl of ice water as soon as you wake up for 30 seconds (Immersion Reflex).
    - **The ROI:** Massive increase in norepinephrine (focus), activation of the vagus nerve, and conversion of white fat to brown fat.

3. **FASTING (Autophagy):**
    - **The Mistake:** Looking for "detox" pills while eating 24/7.

- **The Hack:** 16:8 window. And above all: **Stop eating 4 hours before bedtime**.
- **The ROI:** Deep cellular cleansing (autophagy) and nighttime cardiac rest. You save money on food.

4. **GROUNDING (Earthing):**
    - **The Hack:** Take off your insulated shoes. Walk on grass or dirt for 10 minutes.
    - **ROI:** Discharges static electricity (inflammation/positive protons). Thins the blood for free.

2. THE "POOR MAN'S LAB"

You don't need a laboratory. You've already spent €1,400 on your smartphone. Stop using it just for social media and use it as diagnostic hardware.

1. **PHOTOPLETHYSMOGRAPHY (HRV & Stress Audit):**
    - **Protocol:** Every morning, place your fingertip on the main camera using clinical apps (e.g., *HRV4Training*). The sensor detects changes in blood color with each heartbeat.
    - **Action:** If your HRV is low compared to the average, your nervous system is in turmoil. Rest that day. You have just prevented an injury at no cost.

2. **POSTURAL AUDIT (Biomechanical Analysis):**
    - **Protocol:** Use "Slow Motion" mode or the timer. Film yourself walking or doing a squat.
    - **Action:** Analyze symmetry. Posture affects cortisol. Correcting an imbalance today saves you a trip to the physical therapist tomorrow.

3. **COGNITIVE BASELINE (Neuro-Check):**
    - **Protocol:** Free online reaction tests.
    - **Action:** If your speed drops by 10%, your CNS is overloaded. Stop drinking coffee, you need sleep.

3. RESPIRATORY ENGINEERING (FREE GAS)

Air is free, but how you use it changes your blood pH.

1. **BOLT TEST (CO2 Tolerance):**
    - Exhale, pinch your nose, time until the *first* urge to breathe.
    - **< 20 sec:** Respiratory acidosis (chronic stress).
    - **> 40 sec:** Calm athlete.

2. **APEX PROTOCOL:**

- Nasal breathing 24/7. The nose produces **nitric oxide** (vasodilator) and filters pathogens. It is a free antiviral supplement.

4. AIR ENGINEERING (THE INVISIBLE "FREE DETOX")

Elite biohackers know that indoor environments are often 5-10 times more polluted than outdoor environments.

1. **CROSS-VENTILATION PROTOCOL:**
   - **Action:** Open opposite windows for 5 minutes every 2 hours.
   - **ROI:** Reducing CO2 and VOCs (volatile organic compounds) instantly improves cognitive function (+15% focus). Cost: $0.

2. **FRAGRANCE AUDIT:**
   - **Action:** Eliminate scented candles, spray air fresheners, and hyper-chemical detergents.
   - **Safety Insight:** These are "endocrine disruptors" (phthalates) that you pay for to lower your testosterone and damage your thyroid. Replace with clean air or pure essential oils.

5. THE "MACGYVER EXERCISE" (THE SNACK MOVEMENT)

Your metabolism slows down if you sit for 8 hours, even if you go to the gym afterwards.

1. **INTERSTITIAL TRAINING:** 10 push-ups every time you go to the bathroom. 20 squats while the water boils. Keeps insulin sensitivity high throughout the day.
2. **TACTICAL ISOMETRICS:** Push against a doorframe with all your strength for 10 seconds. This recruits deep fibers and stimulates your bones. Cost: $0.

6. NUTRITION: THE FOOD PHARMACY

Nutrient Arbitrage: *How to get expensive molecules from the supermarket.*

"Poor" Food	Replaces (Supplement)	The Safety Officer's Hack
Liver (1 per week)	Multivitamin, B12, Copper	The most nutritious food on the planet.
Sardines / Mackerel	Omega-3 (Fish Oil)	Small fish = no mercury. They cost 1/10 of the price of salmon.
Bones (Broth)	Collagen and electrolytes	Ask your butcher for scraps. Boil them for 24 hours with vinegar. Great for the gut.
Apple Cider Vinegar	Berberine (blood sugar)	One tablespoon in water before a meal reduces the glycemic peak by 30%.

"Poor" Food	Replaces (Supplement)	The Safety Officer's Hack
Turmeric + Pepper	Curcumin Elite	Black pepper + oil increase absorption by 2000%.
Vortex	Structured Water	Stir the water with a spoon to create a vortex before drinking.

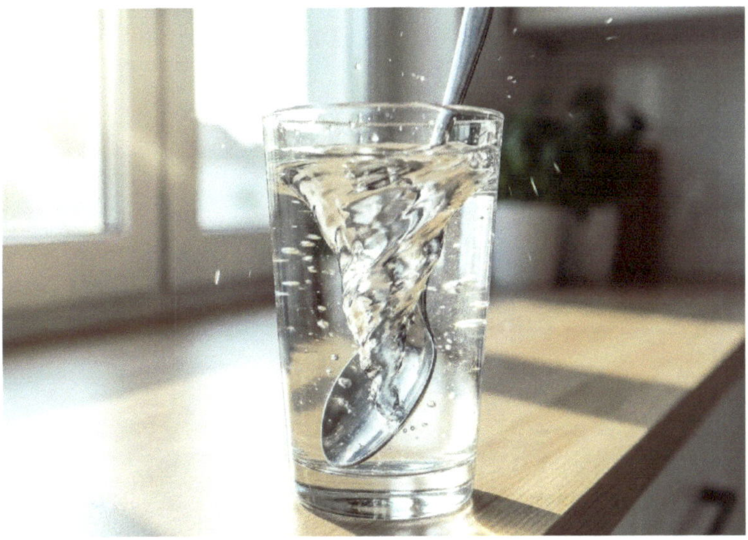

7. THE "BRAIN REBOOT" & DIY GADGET

Replicate expensive technology with biological hardware and tools.

1. **NSDR (Non-Sleep Deep Rest):**

- **Replaces:** €500 Neurofeedback devices (Muse/Sensate).
- **The Protocol:** Search for "Yoga Nidra" on YouTube (free). 10-20 minutes of listening resets dopamine and lowers cortisol better than a nap. Use it during the "4 p.m. slump."

2. **BLUE BLOCKER GLASSES:**
   - Buy **Uvex Skyper** work glasses (orange lenses) at a hardware store (€10). They block 98% of blue light.

3. **MOUTH TAPING:**
   - Use surgical paper tape (€2). A small piece on your lips at night forces you to breathe through your nose.

4. **BLACKOUT:**
   - Use black electrical tape (€1) to cover every single LED in the room.

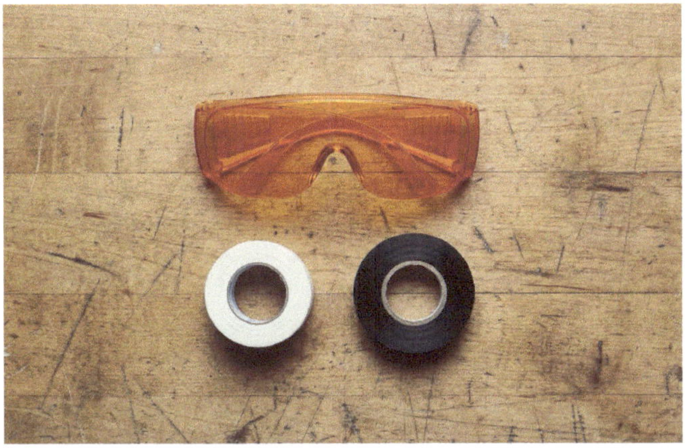

8. THE SOCIAL DIVIDEND (ROI OF CO-REGULATION)

Isolation is a risk factor for mortality greater than smoking 15 cigarettes a day.

1. **"LOCAL MOAI" PROTOCOL:**
    - You don't need an exclusive club. Walking with a friend or talking to your partner without phones activates Vagal Co-Regulation.
2. **THE ROI: The oxytocin** produced is the most powerful free tissue and cardiovascular repairer available to Homo sapiens.

9. SMART BUDGET: WHERE TO PUT YOUR MONEY?

Earnings by subtraction.

Before spending, **cut out the toxins:**

1. **Stop Alcohol & Junk Food:** Save between $50 and $200 per month.

2. **Stop Plastic:** Eliminate bottled water.

Invest your savings here (Absolute Priority):

1. **Magnesium.**
2. **Vitamin D3 + K2.**
3. **Omega-3.**

SAFETY OFFICER'S WORD

"True luxury is not Russian peptide. True luxury is waking up rested, having stable energy, and not depending on drugs.

This is bought with discipline, not with a credit card.

If your biohacking plan causes you 'financial stress', you're doing it wrong.

The basics always win. Money buys the details, discipline buys the foundation.

First, reduce inflammation in your system, then switch to the Elite integration plan to get the most out of it."

PART 7

THE GENDER DIFFERENCE IN BIOHACKING

(Biohacking XX: The Infradian Operating System)

"Men are solar: they live a 24-hour cycle that repeats identically. Women are lunar: they live a 28-day cycle that changes constantly. For decades, medicine and biohacking have made the fatal mistake of treating women as 'little men'. They applied male protocols (extreme fasting, cold, linear loads) to a physiology that was not designed to withstand them in that way. The result was not optimization, but systemic damage: hypothyroidism, amenorrhea, adrenal burnout. This section is the correction of that mistake. Here we give women back their original instruction manual."

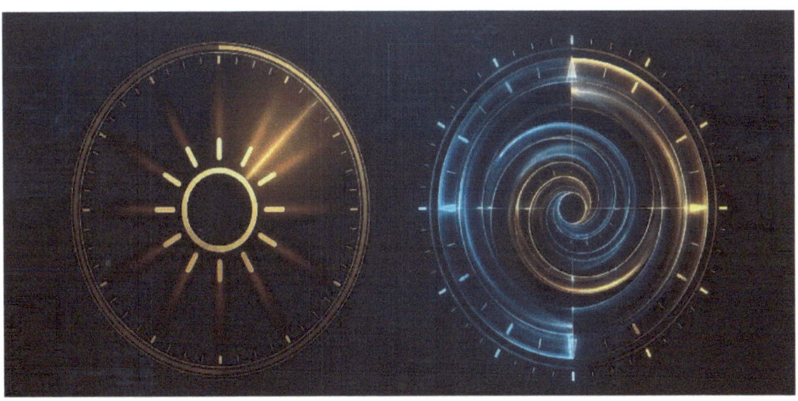

THE EPISTEMOLOGICAL BUG: "PINK IT AND SHRINK IT"

For most of modern history, biomedical research has suffered from a gigantic *Data Gap*. Most clinical studies on drugs, diet, and training have been conducted on **males** (human or animal). Why? Because females are considered "biologically disordered." Their monthly hormonal fluctuations introduce too many variables into the data.

So medicine has adopted the *"Pink it and shrink it"* approach: take the dose for a man, reduce it based on weight, and give it to the woman. As **a Safety- s Officer**, I tell you that this is a violation of safety protocols.

A woman is not a miniature man. She is a completely different operating system.

- Men have stable chemistry.
- Women have **cyclical** chemistry.

THE GOAL OF THIS SECTION

In this Part 7, we will stop fighting female biology and start exploiting it. You will discover that hormonal fluctuations are not a flaw, but a superpower, if you know how to synchronize with them.

We will analyze:

1. **Data Error (Chapter 26):** Why fasting makes your husband lose weight but blocks your thyroid.

2. **Cycle Syncing (Chapter 27):** How to eat and exercise during the four internal seasons to gain an "unfair advantage."
3. **Risk Management (Chapter 28):** The uncomfortable truth about birth control pills and how to mitigate the damage if you decide to use them.
4. **Longevity (Chapter 29):** How to transform menopause from decline to "Second Spring" using bioidentical science.

Welcome to **Bio-Security XX**.

PRELIMINARY SAFETY WARNING

Everything you read in this section is based on one premise: **a woman's health is measured by the regularity and painlessness of her cycle.** If a biohacking protocol (even if it's trendy on Instagram) causes you to skip your period or increases menstrual pain, it is toxic for you. Your cycle is your fifth vital sign. Listen to it.

CHAPTER 26

THE DATA ERROR (Why you are not a "Little Man")

"For decades, medicine has studied human biology while ignoring half the population. The 'male' model as a universal standard has created an epistemological disaster. Women are not men with less testosterone, but a system that operates on a different temporal frequency. Applying male protocols to female physiology is not optimization: it is an uncalculated biological risk."

If you are a woman and have tried to follow standard male biohacking protocols — strict 16:8 fasting every day, cold showers, ketogenic diet, HIIT at dawn — and instead of feeling like a "superhuman," you felt anxious, lost your hair, or missed your period... **it's not your fault.**

You didn't "fail" the protocol. The protocol failed you.

The problem is called **the Gender Data Gap**. Most studies on fasting and cold have been done on young men or male mice. But women are not miniature men. They are a different operating system.

1. SUN VS. MOON: CIRCADIAN VS. INFRADIAN

The first major difference is the temporal rhythm.

- **Men are solar (24-hour circadian cycle):**

Males have a 24-hour hormonal cycle. Testosterone is high in the morning and drops in the evening. Every day is biochemically the same as the previous one. They can follow the same routine 365 days a year and thrive.

- **Women are lunar (28-day infradian cycle):**

Women live according to two rhythms. They respond to the circadian rhythm (24 hours), but their metabolism, immune system, and neurochemistry are governed by **the infradian rhythm** (the menstrual cycle).

A woman is not the same person in the Follicular Phase and in the Luteal Phase. Her brain changes structure, her metabolism speeds up and slows down.

The Biohacker's Mistake: Forcing a body that changes every week into a fixed routine designed for a body that never changes.

2. THE ENERGY AVAILABILITY EQUATION

The math behind why women crash before men.

Why does aggressive Intermittent Fasting (e.g., OMAD) often shut down the female thyroid? The answer lies in **Energy Availability**.

While a man can go below **25 kcal/kg/FFM** (fat-free mass) for short periods without permanent damage, the female hormonal system has a much more sensitive "safety sensor": **Kisspeptin**.

Already below **30 kcal/kg/FFM**, female biology goes into **"Safe Mode"**:

1. It shuts down kisspeptin (stopping reproduction/ovulation).
2. It blocks thyroid conversion (T4 does not become T3) to slow down metabolism.
3. It sacrifices bone density to keep the heart and brain active.

Safety Insight: Male biohacking pushes the accelerator; female biohacking has to manage fuel pressure. If you fall below the safety threshold, your body does not lose weight: it goes into conservative lockdown.

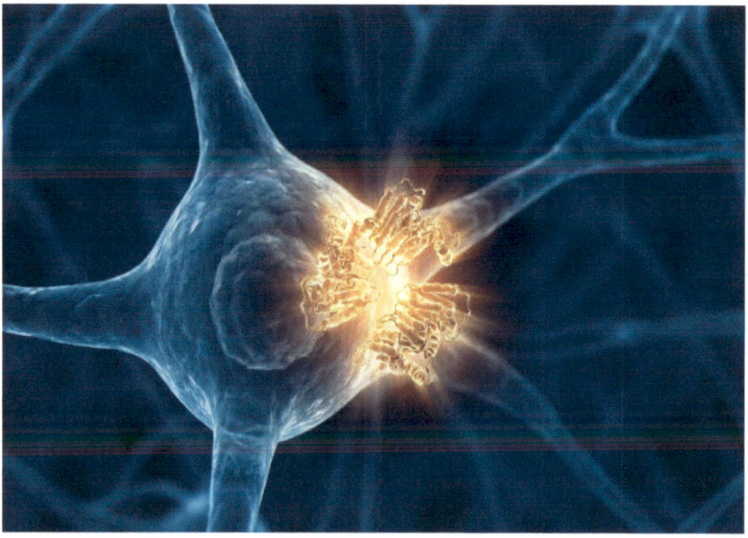

3. HRV DYNAMICS: THE LUTEAL "FALSE ALARM"

How to read wearable data without panicking.

If you use an Oura Ring, a Garmin, or your **smartphone** to monitor stress, you should know that your internal software changes rules in the middle of the month.

- **Follicular Phase (Spring): Parasympathetic** dominance. HRV (Heart Rate Variability) is high, basal temperature is low. The system is ready for hormetic stress (ice, HIIT).
- **Luteal Phase (Fall):** There is **"physiological" sympathetic** dominance. Progesterone raises body temperature by 0.3-0.5°C and increases resting heart rate. As a result, HRV drops.

The Biohacker's Mistake: Seeing HRV drop in the luteal phase, thinking you are "out of shape" or sick, and pushing your training even harder. In reality, it's just progesterone. Ignoring this data leads straight to **adrenal burnout**.

4. THE INFRADIAN SENSOR

Use your hardware to identify the "Seasonal Shift."

Don't just mark the day of your cycle on the calendar. Use technology to identify the **Thermal Shift**.

- **Apex Action:** Monitor your nighttime skin temperature or morning HRV with your smartphone.
- **The Signal:** The day your temperature rises steadily is the signal that you have ovulated and entered the luteal phase ("Metabolic Winter").

- **The Strategy:** From that moment on, the script changes. Reduce fasting, increase complex carbohydrates, eliminate HIIT.

5. THE LOAD OF LIPOPHILIC TOXINS (Endocrine Disruptors)

Why the toxic environment affects her more than him.

While men are more resilient to environmental toxins, women are hypersensitive receivers due to the complexity of their feedback loop.

- **The Concept:** Many endocrine disruptors (BPA, phthalates, parabens) are **xenoestrogens**: they mimic estrogen and bind to receptors, creating "background noise" that distorts the circadian rhythm.
- **Apex Action:** In female biohacking, environmental remediation is not optional, it is vital. "Estrogen dominance" induced by plastics and synthetic fragrances can simulate a perpetual luteal phase, destroying HRV and sleep quality.

6. THE ESTROBOLOME: THE INTESTINAL FIREWALL

We need to talk about how the body expels hormonal toxins.

- **The Concept:** There is a specific set of gut bacteria called **the Estrobolome**. These bacteria produce an enzyme *called beta-* , which can "reactivate" estrogen that has already been discarded by the liver, putting it back into circulation.

- **The Risk:** If the gut is in dysbiosis, toxic estrogens never leave the system, leading to estrogen dominance, inflammation, and circadian rhythm failure.
- **Apex Action:** Female biohacking requires a specific amount of fiber and the use of Calcium D-Glucarate if liver detoxification markers are saturated.

7. THE HORNET WINDOW (Hormetic Narrowing)

The dose makes the poison, but for women, the dose changes.

While men can benefit from extreme stress, women have a much narrower window of tolerance.

- **The Concept:** Stress (ice, fasting, heat) is a U-shaped curve. For women, the base of the U is much narrower.
- **Apex Action:** The "Shock" protocol must be modulated. If a man does 5 minutes of ice, a woman in the luteal phase gets the same beneficial signal (or risks a toxic signal) in just **60 seconds**.

8. MICRONUTRIENT "DRAINAGE" (Contraception Sink)

If you use the pill, you are using software that consumes more battery power.

If the subject uses hormonal contraception, the "software" is partially overwritten, but the hardware suffers from specific deficiencies.

- **The Risk:** The pill and other hormonal contraceptives actively drain Magnesium, Zinc, Vitamins B6, B12, and Folate.
- **Apex Action:** If the "lunar rhythm" is chemically silenced, the supplementation protocol must compensate for this constant drain to prevent mitochondrial decline and depressed mood.

9. TECHNICAL NOTE: CYCLICAL INSULIN RESISTANCE

Why you crave sugar before your period.

In the luteal phase, high progesterone levels make cells temporarily more **resistant to insulin**. The body struggles to push glucose into cells.

Safety Protocol: Don't fight it with fasting (you'll make the equation worse). Increase your intake of healthy fats and complex carbohydrates to stabilize the curve.

10. BIOENGINEERING: THE HPO FEEDBACK LOOP

Mathematical proof of female sensitivity.

To provide definitive scientific rigor, we define hormonal signal stability (Sh) as a function of the pulsatile precision of the hypothalamus (HPO axis - Hypothalamus-Pituitary-Ovary):

Sh = GnRH pulsatility/(Cortisol x Systemic Inflammation)

Safety Insight:

Look at the denominator. If **cortisol** is high (stress, too cold, forced fasting) or **inflammation** rises (toxins, compromised Estrobolome), GnRH pulsatility fragments.

The system no longer "reads" the infradian time and goes into lockdown.

Female biohacking is, first and foremost, **system noise management**.

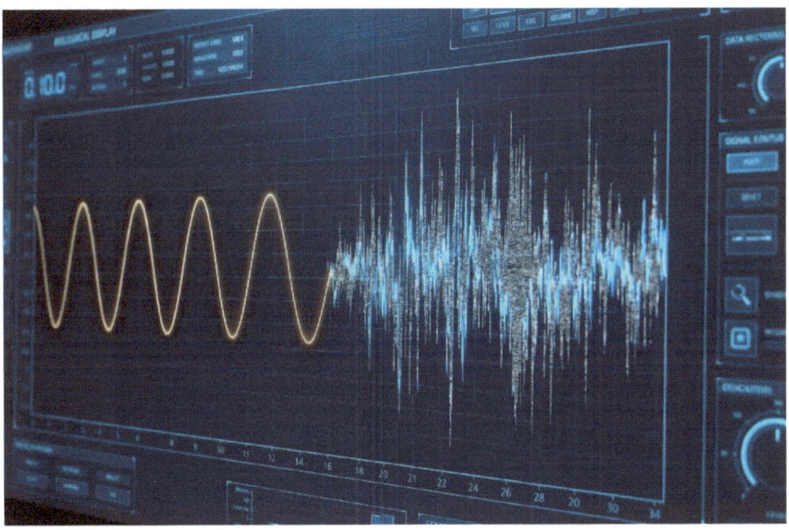

CHAPTER 27

CYCLE SYNCING (Synchronizing the Infradian)

"A man has 24 hours. A woman has 28 days.

Trying to live the same day over and over again is a recipe for hormonal burnout.

Cycle Syncing is not a diet: it is time management based on your biochemistry.

When you stop swimming against the tide, you get what I call the Unfair Advantage."

Your menstrual cycle is not a monthly "nuisance."

It is a continuous biological report on your health and a **Performance Blueprint**.

Hormones (estrogen, progesterone, testosterone) fluctuate in a precise pattern that alters your brain chemistry, metabolism, and physical strength from week to week.

We divide the month into **4 Internal Seasons**.

For each season, here is the **Nuclear Grade** protocol.

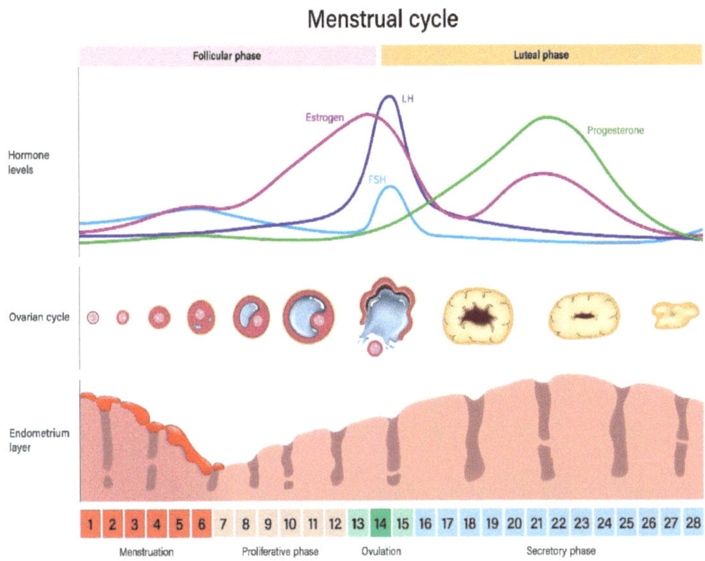

1. MENSTRUAL PHASE: INTERNAL WINTER

- **Duration:** Days 1-6.
- **Hormonal status:** Total reset. Estrogen and progesterone at their lowest. The body is engaged in a controlled inflammatory process (elimination).

OPERATING PROTOCOL

- **Nutrition (Repair):**
  - **Focus:** Iron and zinc (replenishment of blood loss). Cooked and hot foods.
  - **Foods:** Soups, stews, bone broth (collagen), seaweed, red meat. Avoid cold salads and raw foods (difficult to digest).

    - **Seed Cycling:** 1 tablespoon of **flax seeds** + 1 tablespoon of **pumpkin seeds** (ground).

- **Supplementation (Surgical Stack):**
    - **Iron + Vitamin C:** For absorption.
    - **Safety Warning:** No coffee near iron supplements (it blocks absorption).
- **Training (Restoration):**
    - **Activities:** Walking, Yoga Nidra (NSDR), Stretching.
    - **Stop:** No HIIT, no heavy weights.
- **Work & Neurochemistry (Analysis):**
    - The "bridge between the two hemispheres" of the brain is hyperactive. Intuition and analytical skills are at their peak. Great for reviewing strategies and budgets. Bad for big social events.
- **Fasting Algorithm: RED (NO FAST).** Eat when you are hungry. Do not stress a bleeding body.

2. FOLLICULAR PHASE: THE INTERNAL SPRING

- **Duration:** Days 7-12.
- **Hormonal Status:** Estrogen rises. Insulin works better. Energy returns.

OPERATING PROTOCOL

- **Nutrition (Freshness):**
  - **Focus:** Fermented foods (kimchi, sauerkraut) to prepare the gut (estrobolome) to metabolize incoming estrogen.
  - **Foods:** Fresh vegetables, lean proteins, sprouts.
  - **Seed Cycling:** Continue with **flax + pumpkin**.
- **Supplementation (Surgical Stack):**
  - **Fermented Probiotics:** To strengthen the Estrobolome.
- **Training (Neuroplasticity):**
  - **Activities:** Cardio, running, learning new complex sports (coordination improves dramatically).
- **Work (Creativity):**
  - **Acetylcholine Effect:** You are fast, you learn quickly. It's time for brainstorming, starting new projects, and creative problem solving.
- **Fasting Algorithm: GREEN (GO).** You can push to 16:8 or 18:6. The body is resilient.

3. OVULATORY PHASE: THE INTERNAL SUMMER

- **Duration:** Days 13-15 (Short window).

- **Hormonal Status:** Estrogen Peak + Testosterone Peak. You are magnetically attractive, verbally fluent, and energetic.

OPERATING PROTOCOL

- **Nutrition (Elimination):**
  - **Focus:** Raw fiber. The liver must dispose of the massive hormonal peak. You need to "sweep" away the excess to avoid acne and nervousness.
  - **Foods:** Huge salads, raw cruciferous vegetables, berries. Zero alcohol (the liver is already busy).
  - **Seed Cycling:** Last days of **flax + pumpkin**.

- **Supplementation (Surgical Stack):**
  - **NAC or DIM:** Support Phase 2 of liver detoxification. Essential if you suffer from estrogen dominance.

- **Training (Maximum Power):**
  - **Activities:** Maximal efforts in the gym (PR), linear sprints. Testosterone gives you a 10-15% boost in strength.
  - **SAFETY WARNING: THE "LETHAL GAP" (ACL RISK)**

        - **The Science:** Estrogen increases ligament laxity and reduces collagen synthesis for 24-48 hours. Studies show a **4-8 times higher** risk of anterior cruciate ligament (ACL) rupture during ovulation.
        - **Apex Action:** Although testosterone makes you feel invincible, avoid sudden changes of direction or high-impact sports (soccer, tennis, skiing) without specific proprioceptive warm-up. Use power for weights (stability), not for instability.

- **Work (Communication):**
    - The verbal centers are hyperactive. Plan negotiations, public speaking, and first dates here.

- **Fasting Algorithm: GREEN (GO).** Excellent tolerance.

4. LUTEAL PHASE: THE INTERNAL AUTUMN

- **Duration:** Days 16-28 (The critical phase).
- **Hormonal status:** Progesterone dominates. Metabolism accelerates (+200/300 kcal burned at rest), but insulin sensitivity decreases. Cortisol rises easily.

OPERATING PROTOCOL

- **Nutrition (Stabilization):**
    - **Focus:** Complex carbohydrates (slow carbs). Don't cut them out! They help keep cortisol in check and support progesterone.
    - **Foods:** Sweet potatoes, brown rice, oats, root vegetables.
    - **Apex Action:** Increase calories. If you don't eat more, your body goes into "starvation" mode and stores fat.
    - **Seed Cycling:** Change of strategy. 1 tablespoon of **sesame seeds** + 1 tablespoon of **sunflower seeds** (ground).

- **Supplementation (Surgical Stack):**
    - **Magnesium + B6:** Mandatory. Progesterone "washes away" magnesium (causing cramps and chocolate cravings). B6 is needed to synthesize GABA (calming) and progesterone.

- **Training (Endurance):**
    - **Activities:** Weights (slow repetitions), Pilates, walking uphill.
    - **Stop:** No HIIT or extreme cardio after day 20. This would only increase inflammation.

- **Work (Deep Work):**
    - **GABA effect:** Social energy decreases, but focus on details increases. Finish projects, do accounting, organize.

- **Fasting Algorithm: YELLOW -> RED.**
    - *Early Luteal:* 12:12 or 14:10.
    - *Late Luteal (pre-cycle):* **NO FAST.** Eat breakfast within 30 minutes of waking up to calm the adrenal glands.

5. DEEP DIVE: THE LOGIC OF SEED CYCLING

It's not magic, it's lipid modulation.

PHASE	SEEDS (Ground & Raw)	BIOCHEMICAL MECHANISM
1 & 2 (Days 1-14)	**Flax + Pumpkin**	**Flax:** Lignans block excess estrogen. **Pumpkin:** Zinc supports follicle formation.

PHASE	SEEDS (Ground & Raw)	BIOCHEMICAL MECHANISM
3 & 4 (Days 15-28)	**Sesame + Sunflower**	**Sesame:** Lignans block estrogen conversion, leaving room for progesterone. **Sunflower:** Vitamin E and selenium are cofactors for progesterone synthesis in the corpus luteum.

6. DEEP DIVE: THE NEUROCHEMICAL MAP

Why you feel this way (and how to take advantage of it).

1. **The Dopamine Effect (Week 2):** Estrogen protects the brain from fatigue. You are biologically programmed to be curious and outgoing.
   - ***Hack:*** Do the hard things now.

2. **The GABA Effect (Week 4):** Progesterone acts on GABA receptors (like a natural sedative).
   - ***The Problem:*** If you're stressed, progesterone is "stolen" to make cortisol -> GABA crashes -> Premenstrual Anxiety sets in.

- ***Hack:*** If you feel anxious, don't force yourself to meditate. Take **magnesium**, **theanine**, and eat carbohydrates in the evening to raise your serotonin. It's chemistry, not character.

SAFETY OFFICER'S WORD

"Many women think they are 'inconsistent' or 'moody'. The truth is that you are cyclically consistent.

If you try to set a personal record at the gym during your menstrual phase, you'll get injured. If you try to do detailed accounting during ovulation, you'll get bored.

Male biohacking is like flipping a switch and leaving it on.

Female biohacking is knowing exactly which switch to turn on in which week.

Synchronize, and you'll stop fighting your own body."

CHAPTER 28

BIO-SECURITY AND CONTRACEPTION (The Disruptor Software)

Hormonal contraception was a social revolution, but biologically it has a hidden cost. The Safety Biohacker doesn't judge the choice, but manages the risk. If you decide to turn off your natural hormonal operating system, you must manually install the safety drivers that the drug uninstalls. You can't hack a system that has been turned off unless you know how to turn it back on artificially.

Many women use the pill (or ring/patch) not only for contraception, but to "regulate their cycle."

There is an uncomfortable technical truth you need to know: **under hormonal contraception, you don't have a cycle.** You have withdrawal bleeding.

The drug works by suppressing communication between the brain (hypothalamus/pituitary gland) and the ovaries (HPO axis). Technically, you are in a temporary chemical menopause controlled by synthetic hormones.

This has profound systemic impacts. Let's analyze them level by level.

1. BEHAVIORAL LEVEL: THE DISRUPTOR SOFTWARE

A. The Pheromone Radar (Partner Selection)

In nature, women are attracted to the scent of men with a different immune system (MHC) than their own. The pill alters this perception.

- **Safety Insight:** Studies show that women on the pill choose partners with similar MHC (genetically more "related"). If you stop taking the pill, you may find your partner's scent suddenly different.

B. Libido and SHBG (The Chemical Lock)

The pill causes the liver to produce massive doses of **SHBG** (Sex Hormone Binding Globulin). This protein "sequesters" free testosterone.

- **The damage:** decreased desire, dryness, inability to build muscle mass (early sarcopenia), and resistant cellulite.

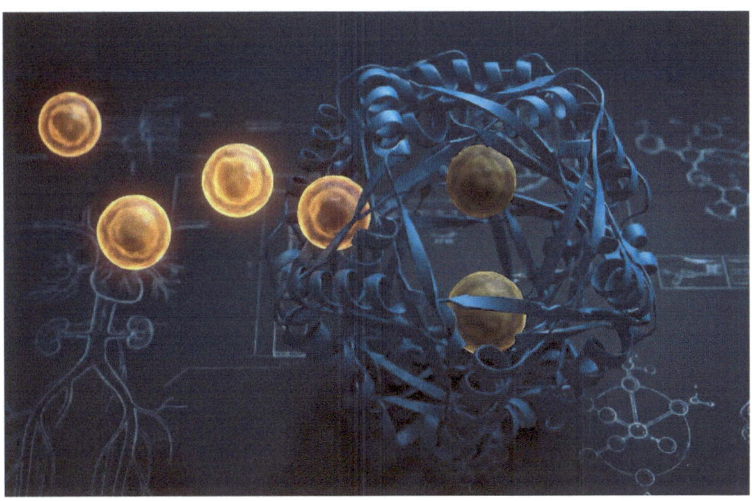

2. NEUROLOGICAL LEVEL: NEURO-EDITING

Why you feel "flat" or anxious (the biochemistry of emotion).

The Collapse of Allopregnanolone

Have you noticed anxiety or "emotional blunting" (life in shades of gray)? Here is the technical cause.

- **The Science:** When metabolized, natural progesterone converts to **allopregnanolone**, a powerful neurosteroid that acts on GABA-A receptors (your endogenous anxiolytic).
- **The Bug:** Synthetic progestins in the pill (e.g., levonorgestrel, drospirenone) do *not* undergo this conversion.
- **Safety Insight:** When taking the pill, the brain experiences an "allopregnanolone famine." You lose your natural tranquilizer.
- **Apex Action:** Support the GABAergic system with **L-Theanine** and **Magnesium Taurate** to artificially compensate for the loss of the neurosteroid.

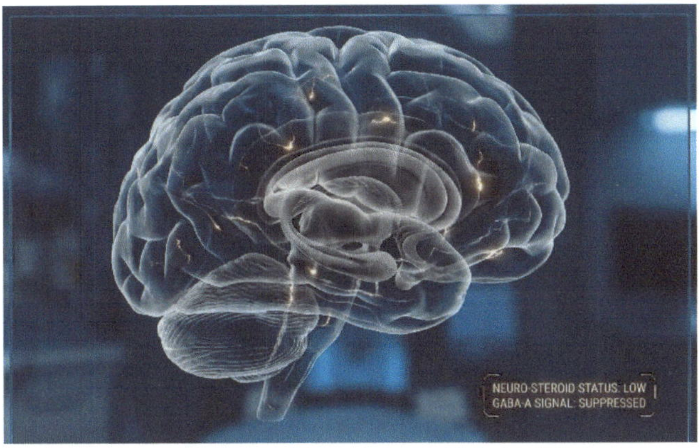

3. PHYSIOLOGICAL LEVEL: BONE & HEART

The silent risks.

A. The "Silent Crash" of Bone

Peak bone mass is reached between the ages of 20 and 30. Natural estrogens are the "builders" of bone.

- **Apex Action:** If you used the pill between the ages of 16 and 25, you are at risk for early osteoporosis. You need to supplement with **Vitamin K2 (MK-7)** and do **high-impact mechanical** training (heavy squats, jumps) to force osteogenesis.

B. Bioengineering: The Endothelial Stability Equation

The pill increases *C-reactive protein* (hs-CRP), creating a basal inflammatory state.

Safety Insight: Ethinyl estradiol raises hs-CRP. If you also have a folate deficiency, homocysteine explodes and stability collapses (thrombus risk).

- **Apex Action:** The mitigation protocol must act by raising the numerator: **Methylated B-Complex** is mandatory to maintain balance.

4. METABOLIC LEVEL: MICROBIOME BREACH

The bacterial war on two fronts.

A. The Intestinal Firewall (Estrobolome)

The Estrobolome is the set of bacteria that manages estrogen.

- **The Risk:** If the intestine is sluggish, an enzyme (beta-glucuronidase) recirculates toxic estrogens instead of expelling them.
- **Apex Action:** Liver support (Calcium D-Glucarate) + **Soluble Fiber** (Psyllium) to ensure daily bowel movements.

B. Vaginal Barrier Breach

Contraception alters glycogen in vaginal cells, reducing the population of *Lactobacillus* (the acid guardians).

- **The Risk:** The pH rises, opening the door to Candida and chronic vaginosis that fuel systemic inflammation.
- **Apex Action:** Cyclical use of specific probiotics (**L. reuteri, L. rhamnosus**) to keep the immune hardware intact despite synthetic software.

5. GENETIC LEVEL: THE MTHFR VARIABLE

If you have the **MTHFR** mutation (40% of the population), the pill drains folate and raises homocysteine.

- **Safety Insight:** If homocysteine rises above **9-10 µmol/L**, you must intervene immediately with methylated folate and ubiquinol.

6. THE NUTRIENT AUDIT (THE NUTRIENT DRAIN)

Not supplements, but spare parts.

Drained Nutrient	Symptom	Compensatory Action
Methylated B-Complex	Depression, Risk of Thrombosis	Significantly reduces risks
Magnesium Taurate/Bisglycinate	Anxiety, Cramps	Compensates for GABA/Allopregnanolone deficiency.
Zinc Picolinate	Immunity, Skin	Essential for thyroid and intestinal barrier.
Selenium	Slow thyroid	Counteracts high TBG.

Drained Nutrient	Symptom	Compensatory Action
CoQ10 / Ubiquinol	Oxidative stress	Vascular mitochondrial protection.

7. THE "EXIT STRATEGY": TECHNOLOGY VS CHEMISTRY

A. The "Post-Pill Rebound" (Crash Management)

When you stop, rebound acne is common.

- **Apex Action: 2 months before** discontinuing, start **Zinc + Vitex (Chaste Tree)**. Zinc calms the androgen receptors on the skin, Vitex gently restarts the pituitary signal.

B. Smartphone + FAM (Fertility Awareness Method)

Instead of shutting down the system, monitor it.

- **Apex Action:** Use your smartphone paired with a basal temperature sensor and algorithms (*Natural Cycles*). 93-98% effective with **zero side effects**.

8. BIO-SAFETY AND CONCEPTION (POST-PILL)

Washout window.

Do not try to get pregnant the month after stopping. Wait **3-6 months**. Load up on **choline, omega-3, and methylated**

folate to regenerate the uterine lining and prevent neural tube defects.

SAFETY OFFICER'S WORD

"Reproductive freedom is sacred. But freedom requires technical awareness.

The pill is not candy, it is hormone replacement therapy.

If you decide to use it, protect your hardware (bones, liver, brain).

If you decide to stop, prepare the ground to avoid a crash.

Your fertility is not just your 'ability to have children', it is a vital sign of your overall health."

CHAPTER 29

THE SECOND SPRING (Perimenopause, Menopause, and BHRT)

In Chinese medicine, menopause is called 'Second Spring'. It is the moment when energy (Qi) stops flowing to the uterus to create external life and rises back up to the heart and brain to create internal wisdom. In Biohacking, we are more pragmatic: it is the moment when your protective hormones say goodbye. If you don't have a contingency plan, your brain and bones remain un . It's not the end, but it is a mandatory fuel change."

There is an unjustified fear surrounding menopause, born of outdated studies (WHI 2002) that confused synthetic hormones with natural ones.

The result? A generation left to suffer from hot flashes, insomnia, brain fog, and osteoporosis without help.

As **Safety Officers**, we are reestablishing the scientific truth: menopause is not a disease, but a **security breach** for your system. Natural barriers are falling. Here's how to rebuild them.

1. PERIMENOPAUSE: THE TURBULENCE ZONE

You don't wake up one day in menopause. You get there by going down a roller coaster.

From ages 40 to 50, ovulation becomes irregular.

- **The first to fall: progesterone**. Since you don't ovulate every month, progesterone plummets, while estrogen remains high or fluctuates wildly.
- **The Result:** Sudden anxiety, insomnia (you wake up at 3:00 a.m.), heavy periods, irritability.
- **Apex Action:** Don't wait for your cycle to end. If you have these symptoms at age 43, you need to supplement with **Bioidentical Progesterone** (micronized) in the luteal phase. It calms the brain and protects the uterus.

2. THE HANDOVER: OVARIES TO ADRENALS

Why stress makes you gain weight in menopause like never before.

When the ovaries shut down, the body tries to delegate residual hormone production to the **adrenal glands**.

- **The conflict:** The adrenal glands also produce cortisol.
- **The Cortisol Steal:** If you reach menopause stressed, your adrenal glands are already depleted ("Pregnenolone Steal"). They don't have the resources to produce your reserve sex hormones.
- **The Result:** Devastating hot flashes and immediate accumulation of visceral fat.
- **Apex Action:** In menopause, stress management is **hormone therapy**. Before estrogen, treat the adrenal glands: **Adaptogens** (Ashwagandha, Rhodiola) and sacred sleep.

3. BIOENGINEERING: THE LEAP OF EPIGENETIC AGING (Aepi)

The mathematics of accelerated decline.

The science of longevity tells us that menopause is not a linear decline, but a real "step" in the biological clock. The loss of estrogen accelerates systemic aging.

We define the rate of aging (Aepi) as a function of hormonal protection (H) and oxidative stress (Os):

$$\mathbf{Aepi = Os/(H \times Myokines)}$$

Safety Insight:

Look at the equation. Without H (Hormones/BHRT), the denominator becomes very small and Aepi explodes.

The only way to balance the equation without hormones (or to enhance them) is to triple the value of **Myokines**. How? With heavy weight lifting and targeted nutrition.

4. CHANGING BRAIN FUEL (Neuro-Metabolism)

Why you have "Brain Fog."

Estrogens are essential for pushing glucose into neurons. When they collapse, neurons go into energy crisis (hypometabolism).

Deep Dive: The APOE4 Genetic Variant

The **APOE4** gene is the main risk factor for Alzheimer's. Women who carry this gene accumulate amyloid plaques quickly when estrogen levels drop.

- **Apex Action:** If you have a family history of Alzheimer's or are APOE4 positive (DNA test), **early BHRT** is not optional, it is neuro-life-saving.

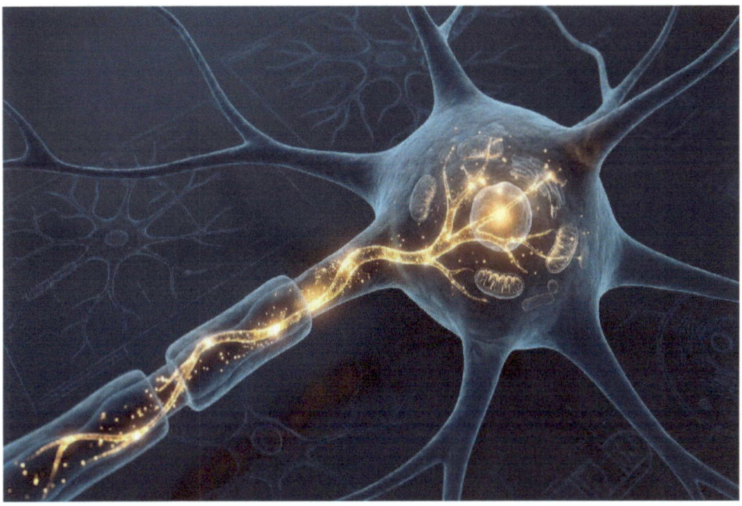

5. INSULIN METABOLISM

You are not eating more, you are burning differently.

Estradiol is an insulin sensitizer. When it drops, cells become resistant.

- **The Paradox:** You eat the same calories as you did 5 years ago, but you gain weight around your belly.
- **Apex Action:** You need to change your macronutrients.

    - **Reduce:** Simple carbohydrates and starches.
    - **Hack:** Use **berberine** or apple cider vinegar before meals.

6. HRT vs. BHRT: THE LIFE-SAVING DISTINCTION

Not all hormones are created equal.

- **Synthetic HRT:** Increased risk of cancer/blood clots.
- **BHRT (Bioidentical):** Hormones that are molecularly identical to your own.
    - **Transdermal Estradiol (Gel/Patch):** Does not pass through the liver, zero risk of thrombosis.
    - **Micronized Progesterone:** Protects the breasts and calms the brain.

The Critical Window:

The therapy is protective *only* if started within 10 years of the last cycle (or before age 60). Timing is everything.

7. THE "OPEN" LIPID PROFILE (Endothelial Security)

Heart and arteries without protection.

Until menopause, estrogen keeps arteries flexible. When estrogen levels drop, women's cardiovascular risk exceeds that of men.

- **The Risk:** Immediate increase in small, dense LDL and collapse of HDL.

- **Apex Action:** Monitoring must be forensic. Don't just look at "total cholesterol."

  Request **ApoB** (number of atherogenic particles) and **Lipoprotein (a)**.

  Transdermal BHRT is the only therapy that stabilizes the endothelium without increasing the risk of blood clots.

8. HARDWARE OVERHAUL: MUSCLE, PROTEIN, AND FASCIA

The physical structure collapses without estrogen. Here's how to rebuild it.

A. Muscle as an Endocrine Organ

Without estrogen, you lose bone and muscle at twice the rate.

- **The Protocol:** Lift heavy weights.

  You must create a mechanical stimulus to produce **myokines** that balance the Aepi equation.

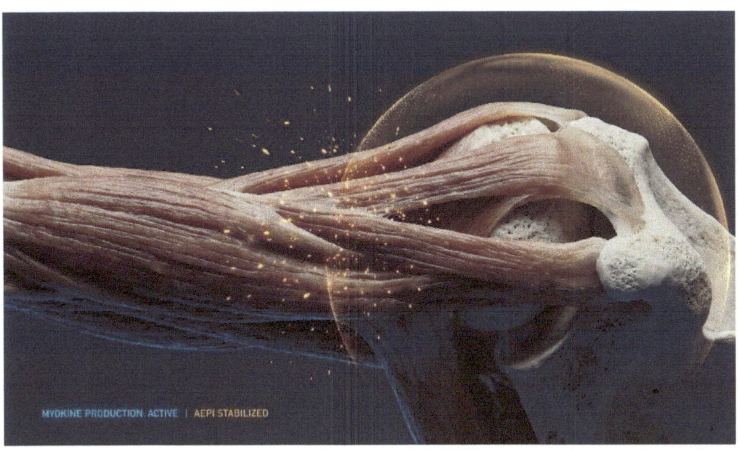

B. Anabolic Resistance (The Protein Threshold)

During menopause, muscles become "deaf" to growth signals. It is no longer enough to "eat protein."

- **The Concept:** Without estrogen, a higher concentration of amino acids (especially leucine) is needed to activate muscle protein synthesis (mTOR).
- **Apex Action:** Don't settle for 1g of protein per kg (standard dose). At this stage, the target should be **1.6g - 2g/kg**, with at least **30-40g of high-quality protein per meal.** This is the only way to overcome the "anabolic threshold" and make heavy training effective.

C. The Collapse of Collagen

The loss of estrogen causes a **30%** collapse **of** skin and fascial **collagen** in the first 5 years.

- **The Risk:** Pelvic organ prolapse, tendon fragility, and joint pain.
- **Apex Action: Collagen peptides (20g/day)** combined with vitamin C and copper. At this stage, collagen is not a cosmetic, it is a structural safety component.

9. APEX SUPPLEMENTATION: THE SURVIVAL KIT

In addition to hormones, non-negotiable nutrients.

1. **Creatine Monohydrate (5g/day):** The "backup battery" for neurons. Clears brain fog.

2. **Elite Molecule: S-EQUOL:** Directly supplements fermented **S-Equol** (super-soy) to act on hot flashes and skin.
3. **Magnesium Taurate:** Cardiac protection.
4. **Vitamin K2 + D3:** To put calcium back into the bones.

10. GENITO-URINARY SYNDROME (GSM)

Vaginal dryness and cystitis are tissue atrophy.

- **Apex Action: Local Estriol (Cream/Ovules).** Local estrogen does *not* enter the systemic bloodstream. It is safe and restores the microbiome and comfort.

SAFETY OFFICER'S WORD

"Menopause is a 'Security Breach' event. Barriers come down.

You have two choices: accept decline as 'natural', or take control of the control panel.

Bioidentical therapy, weights, high-dose protein, and creatine are not vanities. They are tools that allow you to live your Second Spring with the same power as your first, but with twice the wisdom.

PART 8

TOWARDS ZERO INJURIES

(Predictive Maintenance and the Future of the Species)

"We have cleaned up the air. We have filtered the water. We have nourished the mitochondria and synchronized the hormones. Now, let's look up from the microscope and gaze at the horizon. Twentieth-century medicine was the art of repairing broken pieces: it waited for the symptom (the failure) to intervene. It was reactive medicine. Safety Biohacker medicine is predictive. It is the engineering of calculated risk. We don't wait for the system to collapse. We use data to predict wear and tear and intervene when the damage is still invisible. This is the concept of 'Zero Accidents'."

THE PARADIGM SHIFT

We have reached the end of the journey, but the beginning of a new era. Until a few years ago, longevity was a gamble based on genetics and luck. Today, it is an engineering problem that can be solved through data management.

In this final section, we combine biology (wetware) with technology (software).

- You are no longer just a biological body.
- You are a **Cyber-Physical System**.

Thanks to tools such as your smartphone, AI, and wearable sensors, you can now have control dashboards that were once exclusive to NASA . But having the data is not enough. You need

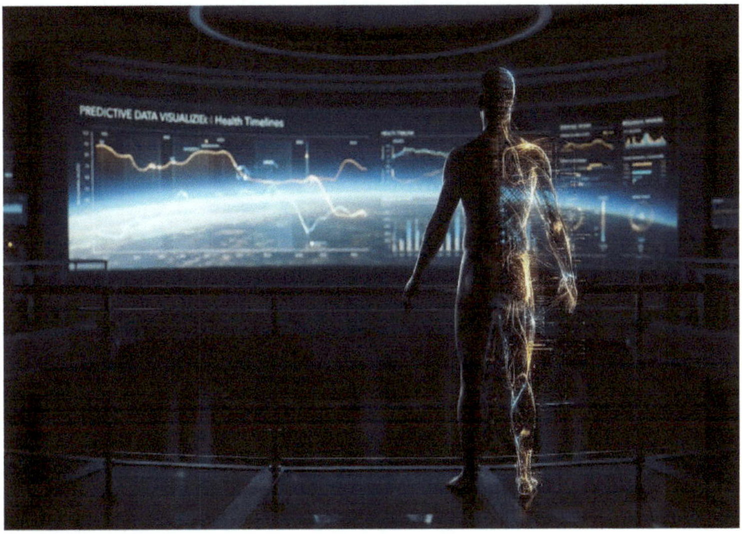

to have the philosophy to interpret it.

WHAT YOU WILL FIND IN THIS SECTION

This is not a formal conclusion. It is the operational launch into the future.

1. **Human 2.0 (Chapter 30):** How to build your **Digital Twin**. You will learn to use AI not to write emails, but as a personal "Safety Guard" that simulates the effects of diet and stress before they affect your real body.
2. **Zero Injury (Chapter 31):** The philosophy of **Predictive Maintenance**. Because the goal is not to live forever, but to live without preventable failures until the end of the operating cycle.

THE FINAL MESSAGE

Biohacking is not about becoming robots. It is about becoming more resilient, more aware, and freer from the fear of disease. Technology is the map. Biology is the territory. You are the pilot.

Let's start the engines for the final lap.

CHAPTER 30

HUMAN 2.0: AI, DIGITAL TWINS, AND THE FUTURE OF THE SPECIES

"We are the last generation of 'blind' human beings. Until yesterday, medicine was reactive: it waited for the failure (the symptom) to intervene. Today it is preventive. Tomorrow it will be predictive. Human 2.0 is not a cyborg full of chips under the skin. It is a human be , who uses data to build a 'Digital Twin' on which to test stressors before they affect the biological body. We are no longer passengers of our biology, we are the pilots. And AI is our safety co-pilot."

Imagine you are a Formula 1 engineer. Would you send your car onto the track without sensors, waiting to see smoke coming from the engine to realize that something is wrong? Absolutely not.

Yet that's how we've been managing the human body for centuries. We drive blindly until we feel pain.

Safety Biohacking introduces a paradigm shift: the construction of the **Digital Twin**.

This technology, developed by NASA to simulate spacecraft failures before launch, is now accessible in your "Poor Man's Lab."

1. THE TWIN'S ARCHITECTURE (Building the Biological Avatar)

Your Digital Twin is a dynamic mathematical model of your metabolism, built on three layers of data.

LAYER 1: THE SOURCE CODE (Static Genetics)

- **Input:** Your DNA "Raw Data" file
- **What it tells the AI:** "This system has an *MTHFR* variant, is *APOE4,* and metabolizes caffeine slowly."
- **The Advantage:** The AI knows in advance which drugs or supplements will be toxic to you (Pharmacogenomics).

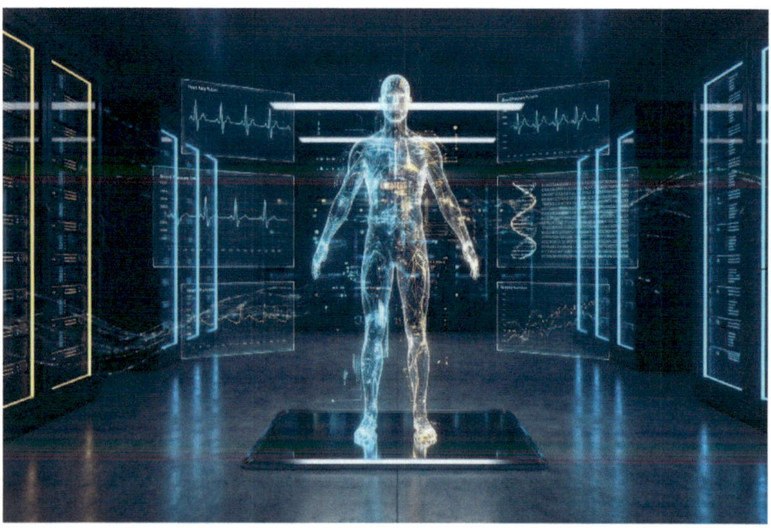

LAYER 2: TELEMETRY (Real-Time Data)

- **Input:** Data from your **smartphone** ecosystem - Wearable

- **Metrics:** HRV, Skin Temperature, SpO2, Sleep.
- **What it tells the AI:** "Right now, the system is under stress. Nighttime recovery was only 40%."

LAYER 3: DEEP DIAGNOSTICS (Periodic Biomarkers)

- **Input:** Quarterly blood tests (PCR, ApoB, HbA1c, Testosterone).
- **What it tells the AI:** "The arteries are slowly becoming inflamed, even though the HRV seems fine."

2. THE BIOREACTIVE FEEDBACK LOOP (The Smart-Cave)

The Digital Twin shouldn't just talk to you via your smartphone; it should talk to your home.

It's not enough to know that you're sleeping poorly; you need an environment that reacts to protect you. This is the integration between Biohacking and IoT (Internet of Things).

- **Operating Scenario:** Your Galaxy Ring detects a +0.4°C increase in skin temperature and a decrease in HRV during REM sleep (early signs of fever or overtraining).
- **Apex Action (Passive):** Instead of sending you a notification that you will only read in the morning (too late), the Digital Twin communicates with your Smart Home:

1. It instructs the smart thermostat to lower the room temperature by 1.5°C to facilitate thermoregulation.
2. It activates the humidifier to optimize the respiratory mucosa.
3. It completely dims the standby LEDs on appliances to maximize melatonin.

This is **Passive Bio-Security**: the environment takes care of you while you sleep.

3. "IN SILICO" TESTING & LONGITUDINAL SIMULATION

Shift the risk from the biological body to the digital body.

A. The "In Silico" Test

Don't try a diet "to see how it goes." Ask your Digital Twin: *"What will happen to my ApoB cholesterol if I switch to a Carnivore diet for 3 months, considering my APOE4 genetics?"*

- **AI result:** *"CRITICAL RISK. Estimated 35% increase in oxidized LDL. Not recommended."*

The best injury is the one that never happened because it was virtually discarded.

B. The 2050 Preview (Longitudinal Simulation)

The test doesn't have to be limited to the next 3 months.

- **Apex Action:** Ask your Digital Twin to simulate your health trajectory until 2050, based on your current rate of telomere shortening and arterial plaque buildup.
- **The Value:** Seeing a rendered video simulation of your 80-year-old self walking frail (sarcopenia) or strong, based on whether or not you choose to lift weights **today**, is the most powerful behavioral driver ever created. AI makes invisible consequences visible.

4. GENERATIVE MICRONUTRITION (Real-Time Compounding)

We move AI from advice to production.

Instead of taking a generic multivitamin (which is a statistical average), Human 2.0 uses "on-demand" delivery systems.

- **The Concept:** AI analyzes the day's telemetry: high stress at work, exposure to PM2.5 in traffic, intense running session.
- **Apex Action:** When you return home, a precision machine (concept "Nutrient Printer") compounds a liquid "shot" containing electrolytes, N-Acetyl-Cysteine (for pollution), and Magnesium, calibrated to the milligram based on what you consumed today.

You don't supplement by guesswork. You supplement by **exact compensation**.

5. BIOETHICS: THE BIOLOGICAL TRUST EQUATION (Bt)

We need to define the relationship between humans and algorithms. We don't want humans to be "slaves," but rather "augmented."

We define your decision-making stability with this formula:

Bt = (Data Accuracy x User Agency) /Algorithmic Dependency

Safety Insight:

If your ability to listen to your body decreases as AI use increases, the denominator grows and your Biological Trust (Bt) collapses.

- **The Golden Rule:** The goal of Human 2.0 is to maintain **Agency**. AI proposes, the pilot disposes.
- **Scenario:** AI says, "Low recovery, rest." But you feel in a creative and energetic "flow" state.
- **The Action:** You must have the courage and sensitivity to ignore the algorithm. AI is the map, you are the territory. If you lose touch with the territory, the map is useless.

6. THE "ORACLE PROBLEM" (Human-Sensor Calibration)

AI is powerful, but sensors can fail or be "noisy." A Safety Officer does not blindly trust telemetry without a validation procedure.

- **The Concept:** If your Galaxy Ring shows a drop in HRV but you feel great, there may be a positioning error or a bug in the firmware.
- **Apex Action (Manual Override):** Every week, perform a **Subjective Perception Audit**. Human 2.0 must be able to "feel" their own heart rate and temperature without looking at the screen. If the discrepancy between Perception and AI Data exceeds 20%, the system must be recalibrated.
- **Safety Insight:** AI trains your sensitivity, it does not replace it. "Feeling" is the last firewall against technological failure.

7. PRIVACY AND SOVEREIGNTY (The Security Protocol)

Biological data is the new oil. Handing over your DNA to insecure clouds is a risk.

- **The "Local-First" Protocol:** The Safety Biohacker stores the Digital Twin locally.

- **Hardware:** Your smartphone or PC acts as a secure server. Health data processing must take place "on-device," not in the cloud. You hold the keys.

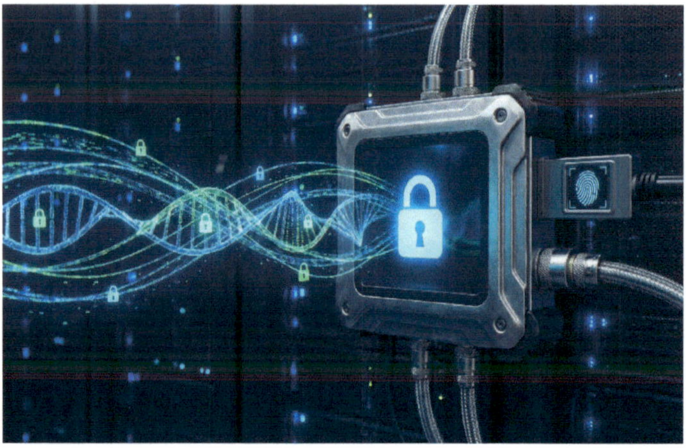

8. BIOLOGICAL CYBER SECURITY (Identity Protection)

Nowadays, stealing your Digital Twin is the ultimate crime. If someone has your genetic code and telemetry, they can simulate (and predict) your every weakness.

- **The "Air-Gap" Protocol:** The most critical data (Layer 1 - DNA) should be stored locally in an isolated partition that never touches the internet, except for specific encrypted queries.
- **Apex Action:** Use apps that support **"Homomorphic Encryption."** This technology allows AI to analyze your data and give you advice without ever "seeing" the raw, unencrypted data. Your biology is your private key; never give it to anyone.

APEX ACTION: BUILD YOUR DATA LAKE

Don't wait for the future. Start collecting the building blocks today.

1. **Centralize:** Use **a Health App** as a central hub to connect your ring, watch, and scale.
2. **Digitize your blood:** Transcribe every blood test into a "Master File" (Excel/CSV).
3. **Visualize:** Use the data to ask the AI: *"Act like a longevity expert. Project my health 10 years into the future if I maintain these blood sugar and sleep trends."*

SAFETY OFFICER'S WORD

" .0 is not a computer made of flesh, but a human being who has finally turned on the light in a dark room. The Digital Twin is not there to tell you how to live, but to show you the consequences of your choices before they become irreversible.

Remember: AI is an exceptional co-pilot in calculating trajectories and analyzing telemetry, but it has no skin to protect and no beating heart. If the sensor says 'rest' but your spirit screams 'action,' trust the territory, not the map. Technology should serve to increase your sensitivity, not replace it. Own your data, protect your privacy, and use the algorithm as a mirror, never as a master."

CHAPTER 31

ZERO ACCIDENTS (The Philosophy of Predictive Maintenance)

"In the factory, zero accidents is a utopian but necessary target. In biology, it is the only sensible strategy for longevity. An accident is not just a torn ligament. Cancer is an accident of DNA. Alzheimer's is an accident of neuronal metabolism. Burnout is an accident of neurotransmitters. The Safety Biohacker does not seek immortality out of fear of death. He seeks total functionality out of respect for life. The goal of is not to live forever, but to die young... as late as possible."

We have reached the end of the manual.

You have the tools (Air, Water, Lights, Digital Twin). Now you need a management strategy.

Contemporary medicine is based on **Reactive Maintenance**: the part breaks (you get sick), we go to the repair shop (hospital).

This approach is expensive, painful, and inefficient.

The Safety Biohacker applies **Predictive Maintenance**. And to do so, they must act like a chief engineer who knows the laws of thermodynamics.

1. BIO-PHYSICS: THE WAR ON ENTROPY (Delta S)

Why do we age? The answer is a differential equation.

In physics, Entropy is the inexorable tendency of every closed system to move from order to disorder. Injury is the moment when Entropy wins over the Energy of the system.

We can define the limit of the system's maneuverability with the **Dynamics of Thermal Death**.

The rate of aging is the speed at which entropy (Delta S) exceeds the capacity for cellular repair (Phi):

Where:

- Delta S is accumulated **disorder** (waste, inflammation, broken DNA).
- Phi is **Repair Capacity** (driven by sleep, autophagy, peptides, and light).

Safety Insight:

When Delta S > Phi, injury is only a matter of time.

The entire Master Plan of this book (from clean air to hormesis) has a single mathematical purpose: to keep Phi constantly higher than Delta S.

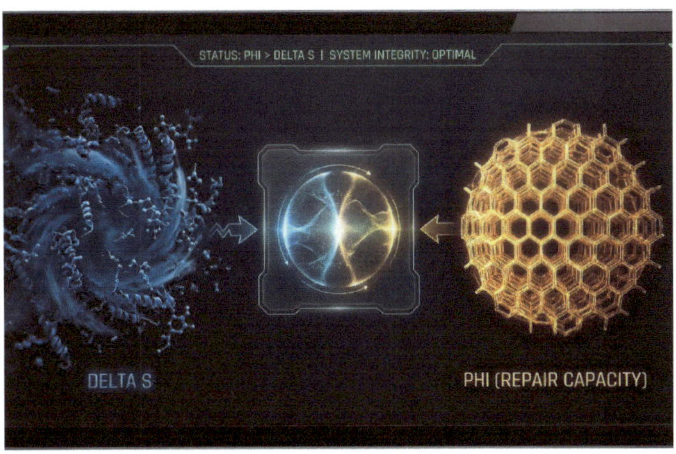

2. ENGINEERING: THE PRINCIPLE OF REDUNDANCY (R sys)

Safety is not just maintenance, it is Reserve.

In aeronautics, a system is only safe if it is redundant: if the main engine fails, there is an auxiliary one.

The human body is naturally redundant (two kidneys, two lungs). But modern stress consumes this reserve.

The elite biohacker builds **Metabolic Redundancy**.

The Redundancy Equation:

R sys = Maximum Capacity/Operating Load

- **If R sys is around 1:** You are fragile. You live on the edge. A mild virus or a sleepless night is enough to cause a crash.
- **If R sys > 3:** You are a crash-proof (antifragile) system.

Apex Action: It's not enough to "feel good." You need to build a buffer.

- If you can fast for 48 hours without losing lucidity, you have energy redundancy.
- If your arteries can withstand a sudden spike in pressure without rupturing, you have vascular redundancy.

3. THE MTBF (Mean Time Between Failures) RULE

The goal is to extend the time between failures to "infinity."

How? With **Daily Micro-Maintenance**.

Many people live in the "Red Zone" for 11 months, hoping to repair themselves in two weeks in August. Biologically, this is impossible.

The "Pit Stop" Protocol:

- Sleep (Module 4) is your mandatory Pit Stop.
- Breathing (Module 9) is the engine cooling system.

If you skip Pit Stops to go faster, you will break the engine on the next lap.

4. THE DIGITAL "BLACK BOX"

When there is a failure, don't guess. Look at the data.

When a plane crashes, the black box is analyzed. When you get sick, tear a muscle, or have an emotional breakdown, you need to perform a **Forensic Audit** using your digital ecosystem (smartphone + wearable).

"T-Minus 14" Protocol:

Don't look at today's data. The injury did not occur when you felt the pain, but in the invisible micro-injuries of the previous two weeks.

Analyze the 14 days before the crash:

1. *Was there a downward trend in nighttime HRV?*
2. *Was your basal temperature slowly rising (inflammation)?*
3. *Was deep sleep fragmented?*

The Black Box tells you why the wing detached. If you don't learn from the data, the mistake will happen again.

5. THE BIOLOGICAL "AIR-GAP" PROTOCOL

Risk Compartmentalization and Baseline Reset.

In computer security, an "Air-Gapped" system is physically isolated from insecure networks. In Biohacking, it means having periods of "Total Cleanup" where the system receives no potentially corrupted external input.

Apex Action: Schedule **3 days of "Biological Air-Gap"** quarterly:

- Zero technology (EMF-free, no notifications).
- Zero processed food (only single ingredients).
- Zero digital stimuli (dopamine detox).

Safety Insight: This is a forced reset of the Black Box. It serves to recalibrate the sensors and your perception of your real baseline, free from everyday "noise."

6. PSYCHOLOGY OF SAFETY: THE PELTZMAN PARADOX

Why feeling safe is dangerous.

Economist Sam Peltzman discovered that seat belts increased accidents because people drove worse, feeling protected.

Apex Action: Don't use biohacking to excuse risky behavior ("I take milk thistle so I can get drunk"). Tools are meant to eliminate the damage of unavoidable risks, not increase them.

7. BEYOND RESILIENCE: ANTIFRAGILITY

Conventional medicine wants to make you *robust* (like a rock). We want to make you **antifragile** (like the immune system).

Zero injuries are not achieved by wrapping your body in cotton wool, but by exposing it to micro-doses of calculated chaos (Hormesis: cold, heat, weights) to teach it to repair itself and increase R sys.

8. EPIGENETIC LEGACY (Legacy Safety)

When you apply Safety Biohacking, you are not just optimizing yourself.

Epigenetics is inheritable. You are "cleaning up the code" for your children. The final act of "Zero Injury" is to break the chain of biological trauma in your family.

9. THE EXIT STRATEGY: THE SQUARE CURVE

The ultimate KPI of your existence.

What is the goal? **Morbidity Compression**.

Most people experience a "slow death" that begins at age 60.

We aim for the **Square Curve**:

Maintain very high **Functional Vigour** (95%) until 90, 100 years or more. Then, when the system reaches its genetic limit (currently estimated at 120 years), it collapses vertically in a matter of days.

Apex Action:

Monitor your physical performance. If at age 80 you can still sprint, lift your own weight, and solve complex problems, you have "squared the curve" and maintained Phi > Delta S.

Live strong, die fast. Don't become a burden, but a resource until your last breath.

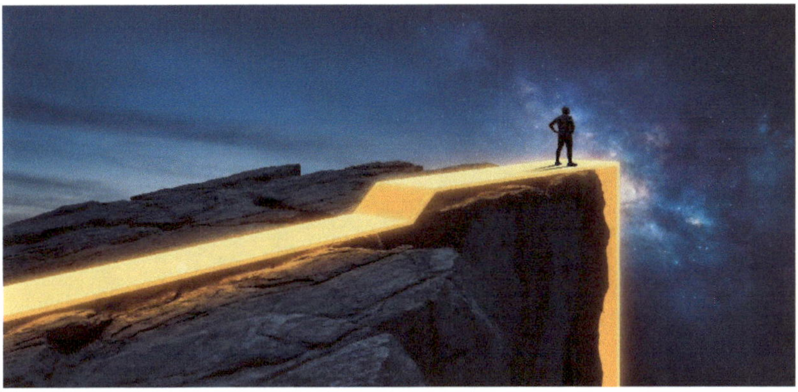

10. THE DEMOCRATIZATION OF SECURITY

The mission is to demonstrate that security is democratic.

Fasting, Sun, Cold, Breathing, and Sleep are free.

Human 2.0 is not the one with the most money. It is the one with the most **Awareness**.

WORD OF THE SAFETY OFFICER

"Zero accidents is a mindset.

It's waking up in the morning and asking yourself, 'Am I increasing my Phi Repair Capacity today, or am I letting Delta S Entropy win?

You don't have to be perfect. You just have to have a margin of safety.

Safety is not the absence of danger. It is the presence of competence."

PART 9

SPECIES HORIZONS: SPECULATIVE BIOSECURITY

(Transhumanism, Exponential Technologies, and the Evolutionary Leap)

Up to this point in the book, we have acted as high-precision mechanics: we have cleaned the filters, changed the oil, and optimized the engine of a vintage car (the human body Sapiens). In this final part, we stop being mechanics and become aerospace engineers. We are no longer trying to make the car last a few more years. We are trying to figure out how to turn it into a spaceship while it is running. This section deals with 'Speculative Bio-Safety': the analysis of the risks and opportunities of technologies that seem like magic today but will be standard hospital practice tomorrow. The Safety Biohacker does not ignore the future. He anticipates it so as not to be overwhelmed by it."

THE BRIDGE STRATEGY

Why should a manual talk about nanotechnology or cryonics?

Because Biohacking also has an unspoken ultimate goal: **survival of the technological gap.**

We are the "Bridge Generation."

- We were born too late to die of trivial infections (thanks to antibiotics).

- We were born (perhaps) too early to benefit from the complete defeat of aging.

The task of this Part 9 is to provide you with a mental map for crossing this bridge. The technologies we will explore (CRISPR, Biostasis, Upload) are not "science fiction."

They are **probabilistic risk scenarios**.

If you apply the protocols from Parts 1-8, your reward is to arrive alive and lucid at your appointment with Part 9.

Welcome to the Event Horizon.

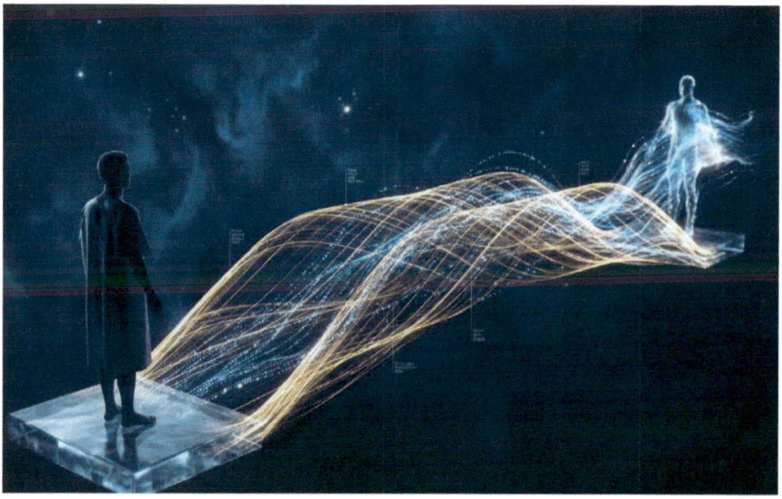

CHAPTER 32

THE EVENT HORIZON (Transhumanism and Future Risk Management)

Natural evolution is slow, cruel, and inefficient. It takes millions of years to make a small upgrade. Technological evolution is exponential. The Safety Biohacker views these technologies not as saviors, but as powerful new tools that require new safety protocols. Hacking death requires 'Root Access' permissions to biology that we do not yet understand. And if the system crashes at that level, there is no reboot."

Here is the **Future Safety Scale**: 6 levels of intervention to manage the transition from Human 1.0 to Human 2.0 (and beyond).

1. THE BRIDGE STRATEGY (Longevity Escape Velocity)

The operational "why."

The key concept is **Longevity Escape Velocity (LEV)**. It is the tipping point where, for every year you survive thanks to current biohacking, scientific progress gains *more* than a year of life expectancy for you.

- **The Risk:** If you reach 2050 with a compromised vascular system or an atrophied brain, you will be too fragile for rejuvenation therapies.

- **Apex Action:** Your lifestyle today is not just about "feeling good"; it's about buying time. You are taking care of the vehicle so that it can cross the finish line into the next era.

2. ACTIVE GENETIC EDITING (CRISPR 3.0 & Prime Editing)

From prevention to code rewriting.

Today we modulate gene expression (epigenetics). Tomorrow we will rewrite the code (genetics).

- **The Promise:** Delete risk variants (such as APOE4 for Alzheimer's) with an injection of viral vectors. A "Find and Replace" for DNA.
- **The Safety Risk (Off-Target Effects):** DNA is a "spaghetti" code. If you cut a piece here, you could activate a fatal error (cancer) elsewhere.
- **The Future Protocol:** The Safety Officer's rule will be **"No Editing without Undo."** We will only accept reversible gene therapies or those equipped with a molecular "kill switch."

3. ENDOGENOUS NANOTECHNOLOGY (Internal Hardware)

Mechanical enhancement of wetware.

Imagine *Respirocytes* (artificial red blood cells) that carry 200 times more oxygen, or nanobots that mechanically clean arteries of plaque.

- **The Promise:** Continuous maintenance and super-physical performance.
- **The Security Risk (Malicious Bio-Hacking):** If your nanobots are connected, they are hackable. Computer malware could cause a physical heart attack.
- **The Future Protocol: Air-Gapped Biological Firewalls**. Internal medical devices should never have a public IP address accessible from the outside.

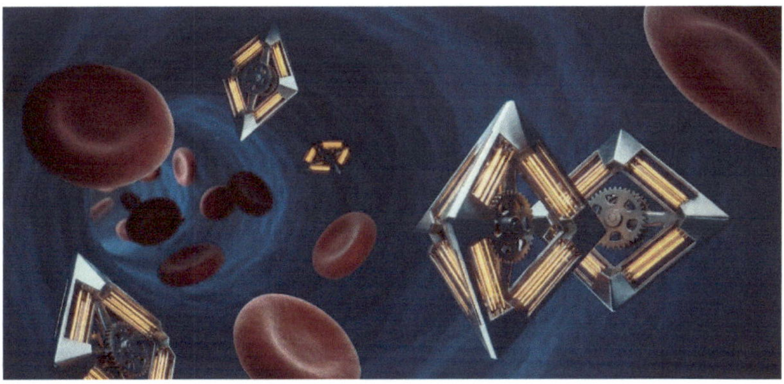

4. SUPPLY CHAIN INDEPENDENCE: 4D BIOPRINTING

On-demand replacement parts.

The current transplant system is fragile (waiting for donors, rejection).

- **The Promise:** Printing new organs using your own stem cells (iPSCs).
- **The 4D Concept:** Tissues that not only have shape (3D), but adapt and grow over time (4D).

- **The Safety Advantage: Total Redundancy**. You will be able to replace a "worn-out" heart at age 90 preventively, like changing an air filter, without waiting for it to fail.
- **The Future Protocol: Autologous Only**. Only organs printed with your DNA for zero risk of rejection.

5. THE CONTINGENCY PLAN: BIOSTASIS AND CRYONICS

The ambulance to the future (Plan B).

If the body gives out before longevity medicine is ready, what is the backup plan?

- **The Concept:** Cryonics (through **vitrification**) is not for the dead, but for "patients who cannot be recovered with current technology." It is a bet on stopping biological degradation while waiting for future cures.
- **Risk Analysis:** It is uncertain, but the odds are mathematically greater than zero (unlike decomposition). For a Safety Officer, it is the emergency fire extinguisher: you hope you won't use it, but you keep it charged.

6. DIGITAL IMMORTALITY (Mind Uploading)

The ultimate backup.

If biological hardware is destined for entropy, the only final solution is to migrate the software (Consciousness) to silicon.

- **The Security Risk (The Copy Paradox):** If you copy your brain onto a computer, is it *really* you, or just a digital clone while you die?
- **The Future Protocol: Continuity of Consciousness.** We reject "Copy & Delete." We only accept progressive integration (e.g., Neuralink), where the brain is enhanced/replaced neuron by neuron over time,

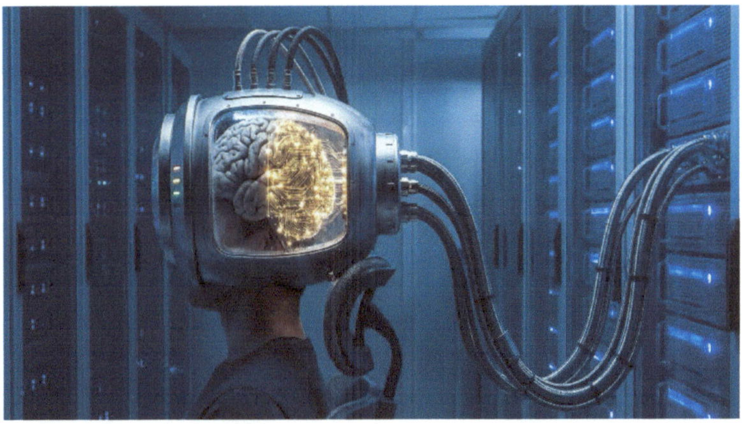

keeping the self intact.

SAFETY OFFICER'S WORD

"Indefinite Lifespan is not vanity. It is the logical consequence of Safety. If we love life, it is our duty to protect it with every means that physics makes available to us. Today we use broccoli and sleep. Tomorrow we will use nanobots and bioprinting. The tool changes, but the mission remains the same: ***Preserve the System.****"*

PART 10

EPILOGUE

"We began this journey with a breath of fresh air and ended it looking digital immortality in the eye. You hold in your hands the operating manual for the most complex system in the known universe: your body. Until yesterday, you were a passenger, often asleep, at the mercy of events. From today, you are the Pilot. And as every Safety Officer knows, the privilege of command comes with the burden of responsibility."

No further technical explanations are needed. What is needed are 10 Rules of Engagement to navigate the chaos of the modern world without losing your way.

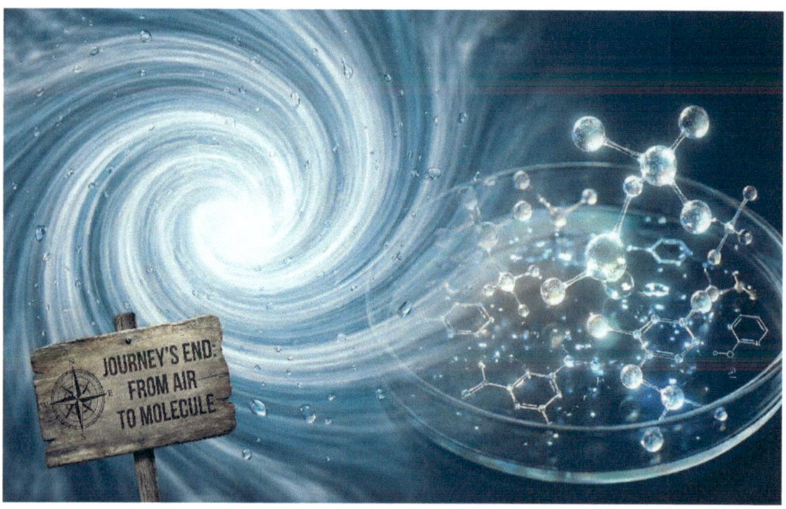

CHAPTER 33

THE 10 COMMANDMENTS OF THE SAFETY BIOHACKER

1. SAFETY FIRST Never follow an Instagram trend if you don't understand the biological mechanism behind it. The first rule is to do no harm to the system. If a protocol makes you feel worse, stop. Your feelings trump any guru.

2. BE THE SCIENTIST, NOT JUST THE GUINEA PIG Measure, test, validate. If you can't measure it, you can't manage it. Don't accept dogma: only accept data.

3. ENVIRONMENT BEATS WILLPOWER Don't rely on your willpower; it's a finite resource. Clean up your environment (air, water, light) so that healthy choices are the default. If your home is toxic, you will be toxic.

4. RESPECT RHYTHMS We are rhythmic beings in an arrhythmic world. Protect your sleep and your circadian cycle as if they were sacred. You can't hack the sun.

5. MICRO-STRESS, MACRO-RECOVERY Use stress (cold, heat, weights, fasting) to grow, but don't live in chronic stress. Stress is the medicine, recovery is the cure. Without recovery, there is only wear and tear.

6. NUTRITION IS CODE Food isn't just calories or fuel. It's information that programs your genes in real time. Every bite is a command: "Inflamm" or "Repair." Write good code.

7. PRECISION SUPPLEMENTATION Supplements are not candy, they are tactical tools. Don't use generic supermarket products full of fillers. Choose only bioavailable (methylated, liposomal, chelated) and certified forms. It's better to take nothing than to take low-quality supplements that intoxicate the liver.

8. PROTECT THE TRIBE An isolated biohacker is a vulnerable system. Share safety. Protect your family. Oxytocin is the most powerful anti-inflammatory.

9. THE GOAL IS FREEDOM Optimal health, muscles, and longevity are not the ultimate goal. They are the means. The goal is to be free to work, love, create, and explore without the body being a limitation.

10. ZERO INJURIES Aim for perfection to achieve excellence. Try to live each day by reducing entropy and increasing energy. Don't die in installments. Live strong, until the end.

Dr. Andrea Bancalà *Safety Officer & The Safety Biohacker*

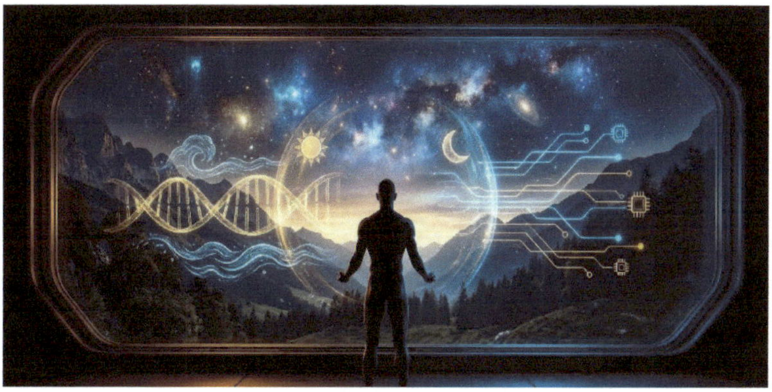

ACKNOWLEDGEMENTS

No complex system, however optimized, can thrive in a vacuum.

As we have explored in these pages, human biology is an architecture of relationships: between cells, between microbiomes, and, above all, between individuals.

Writing this manual was a solitary engineering feat, but its foundations rest on a support network that deserves to be honored.

The Original Tribe: My first thanks go to my family, my primordial "safety net."

Growing up in the Tivoli area taught me that the stability of the territory is the precondition for any evolution.

Thank you for supporting my incessant curiosity, even when my thoughts seemed like obsessions and my questions challenged the tranquility of Sunday dinners.

You are my **System Redundancy**: the certainty of your presence is what allows me to push beyond the horizon.

The Scientific Front: I owe a debt of immense gratitude to my colleagues at the Istituto Superiore di Sanità (ISS) in Rome, Italy.

Working at the heart of occupational safety in healthcare at the national level has been my most valuable training ground.

Thank you for instilling in me a reverence for data, the importance of protocol, and the ethical responsibility that comes with handling information that impacts human lives.

If I can call myself a true **Safety Officer** today, it is because I learned from you how to map the complexity of risk. This book is imbued with the DNA of that research and rigor.

The Masters of the Invisible: Thanks to the pioneers who looked beyond reactive medicine.

To the scientists and bioengineers who transformed biology from a "black box" to open-source software. This manual is a synthesis of your tireless work in mapping the frontiers of Human 2.0.

To You, The Pilot: Finally, the most important thanks go to you, the reader.

Thank you for choosing not to be a "sleeping passenger" on the journey of your life.

Every time an individual takes responsibility for their own biology, the background noise of disease decreases and the frequency of collective health increases.

You are the **Safety Tribe** that will transform biohacking from an elite practice to a new evolutionary standard.

Safety Officer's Note: Gratitude is not just a feeling; it is a biochemical command that instantly reduces cortisol and optimizes vagal tone. Consider these thanks as the final protocol in this book: recognizing the value of your network is the first step in solidifying your new identity.

ABOUT THE AUTHOR

Andrea Bancalà (Tivoli-Rome-Italy 1990) is neither a wellness "guru" nor an improvised biohacker. He is an expert professional in chemical, biological, and radioactive safety, as well as being responsible for specific risk emergencies and an expert in special waste disposal. He currently works **at the Italian National Institute of Health (Istituto Superiore di Sanità - ISS)** in Rome, Italy, as **a Safety Officer**.

Born in Tivoli in July 1990, he has developed a vision based on the integration of rigorous health surveillance methodology and cutting-edge research on molecular longevity.

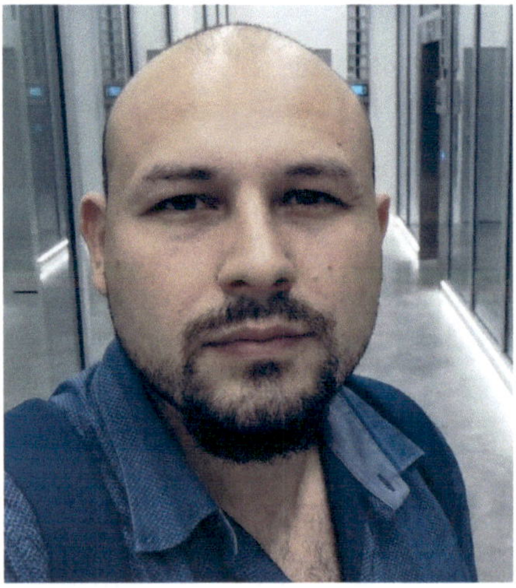

The Bridge between Surveillance and Optimization

Andrea's career in public safety has allowed him to analyze the systemic risks that threaten modern health.

Starting from the data, he identified a fundamental critical issue: a 21st-century environment managed with reactive protocols that only intervene after damage has occurred.

As the founder of **"The Safety Biohacker"** philosophy, he has transposed industrial safety procedures to human biology, making biological optimization a scientific, democratic, and health ROI-oriented practice.

His philosophy is pragmatic: *"Safety is not the absence of danger, but the presence of competence."*

Scientific Validation and Bibliographic Architecture of "The Safety Biohacker" Protocol: Forensic Analysis of Molecular Mechanisms and Clinical Evidence

1. Introduction: The Epistemology of Safety in Complex Biological Systems

This technical report constitutes the scientific validation infrastructure for the work "The Safety Biohacker." The objective of this document is to analyze the operational claims contained in the manuscript and anchor them to specific bibliographic references and randomized clinical studies.

The central philosophy of the text, which applies *Occupational Safety* protocols and the Deming Cycle (PDCA) to human biology, marks a fundamental transition from reactive medicine (symptom treatment) to condition-based predictive maintenance (CBM). This transition is not speculative but is based on a convergence of data from environmental toxicology, molecular biology, chronobiology, and tissue engineering.

The following analysis is structured to mirror the architecture of the book, providing for each chapter the scientific " " necessary to support the proposed biosafety protocols. Every statement regarding environmental toxicity, mitochondrial efficiency, or tissue regeneration is traced back to its primary source, ensuring that the "Class 0" protocol is not a theoretical construct but a documented physiological necessity.

PART 1: FOUNDATIONS AND BARRIERS (Environmental and Internal Remediation)

The first phase of the protocol requires a rigorous risk assessment of the environment in which the biological operator lives. Scientific literature unequivocally confirms that chronic exposure to ubiquitous pollutants is the main driver of *sterile inflammation*, precluding any attempt at subsequent performance optimization.

Chapter 1: Air and Water Engineering

The concept of "Aero-Toxicology" introduced in the text is supported by extensive literature that identifies fine particulate matter and indoor gases as powerful negative modulators of cardiovascular and cognitive physiology.

1.1 Fine Particulate Matter (PM2.5) as an Agent of Vascular Damage

The claim that PM2.5 is not only a pulmonary irritant but also a "vascular killer" is supported by the ability of these ultra-fine particles (<2.5 microns) to translocate through the alveolar barrier directly into the bloodstream.

- **Inflammatory Mechanism:** A critical meta-analysis quantified the acute inflammatory response to PM2.5 exposure, finding a statistically significant increase in systemic markers such as *Tumor Necrosis Factor-alpha* (TNF-α), Interleukin-6 (IL-6), and fibrinogen. Specifically, an increase of only 10 μg/m^3 of PM2.5 is associated with a 3.51% increase in TNF-α levels, a key cytokine in the inflammatory cascade leading to endothelial dysfunction.
- **Direct Cardiac Damage:** Studies in mouse models have shown that exposure to PM2.5 upregulates the expression of mRNA for TNF-α, IL-6, and IL-18 directly in cardiac tissue, suggesting a mechanism of local toxicity that goes beyond a simple systemic response. This validates the HEPA filtration protocol as a measure of cardiovascular protection, not just respiratory protection.
- **Long-Term Impact:** Epidemiological literature confirms that chronic exposure is a major risk factor for ischemic events and heart failure, acting through pulmonary and systemic oxidative stress, autonomic nervous system dysfunction (reduced HRV), and cholesterol accumulation in atherosclerotic plaques.

1.2 CO2 and Cognitive Decline (The COGfx Study)

Indoor ventilation is presented in the book as a "neuroengineering" intervention. This position is directly derived from the results of the *COGfx* study conducted by the Harvard T.H. Chan School of Public Health.

- **Performance Data:** The double-blind study showed that workers in "Green+" environments (low VOC concentration and high ventilation) achieved cognitive scores 101% higher than those in conventional environments. The critical data concerns CO2: levels commonly reached in meeting rooms or unventilated bedrooms (above 1000 ppm) are associated with significant deficits in higher cognitive functions, such as strategic planning and information utilization.
- **Linear Correlation:** A slowdown in response times and a reduction in productivity (throughput) were observed for every 500 ppm increase in CO2, with no apparent minimum safety threshold, validating the need for continuous monitoring using NDIR sensors.

1.3 Radon Gas: The Invisible Risk

The classification of radon as a top priority for home safety is imperative according to data from the EPA and WHO.

- **Carcinogenesis:** Radon is the second leading cause of lung cancer in the general population and the leading cause among non-smokers ( ). The mechanism of action is the release of high-energy alpha particles during radioactive decay, which cause direct damage and double-strand breaks in the DNA of the bronchial epithelium. The risk of cancer increases linearly by 16%

for every 100 Bq/m^3 increase in long-term average concentration.

- **Toxic Synergy:** There is a synergistic, supra-additive effect between radon exposure and cigarette smoking, which exponentially amplifies the risk of cancer. This data underscores the importance of active measurement, as radon is odorless and colorless, making dosimeters the only valid detection tool.

1.4 Water Contaminants and Microplastics

The book's insistence on reverse osmosis filtration and the removal of plastics in contact with food is supported by recent discoveries on the bioaccumulation of microplastics.

- **Infiltration into Atherosclerotic Plaques:** A landmark study published in the *New England Journal of Medicine* identified the presence of microplastics and nanoplastics within human atherosclerotic plaques. Patients with evidence of these contaminants in their plaques had a 4.5 times higher risk of myocardial infarction, stroke, or all-cause death in the following 34 months than those without detectable plastics.
- **Cellular Toxicity:** In vitro and animal model studies indicate that microplastics can penetrate cell membranes, inducing oxidative stress, inflammation, and alterations in endothelial gene expression. This confirms that unfiltered water and plastic containers represent a direct cardiovascular risk vector, not just an ecological problem.

Chapter 2: The Invisible Saboteurs (Systemic Toxicology)

The removal of metabolic interferents is a *prerequisite* for the effectiveness of any subsequent intervention.

2.1 Toxicity of Heavy Metals and Metallothioneins

The concept of "toxic load" can be scientifically quantified through the saturation of endogenous detoxification systems.

- **Mimicry Mechanism:** Metals such as lead, mercury, and cadmium exert their toxicity through "ionic mimicry," replacing essential minerals (zinc, calcium) in the active sites of enzymes, blocking their function. For example, cadmium displaces zinc in "zinc finger" proteins, compromising DNA repair.
- **The Role of Metallothioneins (MT):** MTs are cysteine-rich proteins that act as "sponges" for heavy metals. Their expression is regulated by the transcription factor MTF-1, which responds to metal- ss. However, chronic exposure can deplete MT synthesis capacity or saturate their binding sites, leading to cytotoxicity. This supports the need to nourish MT precursors (zinc, selenium, cysteine) and avoid exposure.

2.2 The Glyphosate Controversy and Glycine Replacement

The warning about glyphosate is based on specific biochemical hypotheses which, although debated, represent an unacceptable risk according to the Precautionary Principle.

- **Replacement Hypothesis:** Researcher Stephanie Seneff has proposed that glyphosate, being a structural analogue of the amino acid glycine, may be mistakenly incorporated into protein chains during synthesis, particularly in glycine-rich proteins such as collagen. This would lead to the production of structurally defective connective tissues.
- **Scientific Controversy:** Other proteomic studies have found no direct evidence of this substitution in actively dividing mammalian cells, suggesting that ribosomal quality control mechanisms are sufficient to prevent the error. However, given the epidemiological correlation between exposure and kidney/connective tissue diseases, the "Safety Biohacker" takes the conservative approach of total elimination (organic foods, detox), treating the hypothesis as a plausible risk to be mitigated.

2.3 Activated Carbon: Tactical Adsorption

The use of activated carbon as a "Safety Kit" for accidental toxin ingestion is based on the physical chemistry of adsorption.

- **Surface Dynamics:** Activated charcoal has an immense specific surface area (800-1200 m^2/g), capable of binding non-polar toxins, drugs, and organic compounds in the gastrointestinal tract by physical adsorption (Van der Waals forces), preventing their systemic absorption and interrupting enterohepatic recirculation.

Chapter 3: The Oral Gateway (Biological Dentistry)

The mouth is presented not as an isolated district, but as the primary interface between the external environment and the immune system.

3.1 Amalgam and Mercury Vapor Release

- **Toxicokinetics:** Studies cited by the IAOMT and published in toxicology journals show that amalgam fillings continuously release elemental mercury vapors. This release is intensified by mechanical events (chewing, bruxism) and thermal events (hot drinks). Inhaled mercury crosses the blood-brain barrier and accumulates in nerve tissue as a neurotoxin.
- **SMART Protocol:** The need for the SMART (*Safe Mercury Amalgam Removal Technique*) protocol is validated by evidence that unprotected removal generates acute peaks of mercury exposure for both the patient and the operator, far exceeding occupational safety limits.

3.2 The Toxicity of Devitalized Teeth

The theory of focal infection has been rehabilitated thanks to modern DNA sequencing techniques.

- **Anaerobic Microbiome:** Genetic analyses (PCR) on asymptomatic devitalized teeth have revealed the persistent presence of pathogenic anaerobic bacteria (e.g., *Fusobacterium*, *Porphyromonas*) within the dentinal tubules, which are impossible to sterilize completely. These bacteria produce powerful enzymatic toxins, such as thioethers and mercaptans.

- **Mitochondrial Inhibition:** Research conducted by Boyd Haley has shown that these toxins (thioethers) can irreversibly inhibit key enzymes in the electron transport chain in mitochondria, reducing ATP production and suggesting a direct link between endodontic pathologies and chronic fatigue or systemic diseases.

3.3 NICO (Necrotizing Inflammatory Cavities) and RANTES

The work of Dr. Johann Lechner has identified cavitations (NICO/FDOJ) as hidden sources of inflammation.

- **Immune Signaling:** Areas of fatty osteonecrosis of the jaw (often at sites of wisdom tooth extraction) show massive overexpression of the chemokine RANTES (CCL5). RANTES levels in these lesions can be up to 30 times higher than in healthy tissue. This cytokine is implicated in the progression of autoimmune (multiple sclerosis), neurodegenerative, and oncological (breast cancer) diseases, acting as an accelerator of metastasis and systemic inflammation.
- **Radiological Blindness:** The confirmation that these lesions are often invisible on 2D X-rays validates the mandatory use of CBCT (Cone Beam) or transalveolar ultrasonography (CaviTAU) for diagnosis.

3.4 Mouthwashes and Blood Pressure

- **The Entero-Salivary Circuit:** The use of antiseptic mouthwashes (chlorhexidine) destroys the commensal oral bacteria responsible for reducing dietary nitrate to nitrite. Since nitrite is the precursor of systemic nitric oxide (NO), the destruction of these bacteria leads to a rapid decrease in the bioavailability of NO and a consequent increase in systolic blood pressure, increasing the risk of cardiovascular events. This mechanism, elucidated by studies such as those by Kapil et al., defines mouthwash as an "anti-drug" for the heart.

PART 2: SYNCHRONIZATION AND ENERGY (The Metabolic Engine)

Once the system has been cleansed, the goal is to maximize energy efficiency through synchronization with natural rhythms and mitochondrial optimization.

Chapter 5: Chronobiology and Sleep

Sleep is not inactivity, but an active process of neurological maintenance.

5.1 The Glymphatic System: The Brain's "Washing Machine"

The discovery of the glymphatic system by Maiken Nedergaard and Jeffrey Iliff revolutionized our understanding of sleep.

- **Fluid Dynamics:** In 2012, it was demonstrated that the brain has a system of paravascular channels (managed by aquaporin-4 on astrocytes) that allows cerebrospinal fluid (CSF) to "wash" the brain parenchyma, removing toxic solutes such as beta-amyloid. This process is active almost exclusively during sleep, when the interstitial space increases by 60% to facilitate flow.
- **Impact of Position:** Subsequent studies (Lee et al., 2015) have shown that glymphatic transport efficiency is maximized in the lateral (side-lying) position compared to the supine or prone positions. This data provides a scientific basis for the postural recommendations during sleep presented in the book.

5.2 Nasal Breathing and Mouth Taping

- **Nasal Nitric Oxide:** NO is produced constitutively in the paranasal sinuses. Nasal breathing allows this gas to be transported to the lungs, where it acts as a vasodilator, improving arterial oxygenation (PaO2) and reducing pulmonary vascular resistance.
- **Effectiveness of Taping:** Clinical studies indicate that the use of *mouth tape* during sleep reduces snoring and the apnea-hypopnea index (AHI) in patients with mild obstructive apnea, forcing nasal breathing and preventing upper airway collapse.

Chapter 6: Photobiomodulation (Solar Logic)

Light is treated as a nutrient that modulates cellular biochemistry.

6.1 Mitochondrial Melatonin

- **Local Synthesis:** Research by Reiter and Zimmerman introduced the concept of subcellular melatonin. Unlike pineal melatonin (regulated by darkness and released into the blood), the vast majority of melatonin is produced within the mitochondria in response to near-infrared (NIR) light. This melatonin has no soporific effects but acts as an in situ antioxidant to protect the mitochondria from free radicals produced during cellular respiration. Exposure to sunlight (rich in NIR) is therefore essential to "recharge" this defense system.

6.2 Mechanism of PBM (Red Light)

- **Photodissociation:** The primary mechanism of *Low-Level Light Therapy* (LLLT) or PBM is the absorption of red/NIR photons by the enzyme Cytochrome C Oxidase (Complex IV) in the electron transport chain. This event causes the photodissociation of Nitric Oxide (NO) which, under stress conditions, binds to the enzyme and blocks it. The release of the enzyme restores oxygen consumption and ATP production, accelerating tissue repair.

Chapter 7: The Metabolic Engine (Zone 2 & VO2 Max)

7.1 Zone 2 Training and Lactate Clearance

- **Mitochondrial Function:** Dr. Iñigo San Millán's work with elite athletes has shown that training in "Zone 2" (intensity eliciting lactate < 2 mmol/L) is the most powerful stimulus for improving mitochondrial function and the density of MCT-1 transporters, which are responsible for lactate clearance. This type of training builds the metabolic "base" that allows for efficient fat oxidation and prevents the accumulation of metabolites that cause fatigue.

7.2 VO2 Max as a Predictor of Mortality

- **The Mandsager Study:** A retrospective cohort study of over 122,000 patients, published in *JAMA Network Open*, found that cardiorespiratory fitness (VO2 Max) is inversely associated with long-term mortality with no observable upper limit. Subjects with "elite" fitness had an 80% reduced risk of death compared to those with low fitness, making VO2 Max a more powerful clinical parameter than smoking, diabetes, or hypertension.

Chapter 8: Thermodynamics (Hormesis)

8.1 Benefits of Sauna

- **Cardiovascular and Neurocognitive Protection:** Data from the *Kuopio Ischaemic Heart Disease Risk Factor Study* (Finland) indicate that frequent sauna use (4-7 times per week) is associated with dramatic reductions in the risk of sudden cardiac death (-63%) and dementia/Alzheimer's (-66%). The proposed mechanisms include improved endothelial function, reduced systemic blood pressure, and activation of *Heat Shock Proteins* (HSP), which prevent protein misfolding.

8.2 Cold and Hypertrophy

- **Anabolic Interference:** Although cold water immersion is powerful for reducing inflammation, studies such as that by Roberts et al. (2015) have shown that immediate post-strength training application attenuates anabolic signals (mTOR, satellite cells), reducing muscle mass gains. This data is crucial for the periodization of cold in the athlete's protocol.

PART 3: STRUCTURE AND DEFENSE (The Hardware)

Maintenance of the body's physical and electrical structure.

Chapter 9: Bio-Electromagnetism and Grounding

9.1 EMF and Calcium Channels (VGCC)

- **Pall Mechanism:** Prof. Martin Pall has identified that low-intensity electromagnetic fields act by activating Voltage-Gated Calcium Channels (VGCC) in cell membranes. This causes a massive influx of intracellular calcium, which in turn triggers the synthesis of nitric oxide and superoxide, leading to the formation of peroxynitrite, a powerful oxidant that damages DNA and mitochondria. This mechanism explains the non-thermal effects of EMFs.

9.2 Grounding (Earthing) and Blood Viscosity

- **Zeta Potential:** Research conducted by Chevalier, Sinatra, and Oschman shows that electrical contact with the earth (grounding) reduces blood viscosity by improving the "zeta potential" of red blood cells (the negative charge that causes them to repel each other). This fluidizing effect improves tissue perfusion and reduces the risk of thrombosis.

Chapter 10: Structural Engineering

10.1 Biotensegrity and Fascia

- **Cellular Architecture:** Donald Ingber has demonstrated that cells use a tensegrity (tension integrity) architecture to stabilize their shape and convert mechanical stimuli into biochemical signals (mechanotransduction). This validates the structural approach to cellular health.
- **Fascia and Inflammation:** Helene Langevin's work has shown that stretching the fascia (connective tissue) actively reduces tissue inflammation levels and promotes injury resolution, linking physical mobility to immune regulation.

PART 4: MOLECULAR OVERCLOCKING (The Software)

Optimization through signaling molecules and advanced diagnostics.

Chapter 15: Molecular Longevity

15.1 Spermidine and Autophagy

- **Induction of Autophagy:** Studies published in *Nature Medicine* (Eisenberg et al.) have identified Spermidine as a powerful inducer of autophagy, capable of extending life in yeast, flies, and mice, and protecting the heart from aging. Human trials indicate benefits on memory in the elderly.

15.2 NAD+ and Sirtuins

- **The Role of NAD+:** David Sinclair and others have clarified that NAD+ levels decline with age, compromising the activity of sirtuins (longevity and DNA repair genes). Supplementation with NAD+ precursors or inhibition of the enzyme CD38 (which destroys NAD+, inhibited by apigenin) are validated strategies for restoring youthful metabolic function.

Chapter 17: Peptides and Bioregulators

17.1 BPC-157: Systemic Repair

- **Angiogenesis and Healing:** BPC-157 (Body Protection Compound) is a stable gastric peptide that has been shown in numerous animal studies to accelerate the healing of tendons, muscles, and the intestine (leaky gut) by promoting angiogenesis through the activation of the FAK-paxillin ro s and the modulation of nitric oxide.

17.2 Epitalon and Telomerase

- **Khavinson Protocols:** The tetrapeptide Epitalon, developed by Prof. Vladimir Khavinson, has been shown to reactivate telomerase production in somatic cells and extend lifespan in animal models, while also acting on the resynchronization of circadian rhythms and pineal melatonin.

17.3 GHK-Cu: Skin Remodeling

- **Gene Reset:** The copper peptide GHK-Cu not only stimulates collagen production, but is also able to reset the expression of over 4000 genes to a more "youthful" state, reducing inflammation and promoting wound healing.

Chapter 18: Bio-Harmony

18.1 Social Genomics

- **Transcription of Adversity:** Steve Cole's work on *Social Genomics* has revealed that loneliness and social stress activate a "Conserved Transcription Response to Adversity" (CTRA), characterized by the upregulation of inflammatory genes (via NF-kB) and the downregulation of antiviral response genes (interferons). This provides molecular evidence that social relationships directly influence gene expression and disease risk.

PART 7: GENDER DIFFERENCE (Gender Safety)

Chapters 26-27: The Gender Data Gap and Cycle Syncing

26.1 The Data Gap

- **Invisible Women:** Caroline Criado Perez's work systematically documents how medical research has historically excluded women from clinical trials, leading to drug protocols and diagnoses (e.g., heart attack) calibrated to male physiology, with consequent iatrogenic risks for women.

27.1 Female Physiology in Sport

- **Stacy Sims:** Dr. Stacy Sims' research ("Women Are Not Small Men") highlights that hormonal fluctuations during the menstrual cycle (estrogen and progesterone) alter substrate metabolism, thermoregulation, and recovery. For example, in the high luteal phase, protein catabolism increases and heat tolerance decreases, requiring specific nutritional adjustments (more protein, targeted hydration).

27.2 Infradian Rhythm

- **The Second Clock:** Alisa Vitti has popularized the importance of the infradian rhythm (the 28-day menstrual cycle) as a biological "second clock" that governs female neurochemistry and metabolism, requiring a "Cycle Syncing" approach to nutrition and training.

PART 8: TOWARDS ZERO INJURIES

Chapter 30: Digital Twins

- **In Silico Simulation:** The use of *Digital Twins* in medicine is emerging as a tool for personalized medicine. Recent reviews confirm the possibility of creating virtual models of patients to simulate their response to drugs or interventions before actual application, reducing the risk of adverse reactions and optimizing therapies.

CONCLUSIONS AND OPERATIONAL SUMMARY

Forensic analysis of sources reveals that "The Safety Biohacker" is not a collection of anecdotes, but an operational summary of distinct and validated lines of research:

1. **Environmental Toxicology:** Validated by data on PM2.5, radon, and microplastics.

2. **Biological Dentistry:** Supported by evidence on amalgam, anaerobic infections, and RANTES.
3. **Chronobiology:** Anchored in discoveries on the glymphatic system and mitochondrial melatonin.
4. **Biochemistry of Longevity:** Based on the pathways of mTOR, AMPK, Sirtuins, and Senescence.

The "Safety Officer" works by integrating this evidence to reduce the entropy of the human system, transforming biology from a stochastic process into a controlled engineering project.

Non-exhaustive summary table of key sources

Area	**Key Concept**	**Primary Scientific Reference**
Air	Cognitive Impact of CO2	Harvard COGfx Study (Allen et al.)
Mouth	RANTES in cavitations (NICO)	Lechner et al.
Sleep	Glymphatic system	Nedergaard & Iliff (Science, 2013)

Area	Key Concept	Primary Scientific Reference
Light	Mitochondrial Melatonin	Reiter & Zimmerman
Metabolism	Zone 2 Training	Iñigo San Millán
Longevity	Spermidine and Autophagy	Eisenberg et al. (Nature Medicine)
Longevity	Plasma Dilution (TPE)	Conboy Lab (UC Berkeley)
Gender	Female Physiology in Sport	Stacy Sims
Structure	Cellular Biotensegrity	Donald Ingber (Harvard Wyss Institute)
Social	Social Genomics (CTRA)	Steve Cole (UCLA)

Below are the main landmark studies that form the foundation of the proposed security architecture.

- 🔬 **“Associations of Cognitive Function Scores with Carbon Dioxide, Ventilation, and Volatile Organic Compound Exposures in Office Workers”** (Allen et al., *Environmental Health Perspectives*, 2016).
- 🔬 **“Fine Particulate Matter Exposure and Inflammation: A Systematic Review and Meta-Analysis”** (Feng et al., *Toxicology Letters*, 2016).
- 🔬 **"Microplastics and Nanoplastics in Atheromas and Cardiovascular Events"** (Marfella et al., *The New England Journal of Medicine*, 2024).
- 🔬 **“Residential Radon and Lung Cancer – A Meta-Analysis of Case-Control Studies”** (Darby et al., *Scandinavian Journal of Work, Environment & Health*, 2005).
- 🔬 **“Cadmium-induced pathologies: where is the oxidative balance lost (or not?)”** (Cuypers et al., *International Journal of Molecular Sciences*, 2010).
- 🔬 **“Glyphosate pathways to modern diseases V: Amino acid analogue of glycine in diverse proteins”** (Samsel & Seneff, *Journal of Biological Physics and Chemistry*, 2016).
- 🔬 **“Metallothioneins: Mercury Species-Specific Induction and Their Potential Role in Attenuating Neurotoxicity”** (Aschner et al., *Experimental Biology and Medicine*, 2021).

- 🔬 **“Peripheral Neuropathic Facial/Trigeminal Pain and RANTES/CCL5 in Jawbone Cavitation”** (Lechner & von Baehr, *Evidence-Based Complementary and Alternative Medicine*, 2015).
- 🔬 **“Physiological role for nitrate-reducing oral bacteria in blood pressure control”** (Kapil et al., *Free Radical Biology and Medicine*, 2013).
- 🔬 **“Association between chronic apical periodontitis and cardiovascular diseases: a systematic review and meta-analysis”** (Berlin-Broner et al., *International Endodontic Journal*, 2017).
- 🔬 **“Toxicities of dental amalgam and mercury vapor”** (Mutter, *Journal of Occupational Medicine and Toxicology*, 2011).
- 🔬 **“Zonulin and its regulation of intestinal barrier function: the biological door to inflammation, autoimmunity, and cancer”** (Fasano, *Physiological Reviews*, 2011).
- 🔬 **“Dietary emulsifiers impact the mouse gut microbiota promoting colitis and metabolic syndrome”** (Chassaing et al., *Nature*, 2015).
- 🔬 **“Urolithin A induces autophagy and mitigates muscle dystrophy”** (Luan et al., *Science Translational Medicine*, 2021).
- 🔬 **“Sleep Drives Metabolite Clearance from the Adult Brain”** (Xie, Nedergaard et al., *Science*, 2013).

- 🔬 **“The Effect of Body Posture on Brain Glymphatic Transport”** (Lee et al., *Journal of Neuroscience*, 2015).
- 🔬 **“Effect of Mouth Taping at Night on Asthma Control”** (Cooper et al., *Respirology*, 2009).
- 🔬 **“Melatonin and the Optics of the Human Body”** (Zimmerman & Reiter, *Melatonin Research*, 2019).
- 🔬 **“Mechanisms of Low Level Light Therapy”** (Hamblin, *Proceedings of SPIE*, 2008).
- 🔬 **“Photobiomodulation for the treatment of retinal diseases: mitochondrial mechanisms and therapeutic potential”** (Eells et al., *Retinal Pharmacotherapeutics*, 2016).
- 🔬 **“Assessment of Metabolic Flexibility in Elite Athletes and Individuals with Type 2 Diabetes”** (San Millán & Brooks, *Sports Medicine*, 2018).
- 🔬 **“Association of Cardiorespiratory Fitness With Long-term Mortality Among Adults Undergoing Exercise Treadmill Testing”** (Mandsager et al., *JAMA Network Open*, 2018).
- 🔬 **“Lactate as a fulcrum of metabolism”** (Brooks, *Redox Biology*, 2020).
- 🔬 **“Association Between Sauna Bathing and Fatal Cardiovascular and All-Cause Mortality Events”** (Laukkanen et al., *JAMA Internal Medicine*, 2015).

- 🔬 **"Post-exercise cold water immersion attenuates acute anabolic signaling and long-term adaptations in muscle to strength training"** (Roberts et al., *The Journal of Physiology*, 2015).
- 🔬 **"Heat shock proteins: linking the immune system to longevity"** (Pockley, *Nature Reviews Immunology*, 2003).
- 🔬 **"Electromagnetic fields act via activation of voltage-gated calcium channels to produce beneficial or adverse effects"** (Pall, *Journal of Cellular and Molecular Medicine*, 2013).
- 🔬 **"Earthing (Grounding) the Human Body Reduces Blood Viscosity—a Major Factor in Cardiovascular Disease"** (Chevalier et al., *Journal of Alternative and Complementary Medicine*, 2013).
- 🔬 **"The effects of grounding (earthing) on inflammation, the immune response, wound healing, and chronic autoimmune and inflammatory diseases"** (Oschman et al., *Journal of Inflammation Research*, 2015).
- 🔬 **"Tensegrity I. Cell structure and hierarchical systems biology"** (Ingber, *Journal of Cell Science*, 2003).
- 🔬 **"Connective tissue: A body-wide signaling network?"** (Langevin, *Medical Hypotheses*, 2006).
- 🔬 **"Induction of autophagy by spermidine promotes longevity"** (Eisenberg et al., *Nature Cell Biology*, 2009).

- 🔬 **“Slowing aging by design: the rise of NAD+ and sirtuin-activating compounds”** (Bonkowski & Sinclair, *Nature Reviews Molecular Cell Biology*, 2016).
- 🔬 **“CD38 dictates age-related NAD decline and mitochondrial dysfunction”** (Camacho-Pereira et al., *Cell Metabolism*, 2016).
- 🔬 **“Pentadecapeptide BPC 157 and its effects on a NSAID-toxicity model: diclofenac-induced gastrointestinal lesions”** (Sikiric et al., *Life Sciences*, 1994).
- 🔬 **“Peptide regulation of gene expression and protein synthesis in bronchial epithelium”** (Khavinson et al., *Lung*, 2002).
- 🔬 **“Regenerative and Protective Actions of the GHK-Cu Peptide in the Light of the New Gene Data”** (Pickart & Margolina, *International Journal of Molecular Sciences*, 2018).
- 🔬 **“Social regulation of gene expression in human leukocytes”** (Cole et al., *Genome Biology*, 2007). **
- 🔬 **“Regulation of the immune system by the autonomic nervous system”** (Tracey, *Nature Reviews Immunology*, 2002).
- 🔬 **“Old plasma dilution reduces human biological age: a clinical study”** (Kiprov, Conboy et al., *GeroScience*, 2022).

- 🔬 **“Women are not small men: Sex differences in exercise metabolism”** (Sims, *Current Opinion in Physiology*, 2020).
- 🔬 **“The effects of menstrual cycle phase on physical performance in female athletes”** (McNulty et al., *Sports Medicine*, 2020).
- 🔬 **“Digital Twins in Health Care: Ethical Implications of an Emerging Engineering Paradigm”** (Braun, *Frontiers in Genetics*, 2021).
- 🔬 **“Personalized Medicine: Time for One-Person Trials”** (Schork, *Nature*, 2015).

LEGAL DISCLAIMER AND BIO-SECURITY PROTOCOL

The work *"The Safety Biohacker"* is a treatise on human engineering and biosafety based on data analysis and exponential technologies. The application of its contents requires a rigorous understanding of the limits of individual and professional responsibility.

1. The information, protocols, and data contained in this manual and its appendices are for educational, informational, and independent research purposes only. Despite the methodological rigor applied, the contents do not represent medical diagnoses, prescriptions, or advice. The work should be understood as a mapping of biological risks and opportunities, not as a clinical action plan.

2. The author, Andrea Bancalà, acts here as an independent researcher and disseminator. As he is not a doctor, dietitian, or licensed healthcare professional, interaction with the text or the author does not establish a doctor-patient relationship. Any changes to your biophysical parameters, dietary regimens, supplementation plans, or use of biomedical devices must be validated and supervised in advance by a licensed physician.

3. The methods and opinions expressed in this work are strictly private and personal. They do not reflect, nor are they intended to represent, the official positions, protocols, or guidelines of **the Italian National Institute of Health (ISS)** or any other public or private entity where the author works or has worked.

The author declines all responsibility for interpretations that associate the contents of the book with institutional activities.

4. Human biology is a highly complex, non-linear system. The application of hormetic techniques (thermal stress, fasting), molecular overclocking (peptides, senolytics) or exposure to light spectra involves intrinsic biological risks. The user accepts full and complete responsibility for any consequences arising from the application of the protocols. The author does not guarantee specific results and declines all responsibility for injuries, medical complications, or damage resulting from the improper or inaccurate use of the information contained herein.

5. References to substances (including peptides and Russian bioregulators) or devices are based on international scientific literature. The reader is responsible for verifying the legality, regulatory status, and availability of such products in their country of residence, assuming all costs arising from the acquisition or use thereof.

Safety Directive: *"Knowledge is a driver of precision. Never 'overclock' your system without active clinical telemetry and a supervising physician who is fully aware of your biosecurity strategy. In biosecurity, the unverified assumption is the primary factor in injury."*

APPENDIX A: SAFETY BIOHACKER TECHNICAL GLOSSARY

Decoding the Molecular Signal

"In bioengineering, miscommunication is the primary driver of injury. Linguistic precision is operational safety. This non-exhaustive glossary helps ensure that every command sent to your hardware is based on rigorous scientific definitions, decoding the technical language used in this manual."

A

- **Adsorption:** A physical (non-chemical) process by which a solid (e.g., activated carbon or zeolite) retains gas or liquid molecules (toxins) on its surface. It is the key mechanism of "binders" for intestinal decontamination.
- **Apheresis/TPE (Therapeutic Plasma Exchange):** A clinical blood "washing" procedure that consists of removing plasma, filtering it, or replacing it with fresh albumin in order to remove inflammatory cytokines, autoantibodies, and circulating "aging factors."
- **AGEs (Advanced Glycation End-products):** Molecular complexes resulting from the covalent bond between sugars and proteins or lipids (without enzymes). They

act as a "molecular glue" that stiffens blood vessels, degrades skin collagen, and accelerates aging.

- **Akkermansia Muciniphila:** A key symbiotic bacterium in the microbiome, known as the "Barrier Engineer." It resides in the intestinal mucus layer and stimulates its turnover, sealing tight junctions and reducing endotoxemia.
- **AMPK (AMP-activated Protein Kinase):** The cell's "energy reserve" sensor. It activates when energy (ATP) drops (fasting, exercise, cold), ordering the cessation of growth processes (mTOR) and the initiation of efficiency, repair, and fat oxidation protocols.
- **Apoptosis:** Programmed and orderly cell death. It is the safety mechanism by which the body eliminates damaged or senescent cells without causing inflammation to surrounding tissues (unlike necrosis).
- **Autophagy:** Literally "self-eating." An intracellular cleaning process in which the cell identifies damaged components (organelles, mis d proteins) and digests them in lysosomes to recycle their materials.

B

- **Blood-Brain Barrier (BBB):** A highly selective filter that protects the brain from harmful substances in the blood. Its permeability can be compromised by systemic inflammation, EMFs, and zonulin.
- **BDNF (Brain-Derived Neurotrophic Factor):** A protein that acts as a "fertilizer" for neurons. It promotes

neurogenesis, synaptic plasticity, and the survival of existing brain cells.

- **Biofilm:** A "slimy" protective matrix produced by bacterial colonies (in the gut, mouth, or on wounds) to defend themselves against antibiotics and the immune system. Enzymes such as Nattokinase are used to break down this barrier.
- **Bio-Individuality:** The principle that every intervention (diet, supplementation, medication) produces different effects based on the individual's genetics (SNPs), microbiome, and medical history.
- **Biotensegrity:** Application of the architectural principle of tensegrity to biology. The body's structure is maintained by discontinuous compression (bones) floating in a sea of continuous tension (fascia).
- **BPC-157 (Body Protection Compound):** Short-sequence peptide with systemic regenerative properties. Accelerates angiogenesis (vessel creation) and collagen synthesis in poorly vascularized tissues (tendons, ligaments, intestines).

C

- **CBM (Condition-Based Maintenance):** An engineering concept applied to biology: intervention is not performed at fixed intervals, but in response to real-time data (telemetry) to prevent failure before it occurs.
- **Cytochrome C Oxidase (CCO):** Enzyme complex IV located in the inner mitochondrial membrane. It is the

primary receptor for red and infrared light photons (PBM), whose activation increases ATP production.

- **Clearance:** The rate at which an organ or the entire body removes a specific substance from the blood. It determines the safe dosage of any molecule.
- **Cortisol Steal:** A phenomenon whereby, under chronic stress, the body diverts the hormonal precursor (Pregnenolone) towards the production of Cortisol, "stealing" it from the production of sex hormones.
- **Chronobiology:** The science that studies biological rhythms. In Biohacking, it is the art of synchronizing nutrition, light, and activity with the internal clock to maximize hormonal efficiency.
- **Cycle Syncing:** The practice of adapting nutrition, training, and lifestyle to the four phases of the female infradian cycle to optimize hormonal response.

D

- **Digital Twin:** A dynamic virtual model of an individual's physiology, built by cross-referencing genetic data and telemetry. It allows the impact of interventions to be simulated "in silico."
- **DunedinPACE:** Third-generation DNA methylation algorithm. It measures the "speedometer" of aging, i.e., the rate at which the system is aging at the present moment.

E

- **EDC (Endocrine Disrupting Chemicals):** Exogenous chemicals (BPA, phthalates, parabens) that "hack" the hormonal system, mimicking estrogen or blocking testosterone.
- **Epigenetics:** The study of heritable changes in gene expression that do not alter the DNA sequence. It is the "software" that decides which genes to turn on or off in response to the environment.
- **Epithalon:** A synthetic bioregulatory tetrapeptide capable of stimulating telomerase activity and restoring the sensitivity of the pineal gland.
- **Estrobolome:** The set of intestinal bacteria responsible for the metabolism and modulation of circulating estrogens.

F

- **Fascia:** Connective tissue that surrounds and permeates every muscle, bone, and organ. It acts as a piezoelectric and sensory communication network.

G

- **Glycocalyx:** A protective "hairy" layer that lines the inside of blood vessels (endothelium). It acts as a filter, barrier, and pressure sensor. Damage to it is the first stage of atherosclerosis.
- **Glymphatic System:** A brain cleansing system active during deep sleep, which uses cerebrospinal fluid to "wash away" metabolic waste (beta-amyloid).

- **Glutathione:** The body's "Master Antioxidant." Essential for phase 2 of liver detoxification and for protecting mitochondria from oxidative stress.
- **Grounding (Earthing):** The practice of connecting the body to the earth. It allows the flow of free electrons, neutralizing static positive charge and reducing blood viscosity.

H

- **Hormesis:** The biological principle whereby exposure to moderate doses of a stressor (cold, heat, hypoxia) stimulates adaptive responses that strengthen the body.
- **HRV (Heart Rate Variability):** The measurement of the time variation (in milliseconds) between one heartbeat and the next. It is the "gold standard" biomarker for assessing the recovery and stress of the autonomic nervous system.
- **hs-CRP (High-sensitivity C-Reactive Protein):** A blood marker of low-grade systemic inflammation. It is the "fire alarm" in arteries and tissues.
- **HSP (Heat Shock Proteins):** "Heat shock proteins." "Chaperone" molecules produced by cells in response to heat stress (sauna). They repair damaged proteins and prevent plaque aggregation.

I

- **IGF-1 (Insulin-like Growth Factor 1):** Insulin-like growth factor. It is the main mediator of GH effects. High levels promote muscle growth but also aging; low levels promote longevity but also fragility.

- **Infradian (Rhythm):** Biological cycle with a frequency greater than 24 hours, typically referring to the 28-day menstrual cycle in women.

K

- **Kisspeptin:** Hypothalamic neuropeptide that acts as the main switch for the reproductive axis (HPG). It is sensitive to energy availability and morning light signals.

L

- **Leaky Gut:** A condition in which the tight junctions of the intestine loosen, allowing bacteria and toxins to pass into the bloodstream.
- **LEV (Longevity Escape Velocity):** Theoretical point at which technological progress extends life expectancy by more than one year for each passing year.
- **LPS (Lipopolysaccharides):** Endotoxins found on the cell walls of Gram-negative bacteria. Powerful triggers of systemic inflammation.

M

- **Methylation:** A biochemical process that involves adding a methyl group ($-CH_3$) to a molecule. It regulates gene expression, detoxification, and neurotransmitter production. It depends on the folate cycle (MTHFR).

- **Molecular mimicry:** A phenomenon whereby the immune system confuses a food protein (e.g., gluten) or toxin with a body tissue due to their structural similarity, triggering an autoimmune reaction.
- **Myokines:** Signaling molecules (such as muscle IL-6 or BDNF) released by muscle fibers during intense contraction.
- **Mitophagy:** A specific form of autophagy that targets and recycles damaged or dysfunctional mitochondria.
- **mTOR:** Protein kinase that acts as a nutrient sensor. When activated, it stimulates cell growth (anabolism). If chronically hyperactivated, it blocks repairs.

N

- **NAD+ (Nicotinamide Adenine Dinucleotide):** Essential coenzyme present in all living cells. Indispensable for energy production and DNA repair (Sirtuins).
- **Neuroception:** An unconscious process by which the nervous system scans the environment for signs of safety or danger.
- **nnEMF (Non-native ElectroMagnetic Fields):** Artificial electromagnetic fields that interfere with human biology by activating calcium channels (VGCC).
- **Nrf2:** A protein that regulates the expression of antioxidant proteins. It is the master switch of cellular

defense against oxidative stress, activated by substances such as sulforaphane.

P

- **PGC-1alpha:** Key transcriptional regulator of energy metabolism. Its activation stimulates mitochondrial biogenesis.
- **Piezoelectricity:** The ability of certain biological materials (such as collagen crystals in fascia and bones) to generate an electrical charge in response to mechanical stress (movement).
- **Polymorphism (SNP):** "Single Nucleotide Polymorphism." A variation in a single letter of the genetic code. Some SNPs (such as MTHFR or APOE4) alter enzyme function.

R

- **ROS (Reactive Oxygen Species):** Reactive oxygen species ("free radicals"). In excess, they cause damage, but in controlled doses, they are essential signals for cellular adaptation.

S

- **SASP:** The toxic cocktail of inflammatory cytokines secreted by senescent ("zombie") cells, which spreads aging to nearby tissues.
- **Senolysis:** A therapeutic strategy aimed at selectively eliminating senescent cells.

- **Symbiosis:** The mutually beneficial relationship between the host (human) and its microbiome. The breakdown of this pact is called *dysbiosis*.
- **Sirtuins (SIRT1-7):** A family of NAD+-dependent enzymes ("longevity genes") that repair DNA and regulate metabolism.

T

- **Telomeres:** The protective "caps" at the ends of chromosomes. They shorten with each cell division, marking biological age.
- **Toxemia:** Presence of toxins in the blood.

V

- **VGCC (Voltage-Gated Calcium Channels):** Voltage-dependent calcium channels located on the cell membrane, sensitive to electromagnetic fields (nnEMF).
- **VO2 Max:** The maximum volume of oxygen that the body can use during maximum exertion. The most powerful biomarker for longevity.

Z

- **Zonulin:** A protein that regulates the permeability of tight junctions in the intestine. Elevated levels indicate a breach in the defensive perimeter.

APPENDIX B: HEMATOLOGICAL AND BIOMETRIC AUDIT PROTOCOL

Technical Guide for the Attending Physician and the Analysis Laboratory

When you go to the doctor, explain clearly that you are not seeking a diagnosis of an acute ongoing condition, but rather an **assessment of your functional reserve** and mapping of silent risks (Medicine 3.0). Laboratory reference ranges indicate the "population average" (often unhealthy); the Target Safety values indicated here represent physiological optimization.

1. INFLAMMATION AND METHYLATION PANEL (Fire Alarm)

Objective: *To detect inflammaging (inflammatory aging) and the efficiency of detoxification processes (Chapters 2 and 15).*

Biomarker	Technical Name / Lab Code	Biohacker Safety Target	Clinical Rationale
hs-CRP	d C-Reactive Protein (High Sensitivity)	**< 0.5 mg/L**	The fire alarm. If >1.0, there is an active outbreak (mouth, intestine, or endothelium). If

Biomarker	Technical Name / Lab Code	Biohacker Safety Target	Clinical Rationale
			>3.0, cardiac risk is critical.
Homocysteine	Plasma homocysteine	**< 7-8 µmol/L**	Primary indicator of methylation cycle efficiency (hepatic phase 2) and neuro/cardiovascular risk. If high, B12/folate deficiency.
Ferritin	Serum Ferritin	**50 - 150 ng/mL**	Marker of iron storage but also acute phase reactant. If too high (>200) indicates hidden inflammation; if low, mitochondrial hypoxia.
Fibrinogen	Functional fibrinogen	**200 - 300 mg/dL**	Measures blood viscosity (Chapter 9). High values indicate "thick" blood and

Biomarker	Technical Name / Lab Code	Biohacker Safety Target	Clinical Rationale
			increased thrombotic risk.
GGT	Gamma-GT	**< 20 U/L**	The most sensitive marker for oxidative stress in the liver and glutathione consumption. Much more predictive than ALT/AST.

2. METABOLIC SUBSYSTEM (The Engine)

Objective: *To map actual insulin sensitivity before glycemic damage appears (Chapters 7 and 13).*

Biomarker	Technical Name / Lab Code	Biohacker Safety Target	Clinical Rationale
Insulin	Fasting Insulin	**< 5-6 μIU/mL**	**The most important data.** Blood sugar may be normal while insulin is skyrocketing

Biomarker	Technical Name / Lab Code	Biohacker Safety Target	Clinical Rationale
			(silent insulin resistance).
HbA1c	Glycated Hemoglobin	**4.8% - 5.2**	The "black box" of the last 90 days. It measures how quickly you are "caramelizing" (glycation/AGEs).
HOMA-IR	Homeostatic Model Assessment	**< 1.0**	Calculated index (Glucose x Insulin / 405). Defines your metabolic flexibility.
Uric Acid	Uricemia	**< 5.0 mg/dL**	Not just gout. It is a proxy for excessive fructose consumption and mitochondrial metabolic stress.
Triglycerides	Triglycerides	**< 80 mg/dL**	Unburned energy. If high, you are accumulating visceral fat and your liver is under stress.

3. CARDIOVASCULAR SUBSYSTEM 2.0 (Advanced Lipid Analysis)

Objective: *To move beyond the outdated concept of "total cholesterol" and count actual particles (Chapter 16).*

Biomarker	Technical Name / Lab Code	Target Safety Biohacker	Clinical Rationale
ApoB	Apolipoprotein B-100	**< 60 mg/dL**	Counts the exact number of atherogenic particles (LDL, VLDL). Much more predictive than calculated LDL cholesterol.
Lp(a)	Lipoprotein (a)	**< 30 mg/dL**	**Safety Alert:** Genetically determined. To be measured *only once in a lifetime*. If high, the risk of heart attack/stroke is elevated regardless of diet.

Biomarker	Technical Name / Lab Code	Target Safety Biohacker	Clinical Rationale
TG/HDL ratio	Triglycerides / HDL	**< 1.0**	The best lipid indicator of LDL particle size. If low, LDL particles are large and fluffy (safe).

4. ENDOCRINE CONSOLE (Thyroid & Sex Hormones)

Objective: *To verify not only the production, but also the conversion and availability of hormones (Chapter 13).*

Biomarker	Technical Name / Lab Code	Biohacker Safety Target	Clinical Rationale
TSH	Thyroid-stimulating hormone	**1.0 - 2.0 µIU/mL**	If > 2.5, the thyroid is struggling (even if the lab says "normal" up to 4.0).
fT3	Free Triiodothyronine	**Upper range**	The only active thyroid hormone that provides

Biomarker	Technical Name / Lab Code	Biohacker Safety Target	Clinical Rationale
			energy. T4 is only stored.
rT3	Reverse T3	**< 15 ng/dL**	The "handbrake." If high, the body is in survival/starvation mode ( ) and blocks metabolism.
Free Testosterone	Free Testosterone (Calc. or direct)	**Upper range**	Total testosterone is useless if we don't know how much is free to act on receptors.
SHBG	Sex Hormone Binding Globulin	**Balanced**	If too high, it sequesters testosterone; if too low, it indicates insulin

Biomarker	Technical Name / Lab Code	Biohacker Safety Target	Clinical Rationale
			resistance or fatty liver.
Estradiol (E2)	17-beta Estradiol	**Physiological Range**	(Men) To be monitored to avoid excessive conversion from testosterone (aromatase). (Women) Essential for the heart and brain.
DHEA-S	Dehydroepiandrosterone sulfate	**400-500 mcg/dL (M) / 250-350 (F)**	The buffer against cortisol. Adrenal reserve marker.
Vitamin D	25-OH Vitamin D	**60-80 ng/mL**	Genomic hormone. Below 40 ng/mL, the

Biomarker	Technical Name / Lab Code	Biohacker Safety Target	Clinical Rationale
			immune system is blind and bones are fragile.

5. FILTERS AND ORGAN SAFETY (Kidneys & Liver)

Objective: *Mandatory monitoring for those using peptides, supplements, or high protein (Chapter 17).*

Biomarker	Technical Name / Lab Code	Biohacker Safety Target	Clinical Rationale
Cystatin C	Serum Cystatin C	**Low**	A much more accurate marker of kidney function than creatinine for people with a lot of muscle mass.
eGFR	Glomerular filtration	**> 90 mL/min**	Renal filtration capacity. It is essential to monitor this if you

Biomarker	Technical Name / Lab Code	Biohacker Safety Target	Clinical Rationale
			are using supplements or peptides.
ALT / AST	Transaminases	**< 20-25 U/L**	If they are at the upper end of the range (e.g., 40), the liver is under toxic or metabolic stress.

6. ADVANCED DIAGNOSTICS (Next-Gen)

Unconventional tests for Biohacker Elite (to be requested from specialized laboratories).

- **Omega-3 Index:** Measures the percentage of EPA/DHA in red blood cell membranes. **Target: > 8**%. (Protection against sudden death).
- **Akkermansia Muciniphila (Fecal DNA):** Metagenomic test of the microbiome. Checks for the presence of the "Guardian of the Barrier" bacterium (Chapter 4).
- **Fecal Zonulin:** Direct marker of intestinal permeability (Leaky Gut).

- **DunedinPACE (Blood/Saliva):** The aging speedometer. It does not measure *how* old you are, but how fast you are aging *now*. **Target: < 0.8**.
- **Metal Toxicology (Mineralogram or Urinary Provocation):** To detect tissue accumulations of mercury, lead, or cadmium that do not appear in the blood (Chapter 2).

APPENDIX C: SUPPLY BRAND HANDBOOK

"If you don't know where the molecule comes from and how it has been tested, you're not supplementing: you're gambling. In biosafety, trust is earned with certificates of analysis (CoA), not with pretty labels. This document is your compass for navigating the unregulated supplement market without taking on board toxins."

1. THE 3 LEVELS OF SAFETY (Validation Protocol)

Before purchasing any product, the *Safety Biohacker* applies this three-stage filter. If a product fails even one level, it is discarded.

LEVEL 1: PURITY (Chemical Defense)

- **HPLC (High-Performance Liquid Chromatography) Audit:** Demand proof that the purity of the molecule is >98% (crucial for peptides).
- **Heavy Metal Analysis:** The product must be tested for Arsenic, Cadmium, Lead, and Mercury. (Critical for marine products, herbs, and medicinal mushrooms).
- **No "Proprietary Blends":** If the label says "Proprietary Blend" without listing the exact milligrams of each component , it is a scam to hide underdoses. Discard.

LEVEL 2: POTENCY (Delivery Technology)

You are not what you eat, you are what you *absorb*.

- **Liposomal/Phytosomal:** Mandatory for water-repellent molecules such as Curcumin, Glutathione, Quercetin, and NAD+. Without this technology, absorption is <5%.
- **Bioactive Forms (Methylation):** B vitamins only as methylfolate/methylcobalamin (no folic acid/cyanocobalamin). Minerals only chelated or bisglycinated (no oxides).
- **Enzymatic Hydrolysis:** Mandatory for collagen and proteins to ensure a low molecular weight (<3000 Daltons) that can be absorbed.

LEVEL 3: PRODUCTION (Industrial Standards)

- **cGMP (Current Good Manufacturing Practice) certification:** Guarantees that the product is manufactured in sterile and controlled environments, not in basements.
- **Third-Party Testing:** The brand must show analyses carried out by *independent* laboratories, not by the manufacturer itself.

2. THE LIST OF BRANDS

These brands have been selected because they consistently comply with the safety protocols described above. This is not an exhaustive list, but a safe starting point.

Category	Recommended Brands	Why They Are Excellent (Technical Specifications)
Essential & Longevity	**Life Extension**	The gold standard. They use patented raw materials (e.g., Kaneka Ubiquinol™, Crominex®) and dosages based on clinical studies, not minimum RDAs. Total transparency on CoAs.
Liposomal technology	**Codeage / Quicksilver Scientific**	Excellence in the encapsulation of fragile molecules (NAD+, Glutathione, Ca-AKG). Quicksilver uses <100nm lipid nanoparticles for immediate sublingual absorption.
Precision Microbiome	**Pendulum**	The only company in the world with a patent for the cultivation and encapsulation of the live and metabolically active

Category	Recommended Brands	Why They Are Excellent (Technical Specifications)
		Akkermansia Muciniphila strain.
Peptides (Research)	**Peptide Sciences**	Certified purity >99% on every batch, freeze-drying under nitrogen and cold chain. They provide mass spectrometry for each vial.
Neuro-Engineering	**MoleQlar / Nootropics Depot**	USP (pharmaceutical) grade for delicate molecules such as Methylene Blue (no heavy metals) and medicinal mushrooms titrated in real beta-glucans.
Enzymes & Fibers	**Doctor's Best**	Strict use of certified raw materials such as Sunfiber® (PHGG) and NattoPhase® (Nattokinase without Vitamin K), ensuring clinical efficacy.
Omega-3 & Oils	**Nordic Naturals / Viva Naturals**	IFOS 5-Star certification for absence of mercury and oxidation (low TOTOX score). Essential for

Category	Recommended Brands	Why They Are Excellent (Technical Specifications)
		avoiding the ingestion of rancid fish oil.

3. THE "BLACKLIST" OF EXCIPIENTS (Label Saboteurs)

A true *Safety Officer* reads the "Other Ingredients" (at the bottom) before the active ingredients. If you find these saboteurs, the product is compromised.

1. **Titanium Dioxide (E171):** Genotoxic carcinogenic whitening agent (banned in the EU for food use, but still present in many US/non-EU supplements). **Action: Discard immediately.**

2. **Industrial Seed Oils (Soybean, Cottonseed, Corn Oil):** Often used as cheap "fillers" in Vitamin D or Omega-3 softgels. They cause inflammation and oxidation. **Action: Look only for extra virgin olive oil or coconut/MCT oil.**

3. **Artificial Colors (Red 40, Blue 1, Yellow 5):** Neurotoxic and destructive to the microbiome. There is no reason to color a pill other than for marketing purposes.

4. **Maltodextrin and Hidden Sugars:** Often found in probiotics or "greens" powders. They sabotage your glycemic curve and fasting.

5. **Magnesium Stearate (in excess):** If it is the first or second ingredient on the list of excipients, it can create an biofilm that reduces the absorption of the active ingredient. Acceptable only if at the bottom of the list.

4. OPERATIONAL MANAGEMENT: STORAGE AND EXPIRY

Biohacking does not end with the purchase. The molecule must remain active until ingestion.

- **The Cold Chain:**
  - ***Refrigerator (43-46°F):*** Reconstituted peptides, live probiotics (Akkermansia, VSL#3), liquid fish oil (once opened), liquid liposomal glutathione.
  - ***Dark and cool:*** Fish oil capsules, CoQ10, fat-soluble vitamins. Oxidation is accelerated by heat.

- **The Smell Test (Omega-3):** If your Omega-3 pills smell strongly of rotten fish as soon as you open the jar, they are oxidized. They have become pro-inflammatory. **Throw them away.**

- **Humidity:** Humidity in the bathroom destroys powders (creatine, pre-workout) and vegetable capsules. Store supplements in a dry place (bedroom or kitchen away from the stove).

Final Note: This list is not sponsored. It is the result of independent audits. Formulations change: always check for the updated label before purchasing. You are the final quality controller before the substance enters your system.

CALL TO ACTION

Follow the Official Channels: To stay up to date on molecular safety and operational micro-hacks.

⚡ **QUICK INSIGHTS (Instagram & TikTok):** Daily micro-hacks, video clips on environmental decontamination, behind-the-scenes footage, and quick explanations.

Follow me on Instagram: Thesafetybiohacker

Follow me on TikTok: Thesafetybiohacker

📡 **REAL-TIME UPDATES (X & Threads):** Breaking news from the world of longevity and quick reflections on institutional biosecurity.

Follow me on Threads: Thesafetybiohacker

Follow me on X: Safetybiohacker

📺 **VISUAL MASTERCLASSES (YouTube):** Tutorials on how to use devices (Red Light, Radon monitors, water filters) and weekly reviews of the various modules.

Follow me on YouTube: Thesafetybiohacker

👥 **COMMUNITY & NEWS (Facebook):** Official announcements, discussions with the Safety Biohackers community.

Follow me on Facebook: The Safety Biohacker – Andrea Bancalà

💼 **PROFESSIONAL PAGE (LinkedIn)** The bridge between Institutional Science and Biohacking. Industry analysis, professional networking, and updates.

Follow me on LinkedIn: Andrea Bancalà

🧠 **DEEP DIVES & PROTOCOLS (Medium & Substack):** In-depth technical analysis, clinical trial reviews, and written guides (in English) for those who want to dive into the molecular details.

Follow me on Medium: Thesafetybiohacker

Follow me on Substack: Thesafetybiohacker

📩 **DIRECT CONTACTS AND SUPPORT**

For requests and collaborations:

thesafetybiohacker@libero.it

Andrea Bancalà - *Safety Officer & The Safety Biohacker*

"Performance is the reward for those who put safety first."

www.ingramcontent.com/pod-product-compliance
Lightning Source LLC
LaVergne TN
LVHW052149210926
848482LV00019B/295
9791224321873